Musculoskeletal Ultrasound for the Orthopaedic Surgeon

ER, OR AND CLINIC

Christopher M. Jobe, MD, RMSK. Dean W. Ziegler, MD

Brian Badman, MD
Central Indiana Orthopedics
Fishers, IN 46037

Alvin Camacho, MD
Assistant Professor, Radiology
University of Texas Medical Branch
Shriners Children's Hospital
Galveston, Texas

Ethan Dean, MD
Hand and Upper Limb Surgery
Piedmont Orthopedics / OrthoAtlanta
Atlanta, Georgia

John R. Fowler, MD
Deputy Chief of Orthopedics, Mercy Hospital
Associate Program Director, Orthopedic Residency
Associate Program Director, Hand Fellowship
Associate Professor, Department of Orthopedics
Assistant Dean, University of Pittsburgh School of Medicine

Tyler W. Fraser, MD
Foot and Ankle Surgery
Ortho South
Memphis Tennessee

Eric Giza, MD
Chief, Division of Foot and Ankle
Director, Orthopaedic Surgery Foot and Ankle Fellowship
Professor, Department of Orthopaedic Surgery
UC Davis

Christopher M. Jobe, MD, RMSK
Professor, Orthopedic Surgery
Professor, Anesthesiology, secondary appointment
Loma Linda University
Orthopaedic Surgeon
Oroville Hospital
Oroville, California

Joseph J. King III, MD
Associate Professor
Dept of Orthopaedic surgery and sports medicine
University of Florida
Gainesville, Florida

Christopher Kreulen, MD
Associate Professor
Department of Orthopaedic Surgery
UC Davis
Davis, California

Kevin Kruse, MD
Texas Orthopaedic Associates
Dallas, Texas

Rosa Magaña, BA
MD Candidate, Class of 2024
University of California Davis School of Medicine
Sacramento, CA

Spencer Moore, MD
Carolina Hand and Sports Medicine
Asheville, NC

Alexander M. Riordan, MD
Aurora Orthopedics
Milwaukee, Wisconsin

Edward Southern, MD
Associate Professor, Uniformed Services University of the Health Sciences
Defense Health Agency Orthopaedic Surgeon
Bayne-Jones Army Hospital
Department of Surgery, Orthopaedic Surgery Section
1585 Third Avenue
Fort Johnson, LA 71459

Alyssa Speciale, MD
Assistant Clinical Professor, Physical Medicine and Rehabilitation
Associate Program Director, PMR Residency
University of California Davis Health System
Sacramento, CA

Robert C. Vercio, MD
Proliance
Puget Sound Orthopaedics
Gig Harbor, Washington

Manaf Younis, MD
1703 Rockhill Rd,
McKinney, TX 75069

Dean Ziegler, MD
Associate Clinical Professor
Orthopaedic Surgery
Blount Orthopaedic Associates
Milwaukee, Wisconsin

CONTENTS

Acknowledgements.......... ix

Chapter 1 Introduction.......... 1

- Dean W. Ziegler, MD;
- Brian L. Badman, MD

Chapter 2 Shoulder.......... 45

- Kevin K. Kruse, MD;
- Brian L. Badman, MD;
- Dean W. Ziegler, MD;

Chapter 3 Ultrasound of the Elbow and Forearm.......... 99

- Ethan W. Dean, MD
- Joseph J. King III, MD

Chapter 4 Hand and Wrist..........185

- John Fowler,MD
- Christopher M Jobe, MD, RMSK
- Robert Vercio, MD

Chapter 5 Hip and Thigh..........291

- Alexander M. Riordan, MD;
- Christopher M. Jobe, MD, RMSK

Chapter 6 Knee

- Christopher M. Jobe, MD, RMSK

Chapter 7 Foot and Ankle

- Alyssa Speciale, MD;
- Tyler Fraser, MD;
- Christopher Kreulen, MD
- Rosa Magana;
- Eric Giza, MD

Chapter 8 pediatrics and Spine

- Edward P. Southern, MD, MBA1
- Manaf H. Younis, MD, MPH2
- Alvin Camacho, MD3

Chapter 9 Practice Integration

- Dean W Ziegler, MD
- Spencer H. Moore, MD

ACKNOWLEDGEMENTS

Family

- Our greatest debt is owed to our wives, Melanie Jobe and Michele Ziegler who not only put up with our dedicating time to writing and editing, but modeled for some of the illustrations
- Our children were also called upon to model.
    - Christina Jobe
    - Zoe Ziegler

Teachers and Mentors

- Jon Jacobson, MD and Marnix Van Holsbeeck, MD are not only the authors of the textbooks which we use in resident and medical student training, but they have been tireless in their dedication to teaching. We never have a conversation with one of them without learning something new and useful.
- Levon Nazarian introduced us to ultrasound guided procedures of the hand, and has lead out in the AIUM
- Three Loma Linda University faculty were very encouraging and generous with their knowledge: Alexander Jesse Chien, MD in radiology, Karina Marianne Torralba, MD, in rheumatology and Vi Dinh, MD in ER medicine.
- Robert E. Markison, MD not only taught one of us (CMJ) but performed a US procedure as well. Thanks again, Bob.

- Rick Matsen, MD who recognized the dynamic utility of diagnostic ultrasound and with the work of Larry Mack, MD pioneered this technology.
- Scott Primack who promoted the use of US in the physical medicine and rehabilitation community and told those of us in orthopaedics: "You have to do this!"

- Inventors

- Much knowledge acquired through experience comes from one technique which is then generalized to other areas of the body. Darryl Barnes, MD and Jay Smith, MD invented a method for releasing the carpal tunnel which is highly effective. Elements of their technique have been found to be effective at the knee and other joints.

Technical Assistance

- Loma Linda University department of radiology was very generous in allowing us to use some of the latest technology. Crystal Mamoulelis, the ultrasound manager, spent a large amount of time helping with recording images and some of her students modeled for illustrations.

Posing for illustrations

- Eventually, in putting together a text like this one, one has to have some images of normal structures. In addition to the people listed above, members of the OR and office staff have been kind enough to pose.

Administrative support

- Special thanks to Robert Wentz, the CEO of Oroville hospital, for seeing the value of ultrasound and investing precious health care dollars.

Colleagues

- Thank you to the members of the Pain Clinic at the Loma Linda VAH
    - Thomas A. Edell, MD, Anne T. Cipta, MD, Gary K. Pang, MD, Shawn Uraine, MD Diep Vuong, MD, Latimer Aguilar, RN, Raelene Del Amen, LVN, Chrissy Payad, LVN, and Ida C Ainley, LVN

Our Inspiration: our residents and fellows who will more fully develop this tool

But, our greatest debt is owed to our authors who spent hours writing text and retrieving images. To them we say thank you, thank you, thank you.

Chapter 1 Introduction

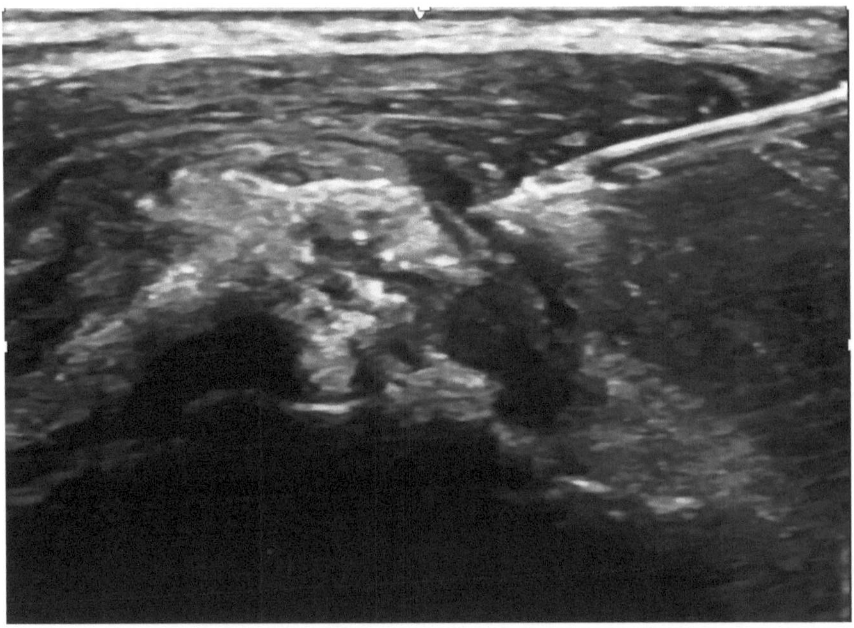

- Dean W. Ziegler, MD;
- Brian L. Badman, MD;

Diagnostic Ultrasound is an important imaging modality in all areas of medicine. Recently, its value in the evaluation and management of musculoskeletal disorders has been recognized. Orthopaedic surgeons can appreciate the utility of ultrasound as perhaps the best way to image structures *in vivo* in their static state, as well as dynamically, functionally and under stress. This allows the practitioner to appreciate not only abnormalities of structure but also how these abnormalities affect the patient functionally. Surgeons also value the ability of ultrasound to precisely guide interventional procedures, assuring that the application is placed exactly where it is intended. The purpose of this book is to present present an efficient and effective way to incorporate ultrasound into your practice. It is written for orthopaedic surgeons, by orthopaedic surgeons who have utilized ultrasound extensively in their practices. It is meant to be an introduction to musculoskeletal ultrasound as well as a quick reference to be used at the point of care while performing diagnosis and interventions. It should be noted that various ultrasound machines were utilized to obtain the images presented. Some are extremely high resolution. Do not be discouraged if your images are not always as sharp or highly detailed, what is important is to be able to adequately image the anatomy and assess the pathology.

Diagnostic ultrasound is most effective and efficient when incorporated into the overall evaluation of the patient's disorder. This includes the past medical history, presenting history, a bilateral physical exam, as well as plain radiographs. Ultrasonic imaging is then indicated either if the patient has failed appropriate non-operative management or has an acute disorder that requires immediate imaging. If this is the case, bilateral exams can be performed, imaging the asymptomatic or least symptomatic side first. This allows the examiner to educate themselves regarding the patient's more normal anatomy while the subject can initially experience the more normal exam. The patients can then better provide feedback during the imaging of the symptomatic side, reporting any discomfort or other abnormalities. This feedback is invaluable in the overall exam. As the examiner becomes more experienced with the structure being imaged, they may feel comfortable only imaging the symptomatic side. However, if there is any question regarding normal anatomy, the evaluation of the opposite side is performed, especially when negative predictability is important.

The best ultrasound images are obtained by an examiner with excellent three-dimensional anatomic understanding of the structures and proficiency with the use of ultrasound. Orthopaedic surgeons with both clinical and surgical experience certainly have an excellent 3-D understanding of the anatomy. Orthopaedists, especially those with arthroscopic experience, can also easily become proficient with the use of ultrasound in obtaining the best image. In arthroscopy, viewing is optimized by moving the arthroscope throughout the joint, rotating the arthroscope to change the viewing direction, and moving the joint with the arthroscope stationary. In similar fashion ultrasound imaging is maximized by moving the probe over the anatomic structure, rotating the probe while maintaining the same position on the structure or moving the structure with the probe held stationary. These similar skills are readily adaptable with hands-on experience and an understanding of the physics of ultrasound.

History of Ultrasound

The development of ultrasound began in 1880 with the work of Pierre and Jacques Curie. The brothers discovered a phenomenon called piezoelectricity, which is the basis of ultrasound technology.[1,2] They discovered the phenomenon that when quartz crystals were subjected to a certain amount of physical stress, the deformed crystals create an electric potential. Likewise, an electric potential can cause the crystals to deform. A rapidly oscillating electric potential can cause the crystals to physically vibrate to create the waves. And likewise, waves returning to the crystals can cause them to generate electric signals sent back to the monitor. Current ultrasound transducers still contain these crystals which allow them to create a diagnostic image.[1,2]

This discovery went on to inspire one of Curie's students to produce the first physical application of the piezoelectricity phenomenon. In 1915, Paul Langevin helped create the first functioning hydrophone, which used piezoelectric quartz crystals to both create and receive sound waves in water. The hydrophone later unveiled the pulse-echo principle, which is the foundation of sonar technology.[2] It was the use of sonar technology that allowed for application in the medical field.

The earliest reported use of medical ultrasound was in 1942. Because of the then recent popularization of sonar technology, Dr. Karl Dussik, a psychiatrist and neurologist, used ultrasound to visualize the brain and diagnose brain tumors.[2,3] Dr. Dussik later published another study in 1958 using ultrasound to visualize different structures that surround joints within the musculoskeletal system.[4] He was able to describe the physical properties of structures such as skin, tendons, articular capsule, articular and intraarticular cartilage, muscle, and bones. He posited that if properties of each structure were known, changes in those properties would then signal an abnormality or pathology. He also believed that with the use of ultrasound, there would be advancements in therapy.[4] In a sense, his team laid the foundation for the use of ultrasound in a musculoskeletal setting.

In 1972, the first B-Scan, which is a two-dimensional ultrasound, was used to visualize a human joint. This enabled researchers to differentiate between the appearance of a baker's cyst and thrombophlebitis.[12] Later, physicians utilized ultrasound to diagnose synovitis in a patient who had rheumatoid arthritis.[3]

Dr. Zweymueller and Dr. Kratochwil pioneered the use of ultrasound in soft tissue tumors and bone.[1,8] They found that ultrasound helped better characterize tumors prior to surgery.[1] In 1979 ultrasound was found to offer additional information to diagnose myositis ossificans.[1]

The technology for ultrasound transducers advanced in the 1970s. In a 1976 case report, physicians used ultrasound to diagnose a rectus sheath hematoma.[1,5] This was monumental at the time, as little was known about rectus sheath hematomas, and upwards of 50% of them were misdiagnosed. This case report demonstrated how ultrasound was able to diagnose a potentially misdiagnosed pathology correctly. The physicians who handled this case utilized a B mode scan with the 2-3 MHz transducer.[5] By the time the study regarding myositis ossificans came out, transducer technology had increased in frequency to 3.5 MHz. [1]

[1,6] In 1984, in Germany, Mayer used ultrasound to characterize a rupture of an Achilles tendon. In the study, 16 patients were suspected of having an Achilles tendon rupture. Out of the 16 cases, ten were confirmed with ultrasound, the remaining six patients had intact tendons. Mayer was able to characterize and localize the rupture by ultrasound, as well as identify an associated hematoma. Technology progressed further to include 5 MHz transducers.[1,7] which allowed visualization of other tendons in the hand, fingers and the foot.[1]

In 1991, Harryman and his team were the first to[3] use ultrasound to determine the integrity of the rotator cuff postoperatively and to draw a correlation between the functionality of the rotator cuffs and different sized tears.[13] In 1999, Primack published a study that explored the cost-effectiveness of ultrasound describing ultrasound as an extension of the clinical exam. He reported that it gave physicians a cost-effective and thorough modality of care.[3,14] A study also showed that the use of ultrasound guidance for injection led to an 8% decrease in cost per patient. Another study by the same group concluded that ultrasound reduces the cost of outpatient treatment by 13%.[15]

Currently, ultrasound has a wide range of musculoskeletal applications and there has been an increase in its efficacy. Ultrasound can give real-time images that are dynamic while avoiding the exposure of radiation. Clinicians have been able to use the musculoskeletal ultrasound to assess fluid collections, joint effusions, soft tissue masses, tendinosis, partial-thickness and full-thickness tendon and ligament tears and even hip injuries.[6,10] It is the preferred method for evaluation of rotator cuff injuries for many as clinicians found that ultrasound is better at visualizing abnormalities than MRI.[9,16] Ultrasound has also been applied to guide injections into joints and tendon sheaths, and it adds the extra convenience of being able to do such interventions in the office rather than the operating room.[3,10] This technology has also been applied towards the guidance of peripheral nerve blocks. Researchers have even proposed that ultrasound has grown more popular amongst doctors who are not radiologists.[16] They have also identified that there has been a 71.7% increase in ultrasound utilization for evaluation and diagnosis in an outpatient setting.[11]

Basic Physics of Ultrasound

Ultrasound consists of mechanical waves with frequencies above those audible to humans (> 20 000 Hz). Usually, diagnostic ultrasound ranges from 2-20 MHz while some probes are now as high as 70 MHz. The waves are generated by inversion of the **piezoelectric effect**. Obtaining an ultrasound image requires sound waves to penetrate tissues and then reflect back to the receiver. A transducer, or probe, first emits high-frequency sound waves into tissues. The tissues then reflect the sound waves back to the probe. The mechanical forces from the sound waves are captured by piezoelectric crystals in the probe and converted to electrical signals, producing an image (Figure 1). The piezoelectric crystal therefore acts as both a transmitter and receiver.

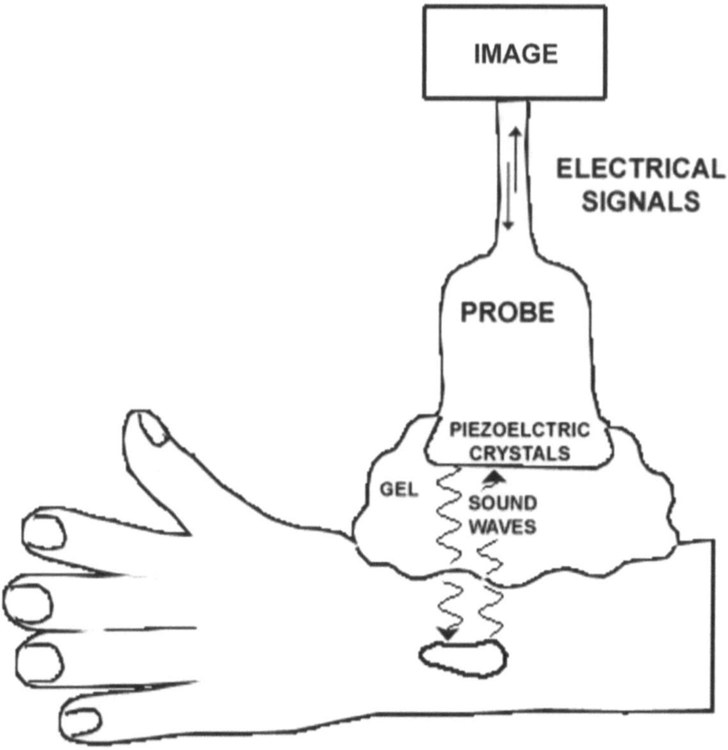

Figure 1-1: Drawing demonstrating the piezoelectric effect. Sound waves created by the piezoelectric crystals are transferred into the tissue through ultrasonic gel, reflected by the structure of interest back to the probe where the crystals covert the waves into electric signals, creating the image.

Ultrasound waves follow the laws of acoustics and therefore can be reflected, refracted, absorbed, and scattered. **Reflection** forms the basis of pulse-echo imaging in which an image is created using energy being reflected back to the source. Reflection of ultrasound waves occurs where there is a difference in the acoustic impedance between two tissues. In tissue, acoustic impedance is based on density and elasticity. The greater the difference in impedance, the more waves will be reflected at the tissue interface. **Refraction** needs to be kept in mind as a structure, such as a needle, passes through one tissue into another. **Absorption** leads to attenuation of the ultrasound waves and increases linearly with frequency. Higher frequency results in less penetration of the ultrasound waves. **Scatter** occurs if ultrasound waves do not travel in a direction perpendicular to an interface. Therefore, the best images are formed when there is a large difference in acoustic impedance between two tissues, while using a transducer whose frequency has a focal region at the depth of the tissue of interest, and whose waves are directed perpendicularly to the structure being imaged.

Resolution of ultrasound images is directly related to the frequency of sound waves used. High-frequency waves (10 - 20 MHz) convert to a high-resolution image, while low-frequency waves (2 - 7 MHz) yield a low-resolution image. Low-frequency waves, however, can penetrate deeper into tissues than high-frequency waves. Fortunately, most musculoskeletal structures are relatively superficial and can be imaged with high-frequency ultrasound. Subcutaneous fat, however, poses a trying issue – it attenuates sound waves and represents a depth barrier to deeper structures. Image resolution is limited due to loss of signal through deeper tissues.

Echogenicity

Tissues that reflect sound well are deemed **hyperechoic** and appear brighter; tissues that reflect little sound are deemed **hypoechoic** and appear darker; tissues that reflect no sound are deemed **anechoic** and appear black. Hyperechoic tissues include bone (brightest), normal tendon, nerves, and fat. Hypoechoic tissues include body fluid (darkest), muscle, and tears of tendons or ligaments. Hypoechoic areas within brighter tissue should key the investigator to pathology. Water and blood minimally attenuate sound waves and pose a unique situation named **acoustic enhancement**. As simple fluids do not absorb, scatter, or reflect waves, more energy passes through the fluid and likewise more energy returns on reflections off structures deep to the fluid. This enhances the signal from the tissues deep to the fluid making them appear brighter than surrounding tissue. An example of an **anechoic** image is the area deep to bone, as ultrasound waves are completely reflected off the bone surface (bright), and this creates an **acoustic shadow** (dark) behind the bone surface. Figure 2 (a & b) demonstrates differences in echogenicity between different structures in the shoulder.

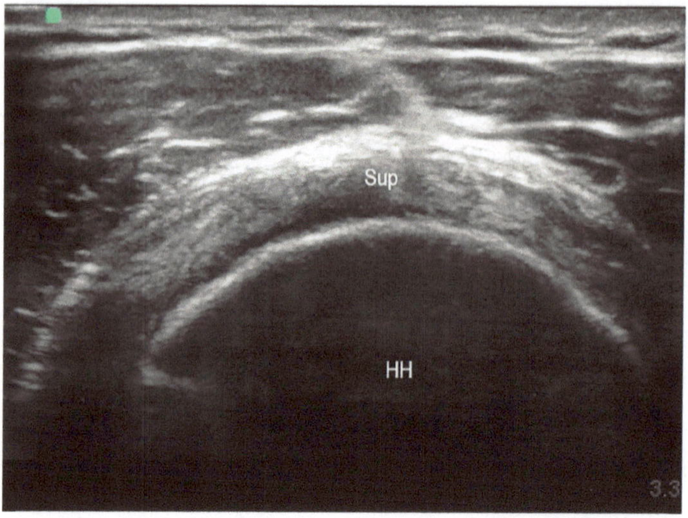

Figure 1-2a

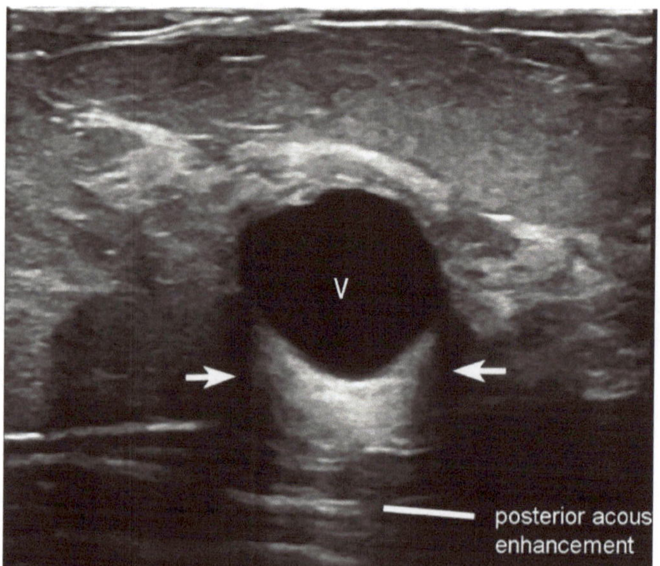

Figure 1-2b

Figure 2: Examples of differences in echogenicity including the (a) hyperechoic humeral head (HH) reflecting all sound waves and an anechoic (b) fluid vacuole allowing all waves to pass through

Anisotropy

Anisotropy is an important cause of artifacts in ultrasound imaging and refers to the phenomenon in which artifacts are produced based on the orientation of the transducer to a structure. This mainly occurs when imaging tendons or ligaments, as sound waves may be reflected off the organized fibers towards or away from the transducer. The result is often a hypoechoic region of a tendon or ligament, which may fool the operator to diagnose a tear or diseased portion (Figure 3 a, b).

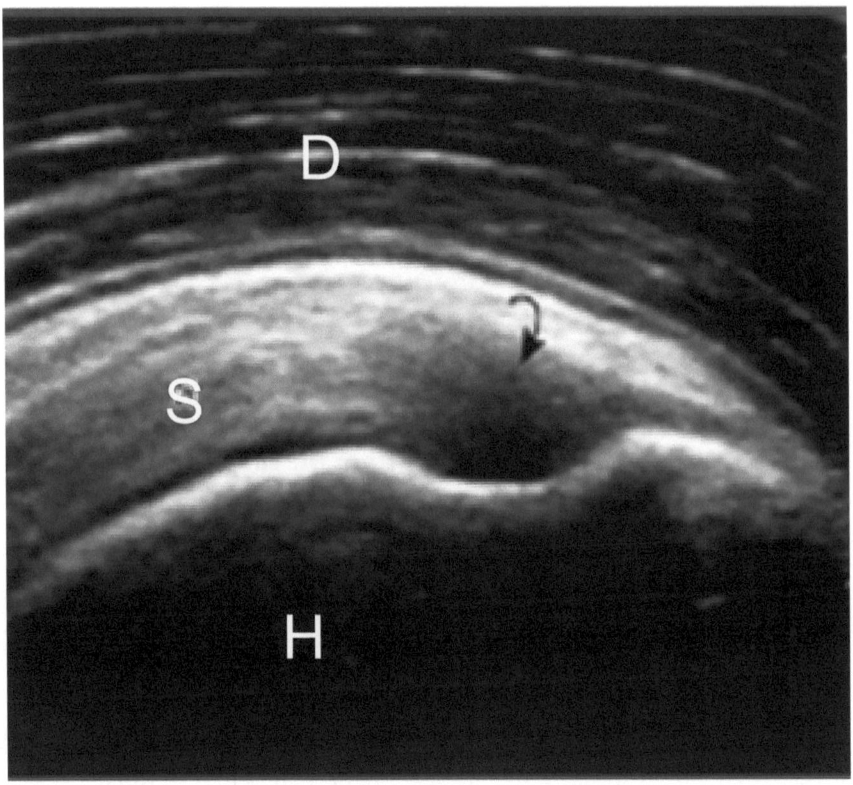

Figure 1-3a

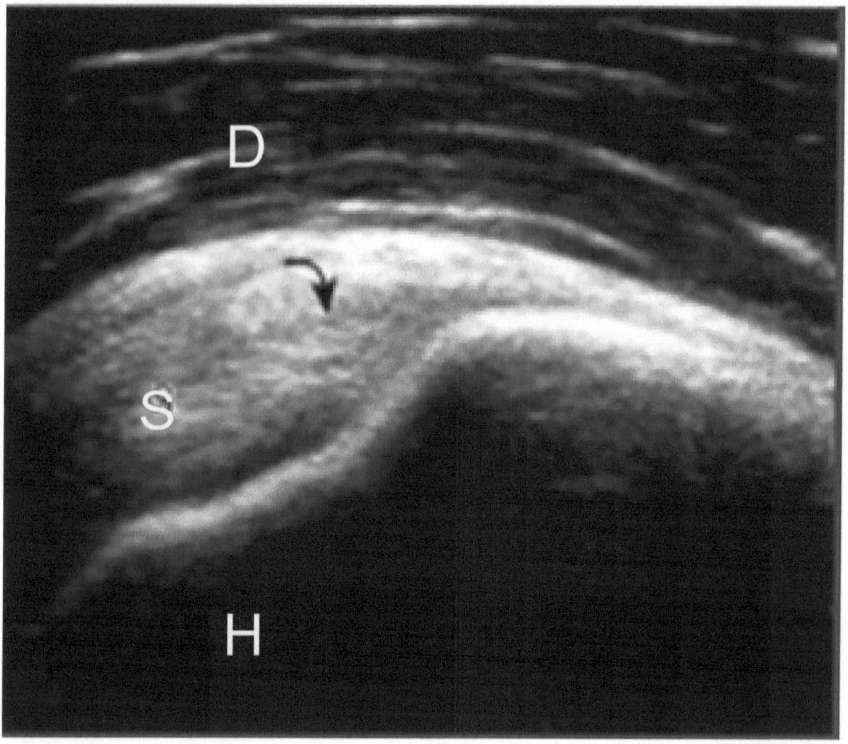

Figure 1-3b

Figure 1-3: Example of anisotropy within the supraspinatus tendon. A potential hypoechoic region near the tendon attachment is seen in (a) which disappears when the probe is moved slightly, eliminating the anisotropy (b).

Anisotropy is minimized in two ways: using a linear array transducer and by placing the transducer perpendicular to the tendon, ligament or other structure being imaged. A **linear array transducer** has a flat surface that allows sound waves to be more perpendicular to the structure of interest. Holding the transducer perpendicular to the structure makes it more probable that sound waves will reflect back to the transducer. As tendons are usually draped over the underlying bone and therefore parallel to the bone, the transducer position that provides the brightest image of the underlying bone is usually the position that provides the best image of the tendon. This is true for the supraspinatus tendon as it passes over the articular cartilage of the humeral head but not the case as it inserts on the greater tuberosity (Figure 4). At its point of attachment, the supraspinatus tendon dives into the bone and is no longer parallel to it.

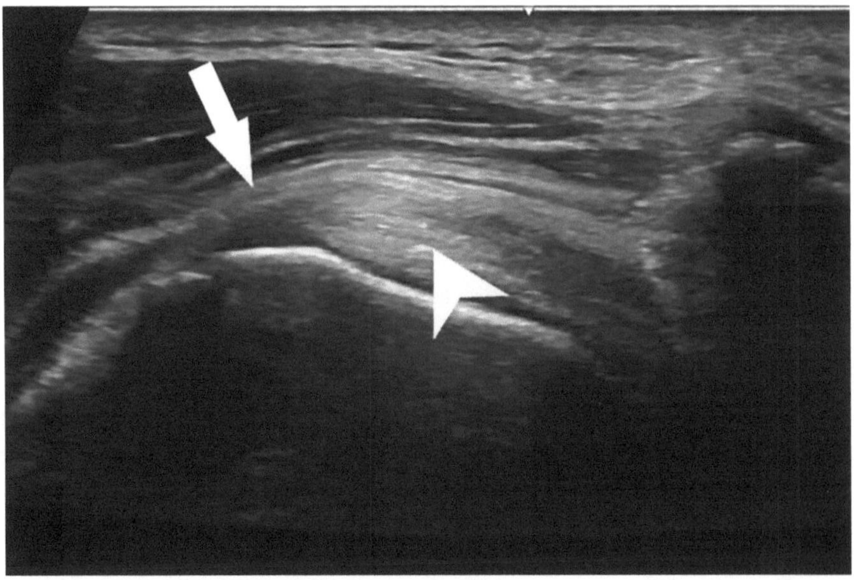

Figure 1-4

Figure 1-4: Supraspinatus fibers seen parallel to the articular surface (arrowhead) changing orientation while inserting to the greater tuberosity (arrow).

The skillset of the ultrasonographer comes into play to combat anisotropy, as the probe must be oriented properly for each structure. Anisotropic artifacts can also be avoided by making sure that any potential pathology is confirmed on both longitudinal and transverse views. Another important point regarding anisotropy is that while ultrasound can make a structure appear worse than it is; it can never make that structure appear better than it is.

Obtaining the Best Ultrasound Image

Diagnostic ultrasound creates two-dimensional images. Unlike plain radiography or advanced three-dimensional imaging that involve obtaining orthogonal views of an entire body part, ultrasound utilizes two views, or axes, to image individual structures. These views are called the **long-axis** (or longitudinal) and **short-axis** (or transverse). These views are entirely dependent on the orientation of the probe relative to the structure of interest. The long-axis view is obtained when the probe is oriented longitudinally to the structure of interest, while the short-axis view is obtained when the probe is rotated 90 degrees and oriented transversely to the same structure of interest (Figure 5).

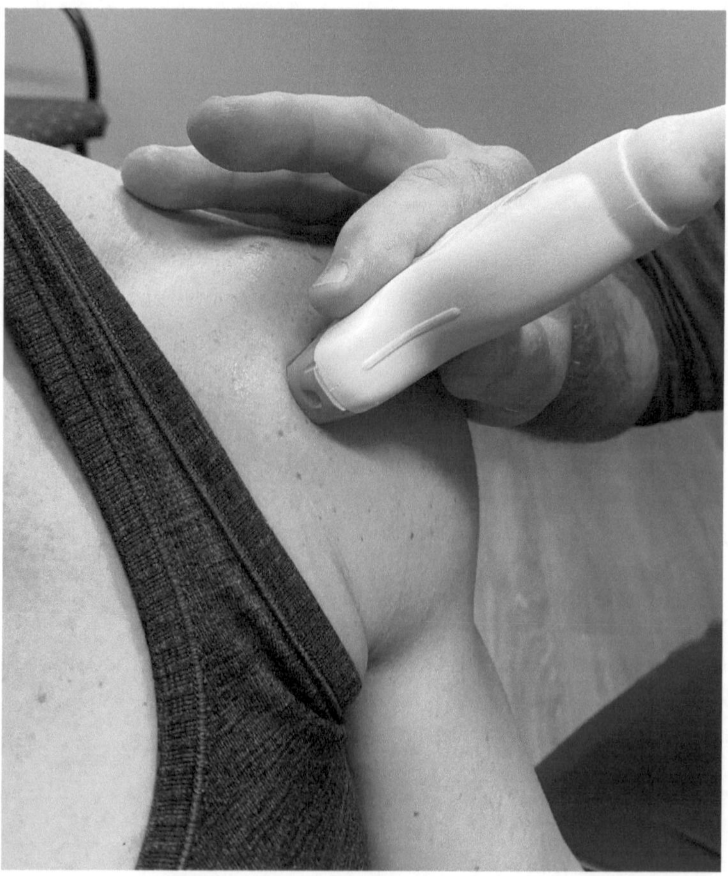

Figure 1-5a

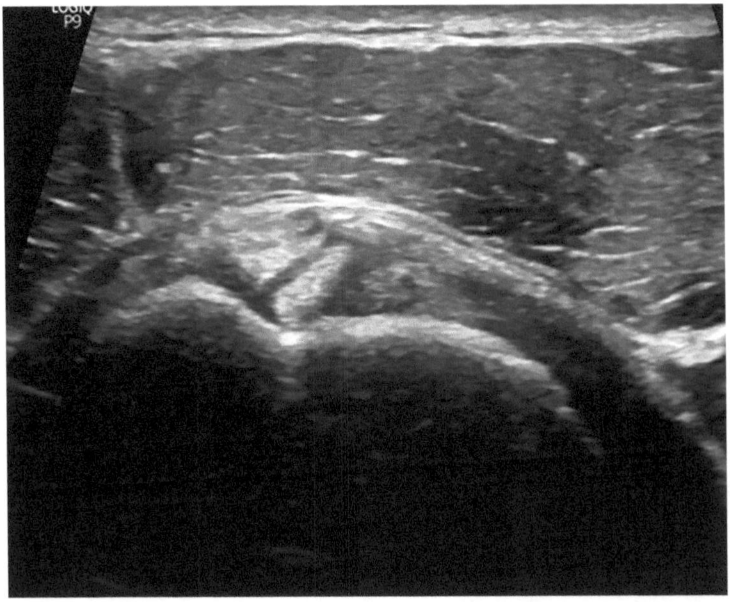

Figure 1-5b

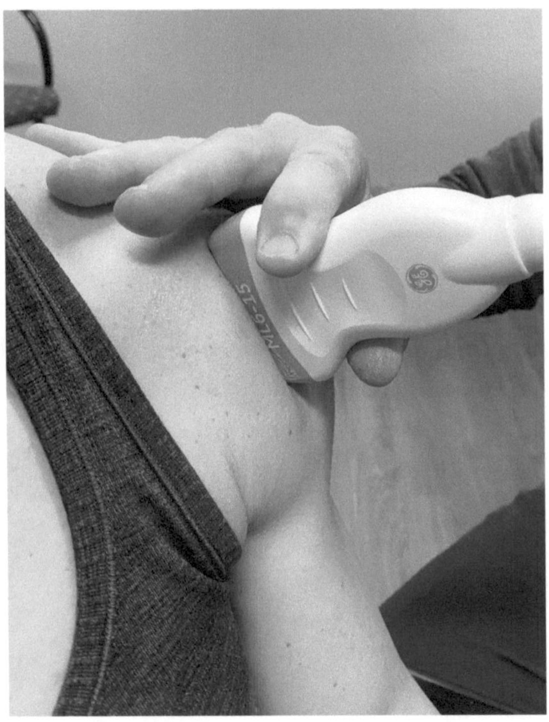

Figure 1-5c

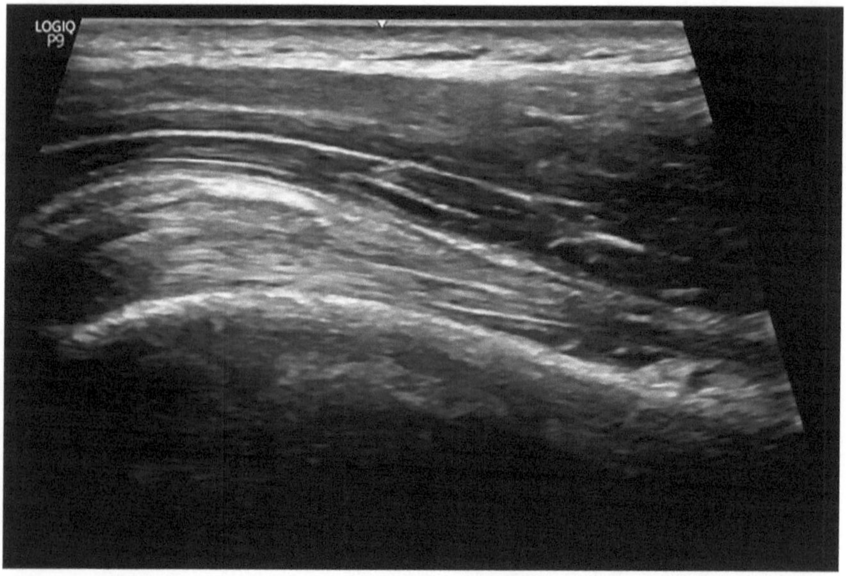

Figure 1-5d

Figure 1-5: Examples of rotation of the probe to change the view from short axis or transverse (a) (b) to long axis or longitudinal (c) (d). In this case imaging the biceps tendon in the bicipital groove

The technique in holding the transducer is also important in obtaining the best image. The transducer should be held in a comfortable manner by the body/head of the probe as opposed to the tail with the hand in contact with the skin to maintain stability (Figure 6).

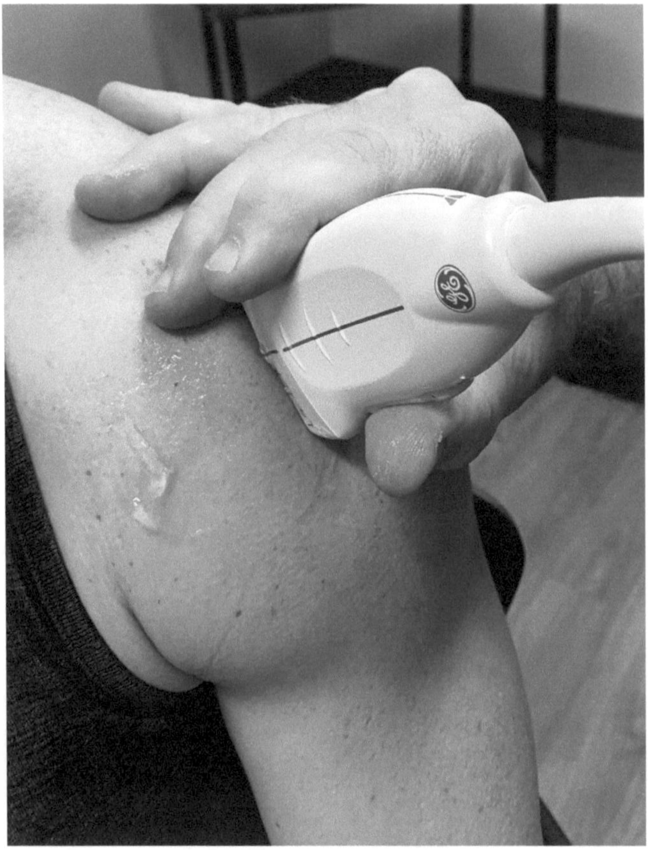

Figure 1-6

Figure 1-6: Proper way to hold the probe. Firmly at its base with a portion of the hand gaining stability on the patient

The transducer can be moved to maximize image quality through rotation (usually 90 degrees) as described above, Toggle/Wag and heel-toe. Toggle/Wag is performed by subtly adjusting the orientation or angle of the probe on the skin while maintaining the same rotation (Figure 7 a-d).

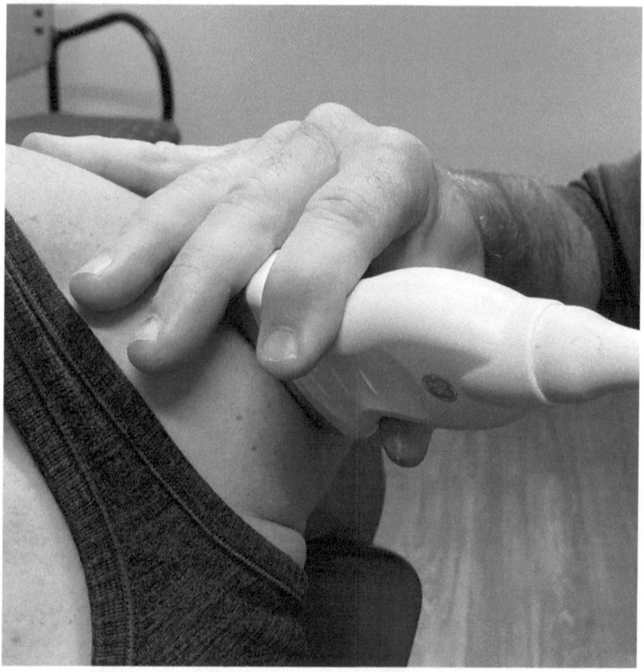

Figure 1-7a

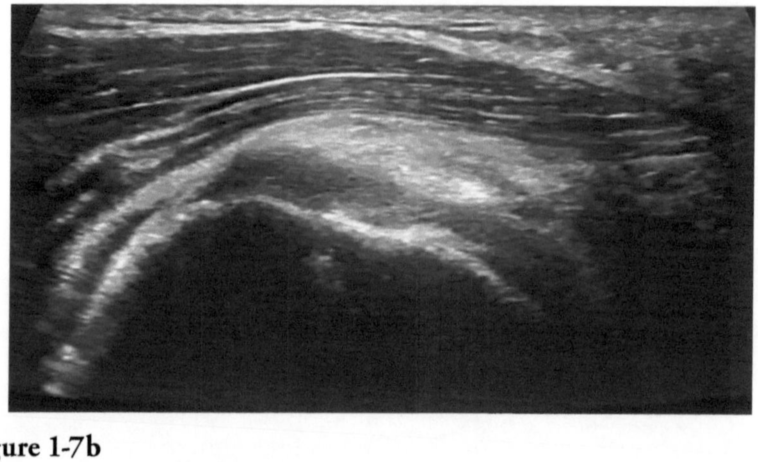

Figure 1-7b

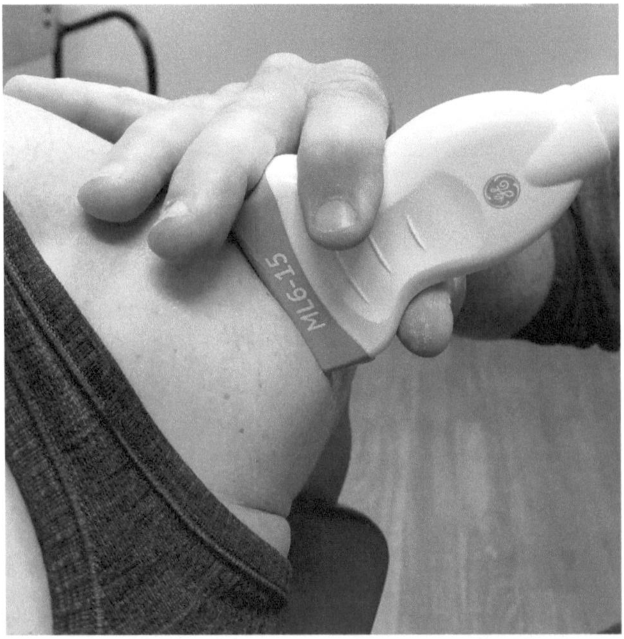

Figure 1-7c

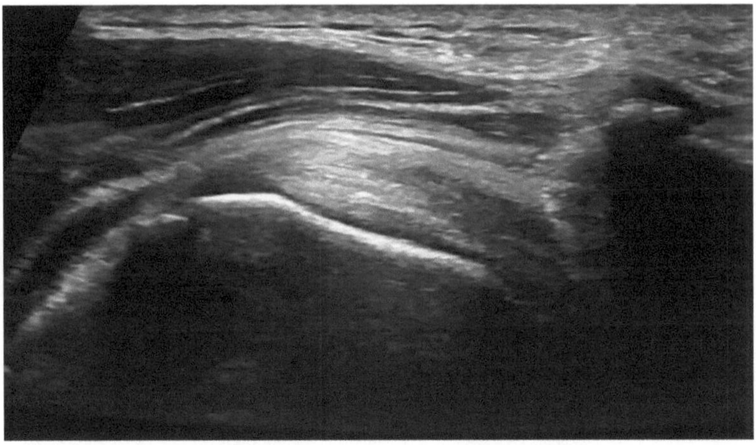

Figure 1-7d

Figure 1-7: Example of Toggle or Wag. While the original position of the probe (a) demonstrates anisotropy within, in this case the supraspinatus attachment (b), minimally tilting the angle of the probe (c) displays normal homogeneous tendon insertion (d).

In a linear probe, Toggle/Wag is a rotation about the long axis of the probe. Heel-toe is a maneuver in which the pressure is applied more to the ends of the probe while maintaining the entire probe on the skin (Figure 8). These maneuvers are performed to assure that the ultrasound waves remain perpendicular to the underlying structure being imaged, minimizing any anisotropic artifact. Both short- and long-axis views for each structure imaged should always be obtained.

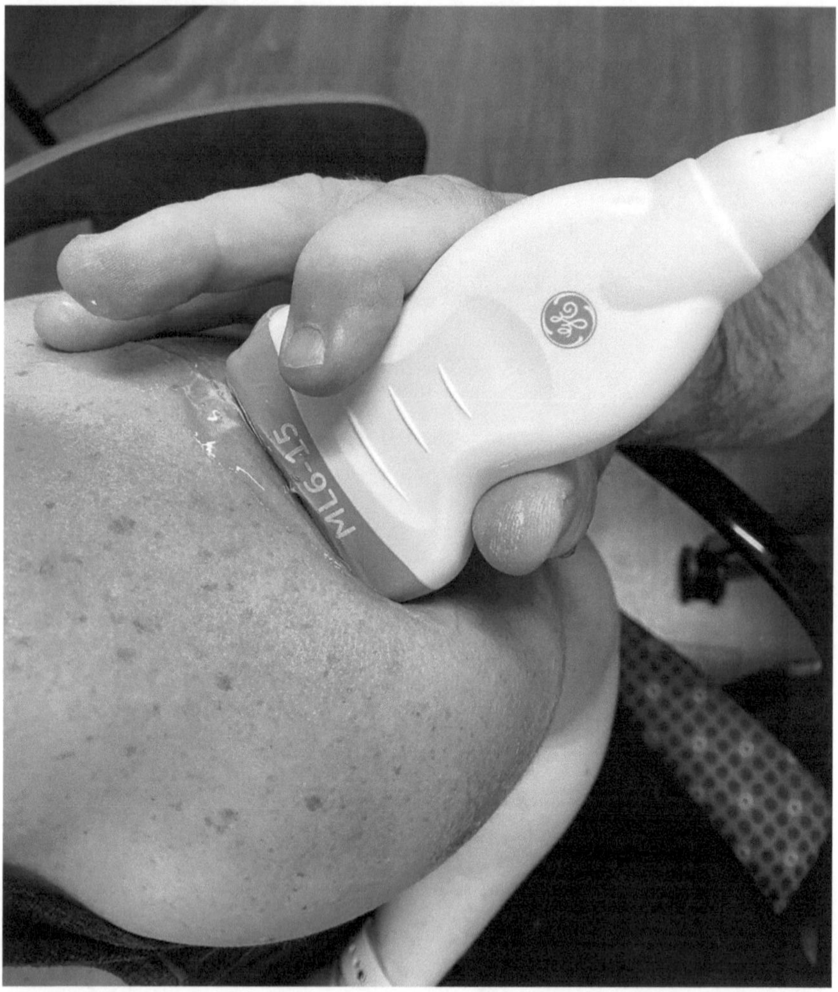

Figure 1-8a

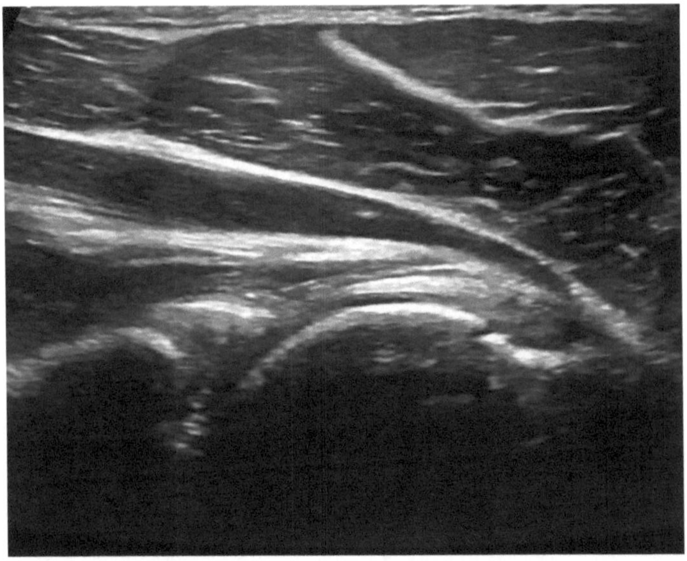

Figure1- 8b

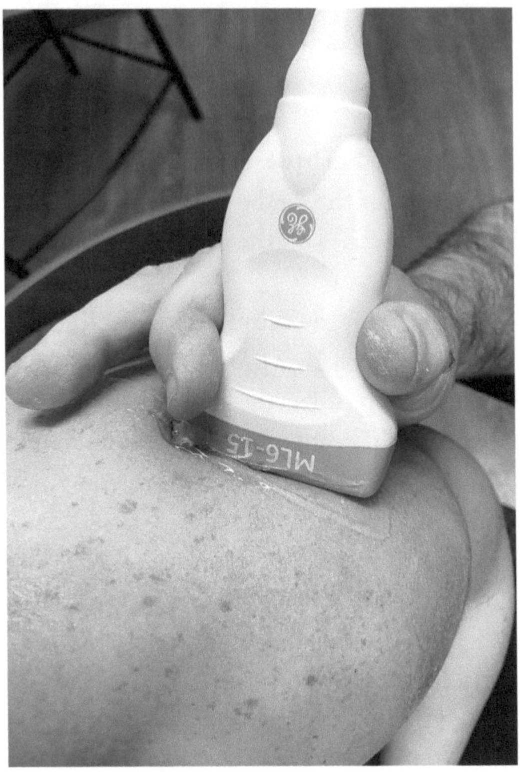

Figure 1-8c

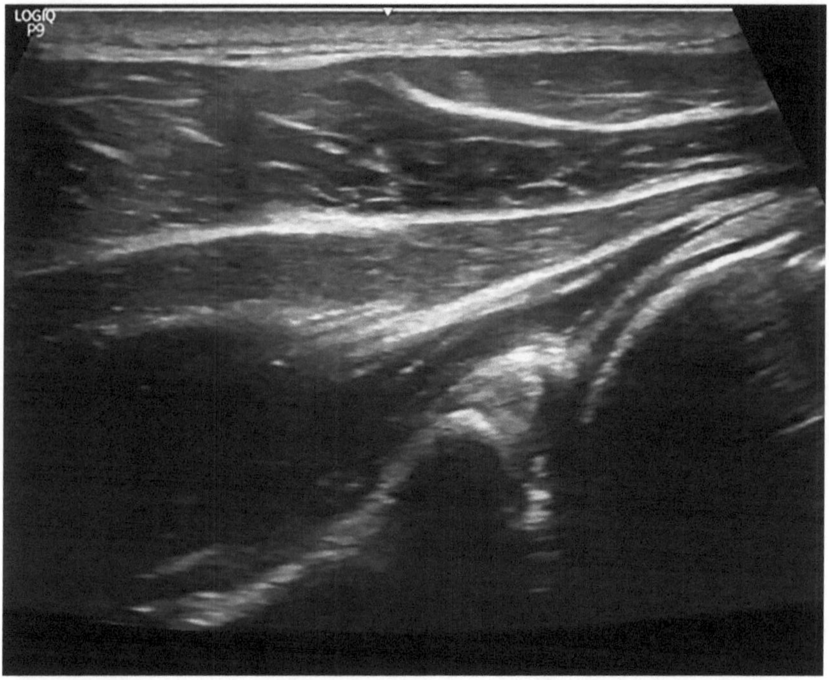

Figure 1-8d

Figure 1-8: Example of heel-toe maneuver. Initial image (a) with pressure on the heel (b) of the probe focuses on infraspinatus tendon. Pressure on the toe (c) focuses on the posterior glenoid and labrum (d).

Optimization of the image occurs by altering the physics/settings of the machine, perfecting, and fine-tuning the images. Functions on the machine itself that can optimize the image include **depth**, **frequency**, **focus, gain** and **time gain compensation**. **Depth** should be adjusted to put the area of interest at ½ - ¾ depth of the screen. A small area should be left in the bottom of the screen to provide structural context. **Frequency** can be altered by either changing the transducer (linear for high frequency, curvilinear for low frequency) (Figure 9) or adjusting the frequency on the machine itself (increase the frequency for better resolution and lower the frequency for more penetration).

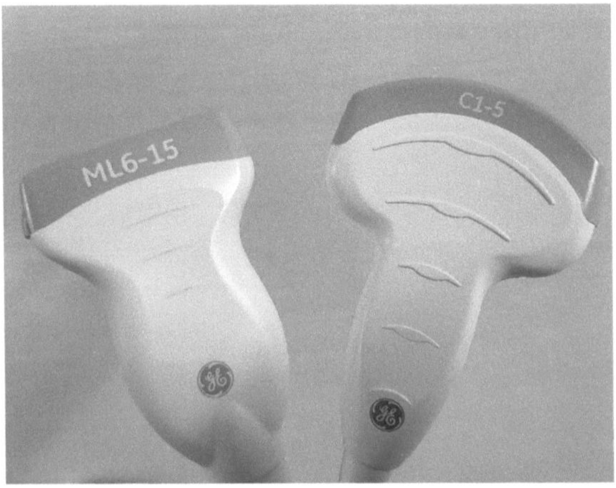

Figure 1-9

Figure 1-9: Types of transducers or probes including linear for high frequency on the left and curvilinear for low frequency on the right.

The ultrasound beam narrows and then widens as it penetrates tissue, with the narrow region being the Focal Zone, where the resolution is best. Therefore, it is best to adjust the **focus** so that the point of interest is centered in the Focal Zone. **Gain** on ultrasound images refers to the brightness of the entire image. Increasing the gain produces a brighter image while decreasing it makes the image darker. The gain should be optimized to provide an image with the most detail (Figure 10).

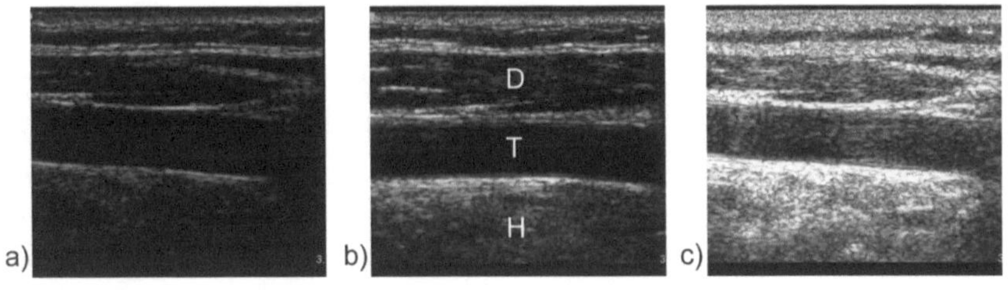

Figure 1-10

Figure 1-10: Example of changes in gain which basically changes the brightness of the signal to maximize the quality of the image seen here as low (a), medium (d) and high (c) when viewing the biceps tendon (T) longitudinally with overlying deltoid (D) and deep humeral head (H).

Time gain compensation is the ability to compensate for attenuation of signal as waves travel through tissues. Depth, frequency, focus and gain can be adjusted with instruments on the control panel of the ultrasound (Figure 11).

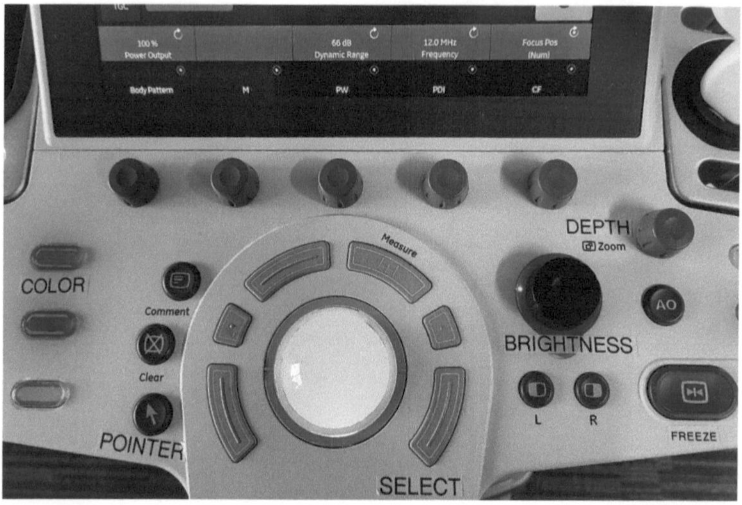

Figure 1-11

Figure 1-11: Example of ultrasound control panel with instruments for adjusting depth, frequency, focus, and gain. Also available are controls for freezing the image, recording image and video, and measuring structures.

On some ultrasound machines there are separate knobs that can adjust each of these individually, while other units may combine several of the functions to simplify the adjustments. For example, increasing the depth of the image will adjust the Focal Zone to place it in the middle of the image on the screen while decreasing the frequency to maximize the penetration and resolution of the image automatically. Other machines will set the frequency based upon your setting the machine for your goal: high resolution versus general versus penetration. There are certain instances however when separating these is necessary to obtain the best information regarding the anatomic structure being studied. While different on different machines, the control panel also allows for other functions including recording images, recording videos, freezing images, and measuring structures on the image to name a few (Figure 11). While this can be intimidating, especially if the physician is new to ultrasound or to the given unit, it is relatively easy to understand with a little use and experimentation.

Another way to optimize the image comes from avoiding artifacts. An ultrasound artifact is any image aberration that misrepresents the correct anatomic structure. Artifacts are intrinsic to ultrasound and while they can lead to falsely calling pathology, they can also be a helpful tool. Common artifacts include shadowing, enhancement, reverberation and as already mentioned anisotropy. Again, **anisotropy** is the property of being directionally dependent, which implies different properties in different directions. Ultrasound anisotropy occurs when the transducer is not parallel to the tissue and therefore the sound beam is not perpendicular to the structure being imaged. When this is the case, fewer sound beams are reflected back to the transducer. As the angle of incidence becomes lower no waves will be reflected back to the transducer and the structure will disappear. Because anisotropy is so dependent on the perpendicularity of ECHO, the denser the structure, the more reflective the structure is and the more susceptible it is to anisotropy. Tendon is more susceptible than ligament, which is more so than nerve, with muscle being least susceptible. This may be helpful when trying to discern nerve from tendon. With slight toggle of the probe tendon will disappear first due to anisotropy leaving the nerve still visible (Figure 12). Anisotropy is a correctable artifact done by adjusting the transducer position using Toggle, Wag and heel-toe maneuvers.

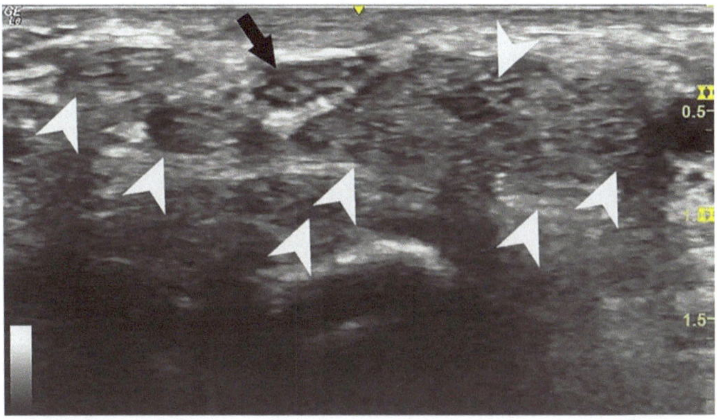

Figure 1-12a

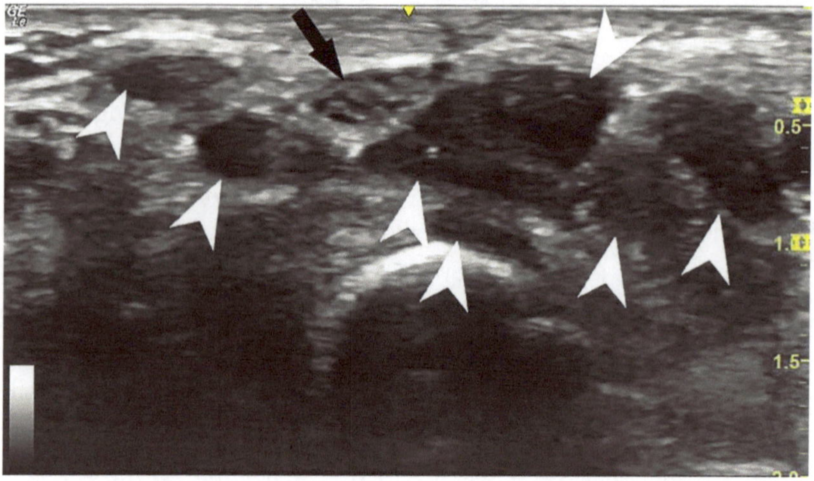

Figure 12-b

Figure 1-12: Example of differences in anisotropy. Tendons (arrowheads) and median nerve (arrow) both visualized with probe perpendicular (a); tendons appear to disappear while the nerve remains with slight toggle of the probe (b).

Shadowing is characterized by a signal void behind structures that strongly absorb, attenuate or reflect ultrasound waves. It occurs most often with solid structures such as bone, dense calcifications including osteophytes, calcifications and loose bodies, and metals (e.g. foreign bodies or implants). It can also occur when refraction seems to direct sound away or alter the reflection. Not all the ultrasound waves coming out of the transducer are parallel. The crossbeams improve our image. If there is a structure just outside of our image it may affect the image on that side without blocking the image being seen (Figure 13).

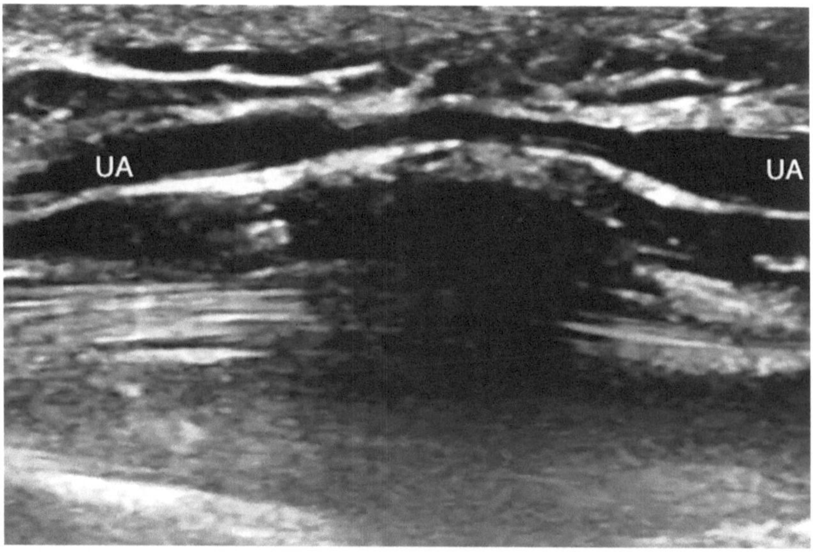

Figure 1-13

Figure 1-13: Example of a structure outside the field of view affecting structure being visualized. In this case the ulnar artery (UA) is imaged longitudinally. While the hook of the hamate is not in the field of view, it creates an echogenic shadow obscuring the image of the underlying tendon.

Enhancement is artificially increased echo signal deep to structures that do not attenuate signal. This is characteristically seen deep to fluid-filled structures such as cysts and vessels and can be used to improve imaging. **Reverberation** occurs when ultrasound waves get 'trapped' between two reflective surfaces, bouncing back and forth, therefore confusing the machine as waves that return, and return at longer intervals, appearing deeper. Example of reverberation include gas bubbles and hollow needles (Figure 14).

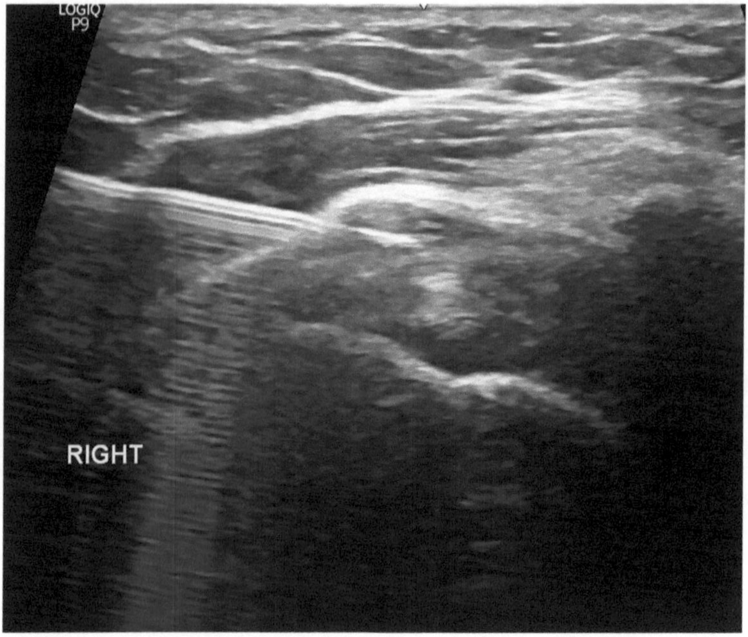

Figure 1-14

Figure 1-14: Example of reverberation artifact imaging a needle during therapeutic injection.

Pitfalls that are inherent to ultrasound can also detrimentally affect the image, while avoiding them is necessary to further optimize the image. The misinterpretation of normal anatomy is a common pitfall. This could include the supraspinatus tendon having similar echogenicity to the overlying deltoid which can occur as the patient ages. Also transitions between structures with different echogenicity such as the anterior supraspinatus where the hyperechoic biceps tendon is adjacent the hypoechoic area just posterior to the biceps could be seen as a defect. The natural thinning of tendons and muscle may be misinterpreted as pathology, as can the mild inhomogeneity in some muscles or tendons. Other pitfalls include soft tissue and bony abnormalities such as calcific nodules, osteophytes, loose bodies, and joint displacement such as subluxation of the humeral head relative to the glenoid. Technical limitations of ultrasound are also pitfalls due to overlying bony structures that limit the ability to image the underlying structures.

Avoiding pitfalls requires an examiner with excellent three-dimensional understanding of the anatomy of the structure being evaluated while also being proficient at using ultrasound. Orthopaedic surgeons who are clinically examining anatomic structures of interest in the clinic and then performing surgery on them in the operating room certainly have excellent anatomic knowledge. Also, given the similarities to arthroscopy, orthopaedists will find that, with a minimal amount of practice, they can also become proficient with ultrasound. Reviewing plain radiographs prior to performing the ultrasound exam helps avoid the misinterpretation of bony and soft tissue calcific abnormalities. Ultrasonically examining the asymptomatic or least symptomatic side of the structure being evaluated initially allows this to be the control to avoid misinterpreting what may be normal anatomy for the patient as pathology. Positioning the anatomic structure being examined to maximize its visibility to the ultrasound probe helps to overcome technical limitations. An example of this would be positioning the shoulder into internal rotation and extension to pull the greater tuberosity and supraspinatus insertion out to length, and out from under the acromion. Pitfalls can also be avoided by using passive and active motion while imaging to dynamically visualize the structure of interest. Further enhancement of the exam can be accomplished by having the patient perform functional movements as well as resisted isometrics during imaging. Imaging can also be performed during typical stress testing to assess for ligament integrity and laxity.

Indications

While initially there is an inclination to ultrasonically image as many patients as possible, indications for diagnostic ultrasound should be the same as those for other advanced imaging. Patients with clinical exam evidence of pathology that can be imaged with ultrasound, who have failed appropriate non-operative management, and have been evaluated with plain radiographs, have indications for diagnostic ultrasound imaging. Indications also include patients with acute, traumatic injuries that require immediate imaging to guide the need for urgent/emergent management. As the surgeon becomes more comfortable with the use of ultrasound in the clinical setting, they may modify these indications, relying on an ultrasound exam earlier than they may previously would have in the case of more expensive advanced imaging.

Standard Exam

Most important during the ultrasound examination is making sure that both the patient and the examiner are comfortable and stable, in a position that allows complete examination of the anatomic structure in question. This may require repositioning or switching positions during the exam. If possible, it is best to position the monitor so that both the examiner and the patient can easily see it. This allows the patient to better understand their condition. It is also important to know your subject and adjust accordingly. For example, while it may be best to examine the shoulder with both examiner and subject on rolling, backless stools, some patients may need more support including stable-backed chairs with arms or even lying supine for a potential injection (Figure 15 a-c). Just as during physical exam or in surgery, the best position for the patient is dependent on what works best in the hands of the surgeon performing the examination.

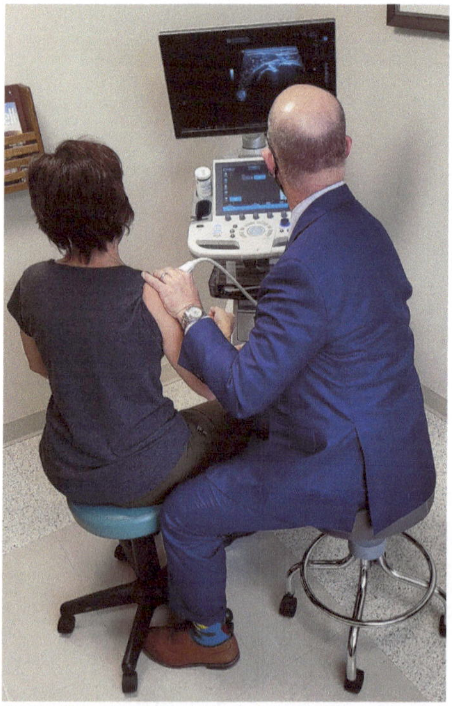

Figure 1-15-a

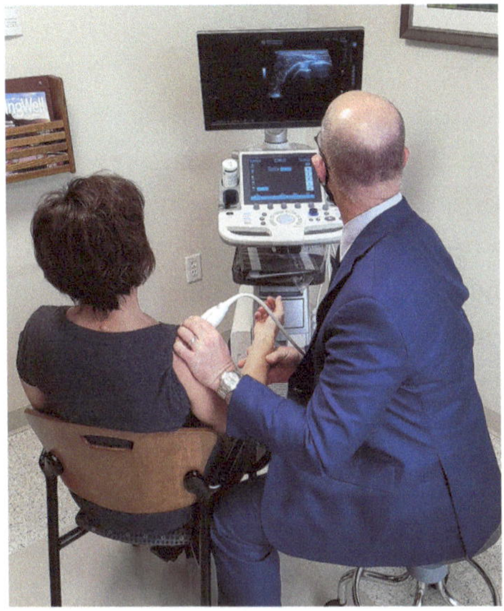

Figure 1-15b

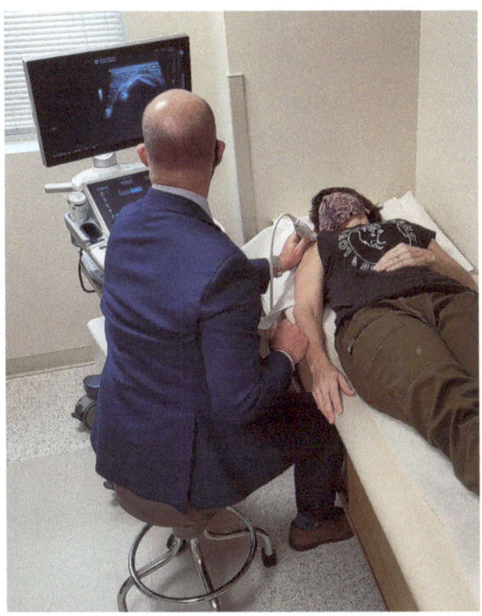

Figure 1-15c

Figure 1-15: Adjust positioning of the patient as needed. While it may be best to examine a shoulder with examiner and subject on rolling, backless stools (a), some patients may need more support (b) & (c).

Bilateral exams should be performed whenever possible, especially early in the learning curve, imaging the least symptomatic side first. This allows the examiner to define the "normal" anatomy of the patient. While there is a wide range of normal values between patients, the values tend to be symmetrical side-to-side in each patient. Examining the least symptomatic side first also educates the patient regarding the structures being evaluated and allows the patient to experience what a "normal" exam feels like. This gives the patient the ability to give proper feedback when the symptomatic structure is being evaluated (e.g., reporting tenderness when imaging over an area of potential pathology). Depending on the payer and contracting, reimbursement may not be made for the second (bilateral) exam. Indications for imaging the opposite side should be included in the dictation, which can simply be for comparison purpose to determine chronicity of the pathology. Regardless of payment, imaging the contralateral side can be well worth the time spent, especially early in your learning curve.

All structures of interest should be evaluated both longitudinally and transversely with measurements being made when applicable. This should initially be done statically. Dynamic imaging should also be performed when possible or beneficial. This should first be passive, moved by the examiner, followed by active or functional movement performed by the patient. Movement of the tissues should be compared to the normal/asymptomatic side and the patient should report any roughness or discomfort with movement whether passive or active. Isometric contraction can be utilized to assess muscle quality and function and tendon integrity. Varus, valgus, and rotational stress can be applied to assess ligamentous integrity. Again, evaluating the asymptomatic or least symptomatic side first allows for excellent control and comparison, while patient feedback further enhances the value of the exam.

Locating Pathology

Evaluating tendon pathology is one of the strengths of ultrasound of the musculoskeletal system. Normal tendons have homogeneous echogenicity. There may be some areas of abnormality in the signal, but in the normal tendon these abnormalities are usually mirrored in the opposite side. Disruption of a tendon may present itself in a variety of ways. Findings in *complete tears* include focal thinning of the tendon; complete non-visualization of the tendon (Figure 16), which is similar to focal thinning, but there is no normal tendon tissue identified; focal discontinuity in the homogeneous echogenicity of the tendon without focal thinning (Figure 17); inversion of the superficial bursal contour of the tendon (going from convexity to concavity) (Figure 18 a, b); and hyperechoic material in the location of the tendon that fails to move during real-time dynamic imaging. Findings in *partial tears* of tendons include a hypoechoic discontinuity in the tendon in which the lesion involves either the superficial or deep side of the tendon; or a mixed hyperechoic and hypoechoic region within the tendon which is thought to be due to a separation of the torn edge from the rest of the tendon, resulting in a new interface within the tendon. Often when imaging over an area of a partial tear (and at times over a complete tear) patients report tenderness as the transducer moves over the defect and pressure is applied to visualize the tear. This sensation should be compared with that experienced during imaging of the asymptomatic side to ensure that the tenderness is not normal for that patient.

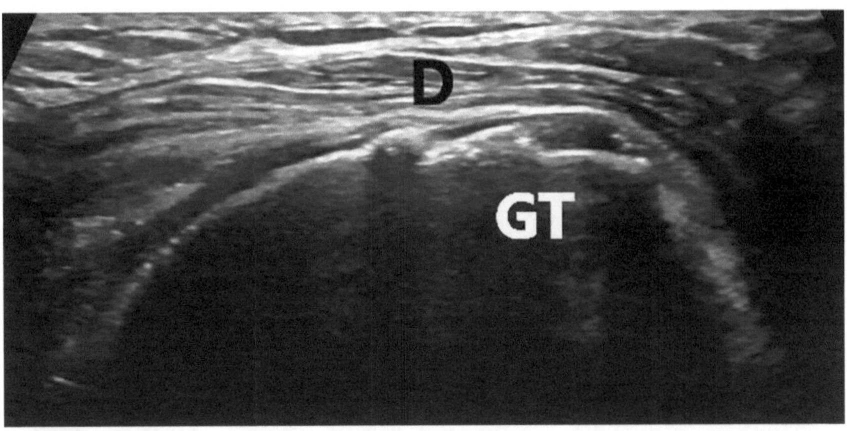

Figure 1-16

Figure 1-16: Example of complete tear of the supraspinatus demonstrated by non-visualization of the tendon with the overlying deltoid (D) directly adjacent to the greater tuberosity (GT).

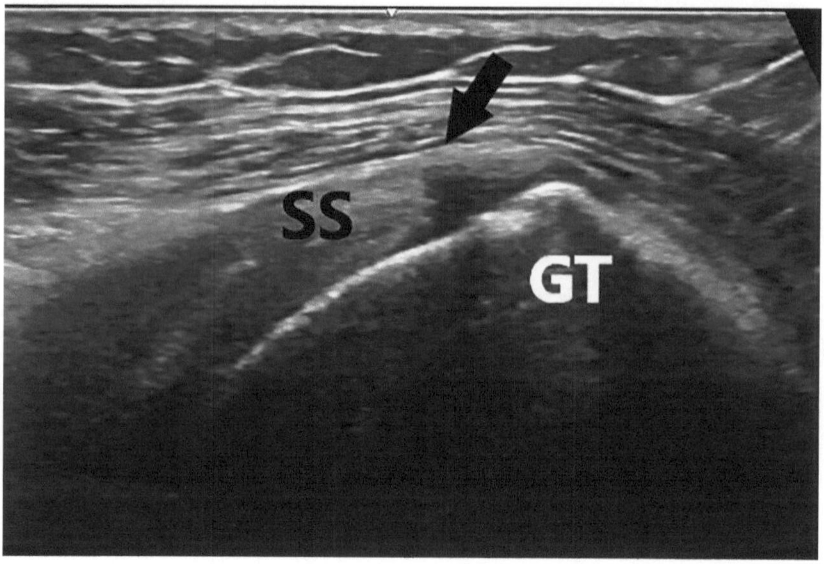

Figure 1-17

Figure 1-17: Full-thickness tear of the supraspinatus tendon (SS) demonstrated by focal discontinuity in the homogeneous echogenicity of the tendon (arrow) without thinning of the tendon as it attaches to the greater tuberosity (GT).

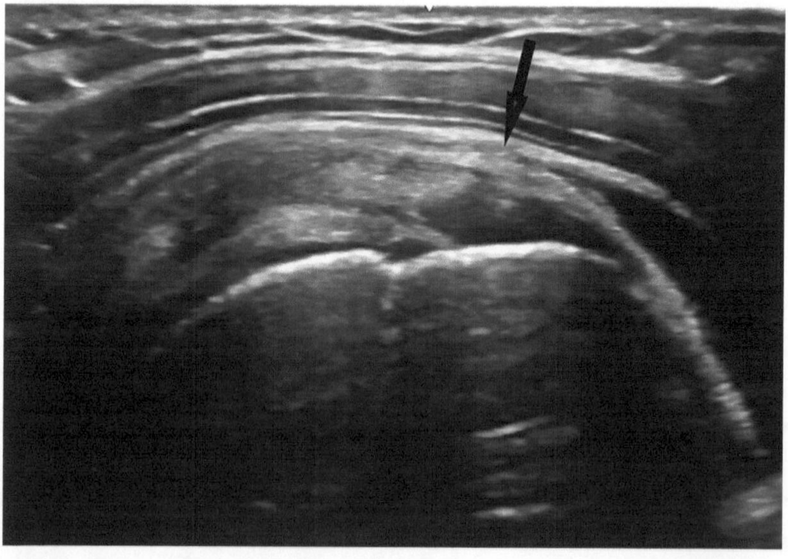

Figure 1-18a

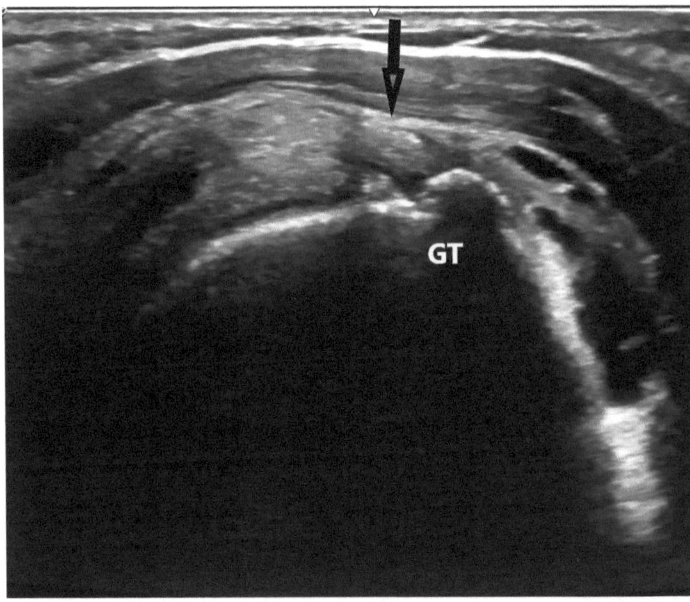

Figure 1-18b

Figure 1-18: Example of full-thickness tear of the supraspinatus tendon by inversion of the normal superficial tendon convexity (arrow) (a) in the more posterior portion of the tendon attachment to concavity (arrow) in the anterior tendon (b).

It is important to have an excellent understanding of the normal sonographic anatomy of the structure being evaluated in general and of the patient's "normal" anatomy. Together with this, application of the above criteria has been documented to enhance the results of diagnostic ultrasonography. Some authors have stressed the value of a two-criteria model in which a defect is only diagnosed if a criterion is reproducible either in different joint positions or in different transducer positions, or if a second criterion (e.g., a static along with a dynamic criterion) is present in different positions. Finally, it is important to understand that the "formal" criteria of thinning, non-visualization, discontinuity of the tendon or disruption, or inversion of the superficial bursal contour are not prone to artifacts, in complete contrast to the criteria of echogenicity. Variations in tendon echogenicity should be recorded, but care is needed in making a diagnosis solely based on this criterion.

Muscle can also be readily evaluated with ultrasound. Muscle tears can be assessed using the same or similar criteria as with tendon tears including discontinuity, disruption, or focal thinning of the muscle. Atrophy can be assessed, especially with comparisons to the opposite side. Quality of the muscle can also be evaluated. The architecture of the superficial and deep surfaces, pennate pattern of the muscle fascicles and structure of the central tendon can be assessed. The echogenicity of the muscle itself should be homogeneous and can be compared either to the opposite side or any other adjacent muscles that are not involved in the pathology (e.g., the trapezius overlying the supraspinatus muscle). Fatty infiltration on ultrasound can be detected by increased echogenicity (similar to hyperechoic fat) within the muscle substance, loss of normal pennate pattern, superficial, deep and central muscle architecture, and overall muscle volume loss. Quality of the muscle can also be assessed with dynamic imaging during an isometric contraction of the muscle. This allows for an assessment of what portion of the muscle is contractile and the contractility can be compared to the opposite side.

Ligamentous tears also have findings like tendon tears. Partial-thickness tears demonstrate a hypoechoic area of incomplete fiber disruption. Full-thickness tears demonstrate a hypoechoic or anechoic region of fiber discontinuity.

Effusions are typically hypoechoic or anechoic, although heterogenic joint fluid caused by hemorrhage or infection may vary from hypoechoic to hyperechoic and possibly heterogeneous (Figure 19).

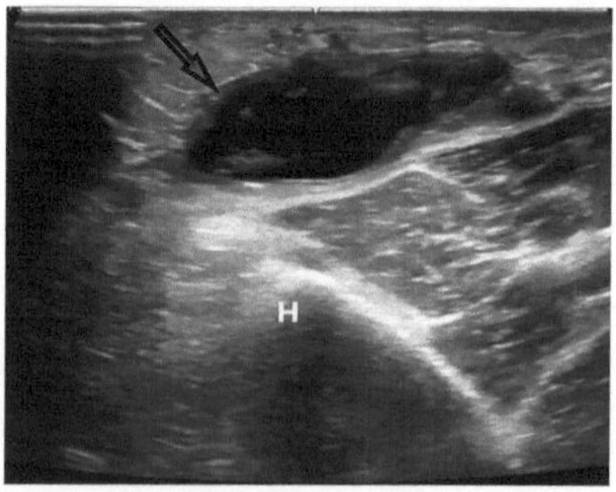

Figure 1-19

Figure 1-19: Ultrasonic evaluation of heterogenous fluid collection (arrow) with areas that are hypoechoic as well as hyperechoic.

Synovial hypertrophy, seen on active infection or inflammatory response, is often diffuse with extension into the joint recesses and a hypoechoic appearance relative to subcutaneous fat. Doppler can be very helpful in identifying inflammation and determining its severity.

Intra-articular loose bodies if mineralized appear hyperechoic superficial to the cartilage with posterior shadowing (Figure 20 a, b). Cartilaginous loose bodies are more difficult to see as they appear hypoechoic and are often obscured by the surrounding hypoechoic effusion.

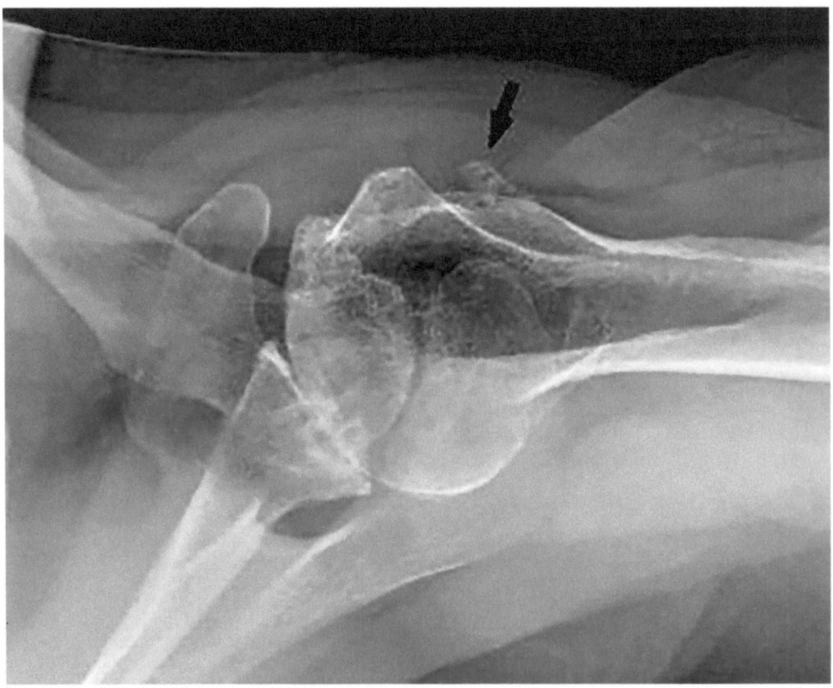

Figure 1-20a

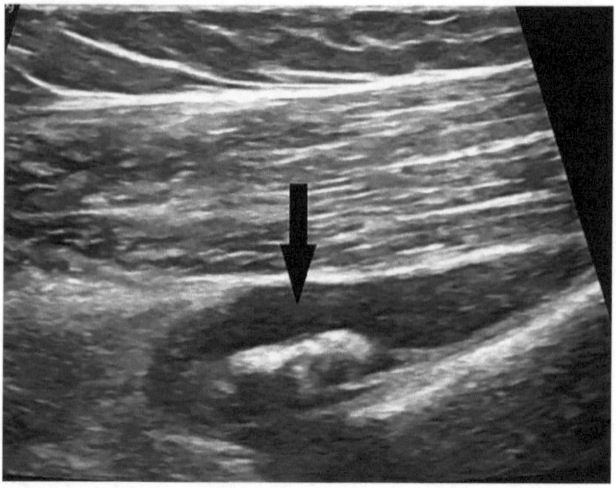

Figure 1-20-b

Figure 1-20: Calcified loose body (arrow) within the biceps sheath on plain radiograph (a) and longitudinal ultrasound view (b) with hyperechoic superficial surface (arrow) and anechoic shadow deep.

For diagnostic evaluation of nerves, high frequency linear array transducers are preferred as they allow best resolution, tissue differentiation, and identification of morphological structure. However, depth of structure, body habitus, or tissue composition may make this infeasible. Use a combination of both high and low frequency transducers for complete evaluation as needed. A nerve in short axis has a typical honeycomb appearance. It often helps to use a fair amount of gel and pay attention to the transducer pressure. Make use of anatomic landmarks and follow the nerve into different locations, proximal going to distal of the location of interest. Alter the speed of scanning. At times, moving the probe faster makes the identification of the nerve more obvious as you follow it anatomically proximal to distal and back to proximal again. As with all structures, most accurate images are obtained by orienting the transducer perpendicular to the nerve and imaging in both the short and long axis. Viewing the nerve longitudinally is certainly more challenging, though important. In the case of focal neuropathies, the nerve should be inspected for overall swelling or notching. The fascicular architecture should be evaluated looking for enlargement of individual fascicles. The course of the nerve should be followed looking for overall enlargement and individual fascicle swelling. Comparisons can be made to the contralateral side. Increased Doppler flow in nerves tends to imply chronic problems. Dynamic ultrasound should be performed as indicated looking for abnormal movement, including ulnar nerve subluxation over the medial epicondyle and encroaching lumbricals on the median nerve in the carpal tunnel.

Interventional Ultrasound

Ultrasound can also be extremely helpful in guiding interventions. Usually this involves needle placement for injection or aspiration, but ultrasound can also be useful for other interventions including portal placement for arthroscopy and location of loose or foreign bodies. Orthopaedic surgeons are often confident that they can place a needle in any joint, bursa or other space. However, using ultrasound allows the surgeon to know exactly where the intervention is applied. This certainly not only increases the confidence of the physician but also the confidence of the patient, that the intervention is placed precisely where intended. This includes precision in determining the location of the insertion site, the direction of insertion and any necessary adjustment during advancement which is visualized under live dynamic ultrasound imaging.

Just as in diagnostic imaging it is important that both the physician and the patient are comfortable, and if possible, positioned so that both can see the monitor. Some patients may not want to see the needle, even as an ultrasound image, and their wishes should certainly be complied with. However, many patients are intrigued with the process and while watching will often be distracted to the point that they will find the intervention only mildly uncomfortable, if at all.

If a full ultrasound exam was not performed prior to the intervention, the structure involved should be imaged both transversely and longitudinally to define the space and pathology and recorded. Then at the discretion of the surgeon, the probe is positioned either longitudinal (long axis) or transverse (short axis) to the structure. The intervention can also then be performed either longitudinal, in the same plane as the probe (in-plane) or transverse (out of plane) to the probe. For the in-plane technique, as the needle is inserted longitudinal to the probe it is visualized initially as it passes under the near edge of the probe, with the entire needle observed advancing through the tissue toward its target (Figure 21 a, b).

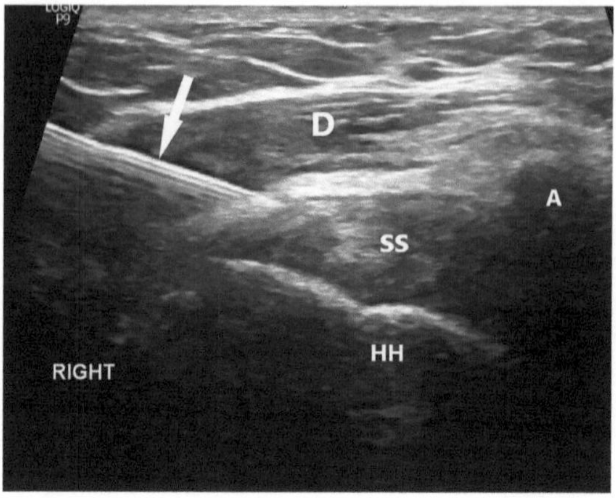

Figure 1-21a

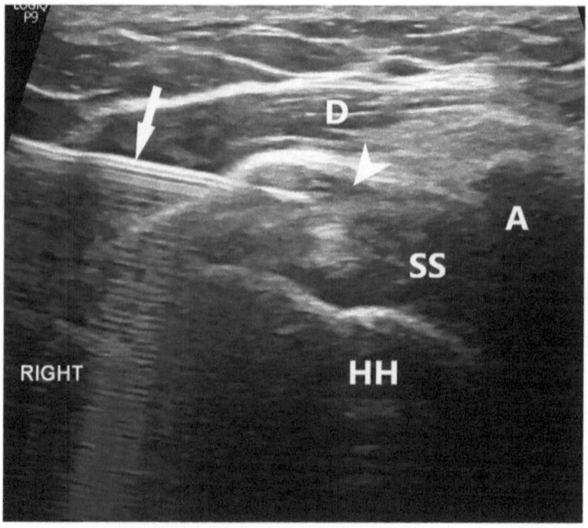

Figure 1-21 b

Figure 1-21: Ultrasound guided injection of the subdeltoid bursa performed with needle (arrow) inserted longitudinal to the probe (a) imaging the humeral head (HH), deltoid (D), acromion (A) and supraspinatus tendon (SS). The entire length of the needle is visualized as it is advanced to the target. With injection (b) the subdeltoid bursa (arrowhead) expands as the needle is advanced

For the out-of-plane approach the needle is advanced transverse to the probe, being seen only as a hyperechoic dot as it passes through the probe's plane of imaging (Figure 22).

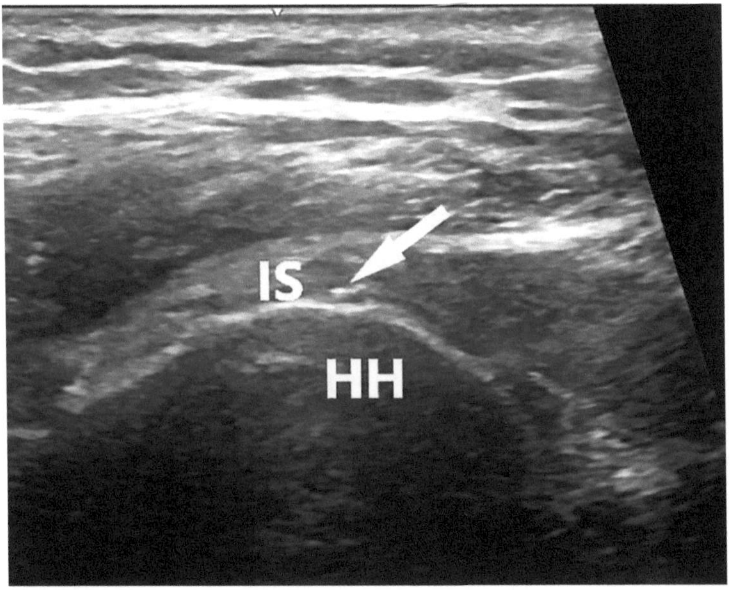

Figure 1-22

Figure 1-22: Ultrasound guided injection of the posterior glenohumeral joint performed with needle inserted transverse to the probe. Only the tip of the needle (arrow) is seen as a hyperechoic dot as it passes through the plane of the transducer deep to the infraspinatus (IS) in the capsule just superficial to the humeral head (HH).

The technique utilized varies based on the anatomic structure involved as well as the experience of the surgeon. The exact location and angle of needle insertion is calculated based on the position under the probe of the structure involved in the intervention and the technique utilized. The angle of insertion can be adjusted in real time by the surgeon based on the live image. This is easier to do with the in-plane technique as the entire needle is visualized throughout the intervention. However, adjustments can also be made in real time when injecting transverse to the probe by observing the soft tissue disturbance as the needle passes adjacent to the plane of imaging.

The image should be recorded as the actual intervention is performed documenting the proper placement of the needle. Post procedure images can also be recorded demonstrating the effects of the intervention including placement or removal of fluid. The patient's comfort level during and after the procedure and tolerance to the procedure should be noted in the record.

An alternative injection or aspiration technique involves the needle inserted slightly off axis to the plane of the probe. For this technique, the identified structure or area is placed in the center of the probe using the plane that helps demonstrate the structure the best. The needle is then inserted adjacent to the centerline on the screen (line is present on the side of the probe) and then passing the needle slightly off axis (nearly parallel) to the plane of the probe. The examiner will see the tissues move adjacent to the needle to know if the needle is passing in the correct trajectory. When the tip of the needle passes the plane of the probe, it can also be seen, but only as a small hyperechoic structure. This technique works well for superficial structures, especially with the small probe.

Conclusion

Ultrasound markedly enhances the efficiency and effectiveness of evaluating and managing musculoskeletal disorders. It is a modality that orthopaedic surgeons can easily master to add value to their practices. While there is obvious variation depending on the anatomic structure being evaluated, ultrasound principles are the same. If there is an excellent understanding of the anatomy, surgeons will find diagnostic and interventional ultrasound a powerful tool for all their patients. However, just as "the surgeon is the method" when it comes to operative procedures, it is extremely important that the physician making the therapeutic decisions and performing any surgical procedures be the one performing the diagnostic and interventional ultrasound. It is fine for residents and fellows to initiate the examination to gain experience or for mid-level providers to facilitate the procedure, but ultimately the attending surgeon needs to perform and experience the exam with the patient to maximize the value of in-office ultrasound.

References

1. Mcnally EG. The development and clinical applications of musculoskeletal ultrasound. *Skeletal Radiology* 2011;40:1223–31. doi:10.1007/s00256-011-1220-5.

2. Man K, Sabourin VM, Gandhi CD, Carmel PW, Prestigiacomo CJ. Pierre Curie: the anonymous neurosurgical contributor. *Neurosurgical Focus* 2015;39. doi:10.3171/2015.4.focus15102.

3. Primack SJ. Past, present, and future considerations for musculoskeletal ultrasound. *Physical Medicine and Rehabilitation Clinics of North America* 2016;27:749–52. doi:10.1016/j.pmr.2016.04.009.

4. Dussik KT, Fritch DJ, Kyriazidou M, Sear RS. Measurements of articular tissues with ultrasound. *American Journal of Physical Medicine & Rehabilitation* 1958;37. doi:10.1097/00002060-195806000-00013.

5. Hamilton JV, Flinn G, Haynie CC, Cefalo RC. Diagnosis of rectus sheath hematoma by B-mode ultrasound: a case report. *American Journal of Obstetrics and Gynecology* 1976;125:562–5. doi:10.1016/0002-9378(76)90379-3.

6. Forney MC, Delzell PB. Musculoskeletal ultrasonography basics. *Cleveland Clinic Journal of Medicine* 2018;85:283–300. doi:10.3949/ccjm.85a.17014.

7. Mayer R, Wilhelm K, Pfeifer KJ. Sonography of Achilles tendon rupture. {Translation from German] *Digitale Bilddiagnostik.* https://pubmed.ncbi.nlm.nih.gov/6394193-sonography-of-achilles-tendon-rupture/ (accessed February 16, 2020).

8. Zweymüller K, Kratochwil A. Ultrasound diagnosis in bone and soft tissue tumors (author's transl). *Archiv Fur Orthopadische Und Unfall-Chirurgie* 1977. https://www.ncbi.nlm.nih.gov/pubmed/871267 (accessed February 16, 2020).

9. Okoroha KR, Fidai MS, Tramer JS, Davis KD, Kolowich PA. Diagnostic accuracy of ultrasound for rotator cuff tears. *Ultrasonography* 2019;38:215–20. doi:10.14366/usg.18058.

10. Wilson CPDJ, Scully MWF, Rawlings CJM. Evolving role of ultrasound in therapeutic injections of the upper extremity. *Orthopedics* 2015;38. doi:10.3928/01477447-20151020-11.

11. Lin CY, Ooi CC, Chan E, Chew KT. Emerging technological advances in musculoskeletal ultrasound. *Pm&r* 2018;10:112–9. doi:10.1016/j.pmrj.2017.08.444.

12. Mcdonald DG, Leopold GR. Ultrasound B-scanning in the differentiation of Bakers cyst and thrombophlebitis. *The British Journal of Radiology* 1972;45:729–32. doi:10.1259/0007-1285-45-538-729.

13. Harryman DT, Mack LA, Wang KY, Jackins SE, Richardson ML, Matsen FA. Repairs of the rotator cuff. Correlation of functional results with integrity of the cuff. *The Journal of Bone & Joint Surgery* 1991;73:982–9. doi:10.2106/00004623-199173070-00004.

14. Primack SJ. Diagnostic ultrasound of the shoulder. *Journal of Occupational and Environmental Medicine* 1995;37:517. doi:10.1097/00043764-199504000-00099.

15. Block J, Berkoff D, Miller L. Clinical utility of ultrasound guidance for intra-articular knee injections: A review. *Clinical Interventions in Aging* 2012:89. doi:10.2147/cia.s29265.

16. Bureau NJ, Ziegler D. Economics of musculoskeletal ultrasound. *Current Radiology Reports* 2016;4. doi:10.1007/s40134-016-0169-5.

Chapter 2 Shoulder

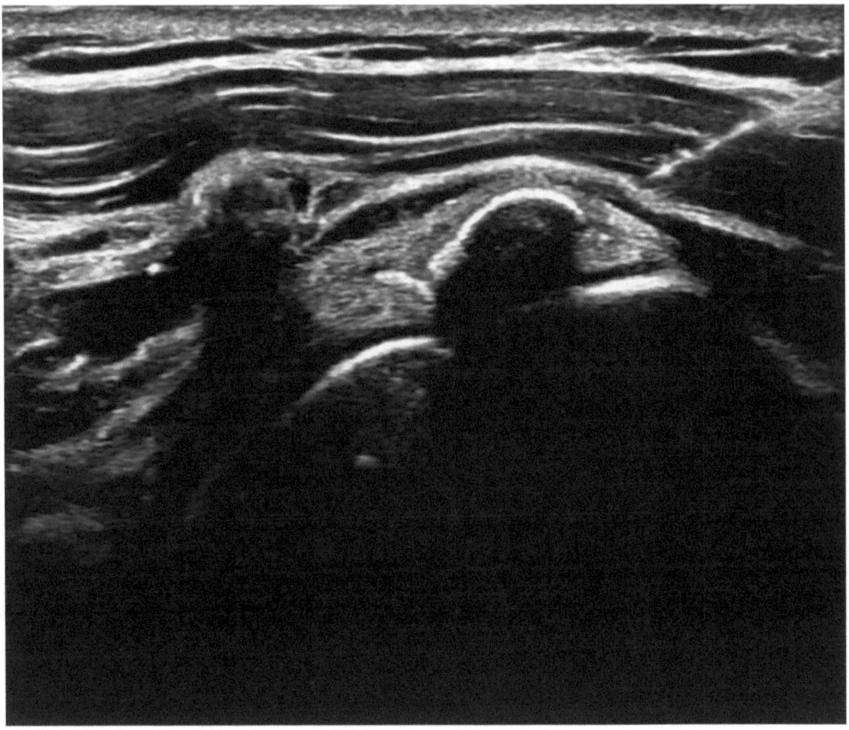

- Kevin K. Kruse, MD;
- Brian L. Badman, MD;
- Dean W. Ziegler, MD;

Ultrasound in the Shoulder

Introduction

Ultrasound is well established as a modality for the evaluation and management of shoulder disorders. The first published report documenting the use of ultrasonography in the shoulder was by Mayer in 1977[1]. In 1983 Farrer et al, at the American Academy of Orthopedic Surgeons Annual Meeting, described using dynamic sonography to evaluate the shoulder in 48 patients[2]. They found 91% sensitivity and 76% specificity for diagnosing complete rotator cuff tears. In 1984 Middleton described the normal ultrasonic shoulder anatomy[3], in 1985 the criteria for diagnosing rotator cuff tears[4], and in 1986 the pitfalls that may lead to poor results[5]. In 1985 Mack et al. described a technique for ultrasound shoulder examination, stressing dynamic sonographic shoulder evaluation[6]. Multiple studies have been published, with variable results regarding the usefulness of ultrasound in diagnosing rotator cuff tears and other shoulder disorder[2,4,6-22]. These reports and others stress the importance of the role of the operator[23-27]. Most important, the sonographer must be present during both static and dynamic imaging, have an excellent three-dimensional understanding of shoulder anatomy and function[28], and be proficient with the imaging techniques of diagnostic ultrasound. If these criteria are met, ultrasonography provides an effective method for evaluating the soft tissues of the shoulder and allows efficient implementation of the management plan.

Diagnostic examination of the shoulder

Positioning

For ease of spatial orientation and to allow evaluation of both the anterior and posterior aspects of the shoulder, patients should be positioned by sitting upright on the exam table. Alternatively, the patient and examiner can sit on adjacent, rotating stools positioned so that both can face and easily see the screen. It is ideal to have the examiner slightly higher than the patient. In addition, the shoulder should be free to extend and rotate.

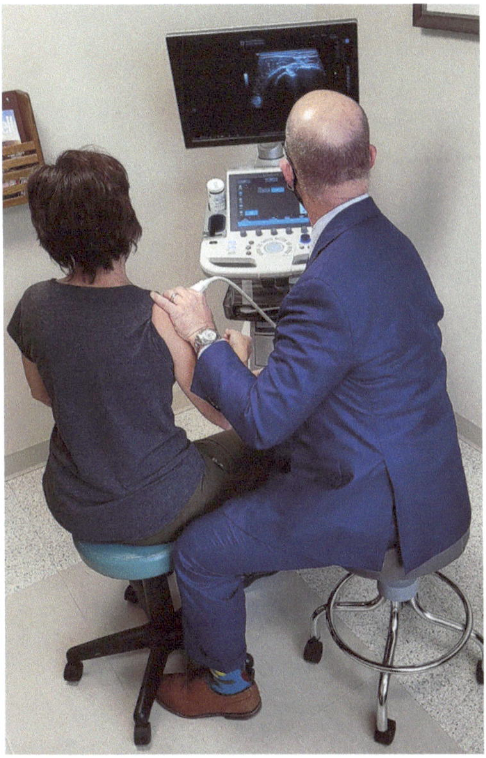

Figure 2-1: Position for imaging shoulder with patient and surgeon seated on rolling stools, allowing for full, free movement of the shoulder during examination.

If the opposite shoulder is examined the examiner and patient can simply switch positions (Figure 1). The shoulder and arm should be free of clothing, ideally with the patient in a sleeveless garment.

Obtaining an image:

The ultrasound machine should be powered on, and patient information should be entered to allow for archiving of selected images. In our experience, the depth of field should be set to 3.3 cm for most patients. For larger patients, a deeper depth (i.e., 4.0 cm) may be necessary to obtain quality images. Figure 2 shows an example of a labeled ultrasound interface for this purpose.

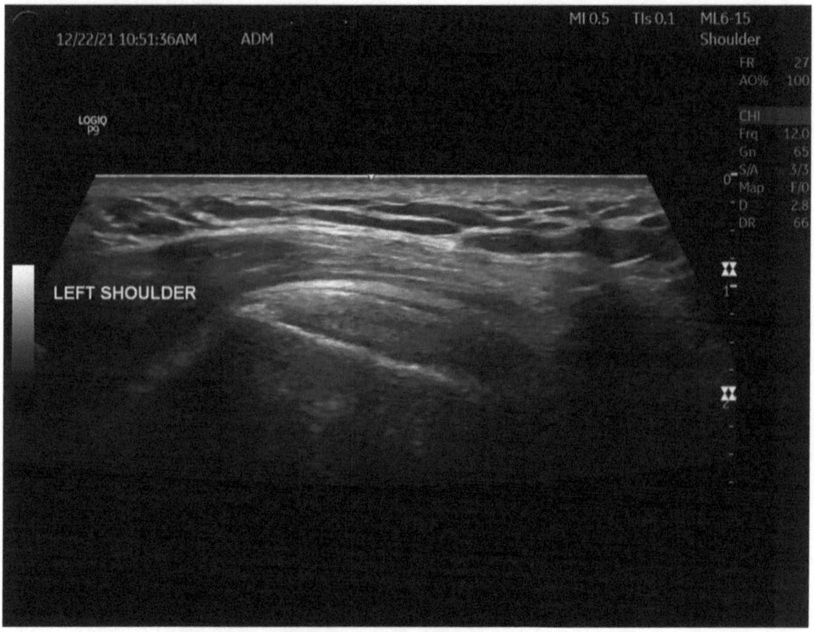

Figure 2-2: Example of a labelled ultrasound interface. Surgeons put up an image that is close to how they are looking at the shoulder rather than the standard view from below. In this view left is on the left rather than on the right as would be the standard view in radiology.

For each structure within the shoulder, both short (transverse) and long (longitudinal) axis views should be obtained. These views are named based on the position of the probe relative to the anatomic structure. Always have an adequate layer of ultrasound gel between the probe and patient.

Normal anatomy:

There are many ways to progress through the ultrasound exam of the shoulder. While there is no correct order, for a complete exam it is best to have a consistent order so that all structures are evaluated appropriately. One example is to follow the anatomic sequence evaluating each structure both longitudinal and transverse: long head of biceps tendon, subscapularis, infraspinatus and teres minor, glenohumeral joint, supraspinatus, and acromioclavicular joint. Another example is a sequence that is based on the most efficient probe movement: transverse view biceps tendon in the groove, longitudinal view subscapularis tendon, transverse view supraspinatus, longitudinal view infraspinatus tendon, longitudinal view teres minor tendon (if indicated), transverse view glenohumeral joint/posterior labrum, longitudinal view infraspinatus muscle belly, longitudinal view teres minor muscle belly (if indicated), transverse view infraspinatus muscle belly, transverse view teres minor muscle belly (if indicated), longitudinal view biceps tendon in groove, transverse view subscapularis tendon, longitudinal view supraspinatus tendon attachment to greater tuberosity, longitudinal view supraspinatus muscle belly, transverse view supraspinatus muscle belly, longitudinal view supraspinatus-infraspinatus tendon attachment with arm in internal rotation and extension, transverse view supraspinatus-infraspinatus tendon attachment with arm in internal rotation and extension.

For surgeons who routinely look at magnetic resonance imaging (MRI) scans of the shoulder rather than ultrasound images, it often helps to correlate the ultrasound images with what an MRI scan of the same shoulder would reveal. For the biceps tendon, the short and long axis views would correlate to axial and sagittal MRI images, respectively. For the subscapularis, the long axis view would correlate with an axial image. For the supraspinatus, the short and long axis views correlate with sagittal and coronal MRI images, respectively.

Figure 3 shows single images during each step of the examination to aid in correlation.

1) Biceps tendon (short axis)

With the elbow flexed to 90 degrees, the forearm fully supinated, and shoulder rotation to neutral, orient the ultrasound first transverse to the arm and place the probe on the anterior shoulder. Localize the bicipital groove containing the long head of the biceps tendon by either translating the probe medially/laterally with the shoulder in neutral rotation or internally/externally rotating the shoulder with the probe held stable. The tendon itself should be round on this view and hyperechoic (Figure 3.1). If it is not visible as such, toggle the probe to make sure that the absence of the tendon is not due to anisotropy. Translate the probe superior and inferior in the groove to thoroughly image the tendon. If there is any fluid or effusion surrounding the biceps sheath, it will appear hypoechoic or anechoic. Fluid in the sheath may represent biceps tendon pathology but is more likely due to a glenohumeral joint effusion implying intra articular pathology. Absence, splitting of the tendon or tenderness when imaging over the tendon should be noted. Absence of tenderness when imaging over the tendon should also be noted, especially in the case where is a concern for biceps tendon pathology.

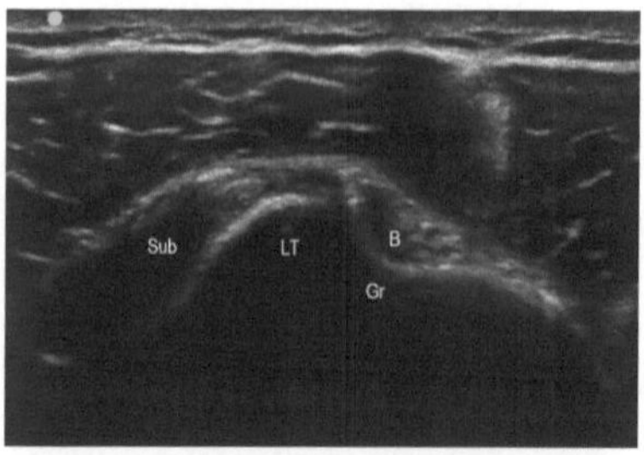

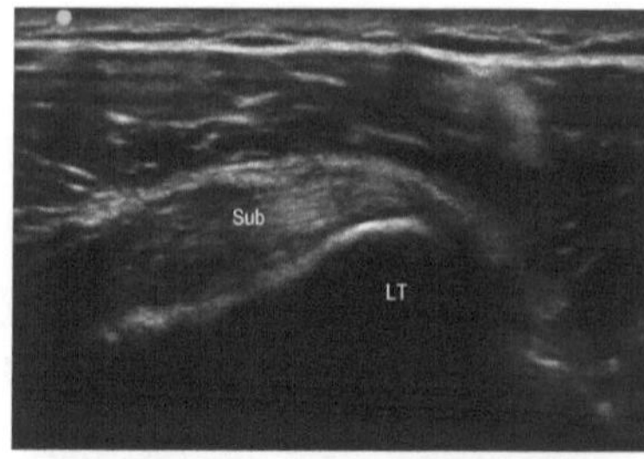

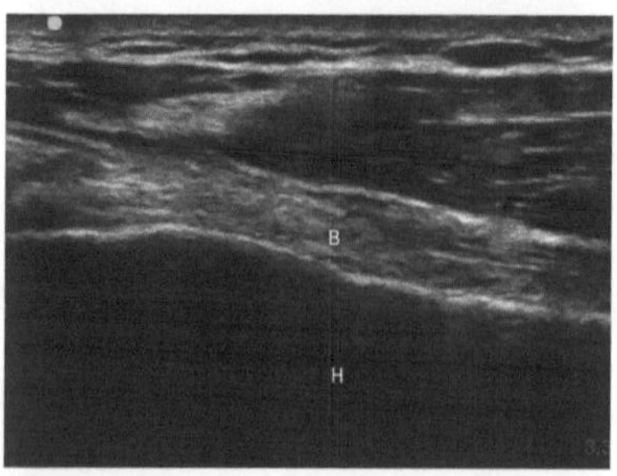

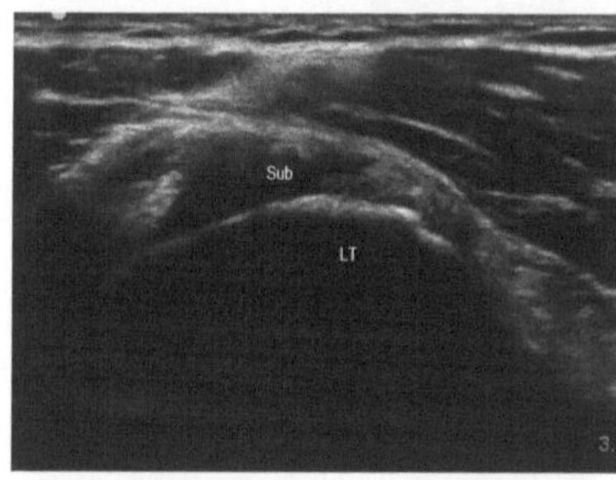

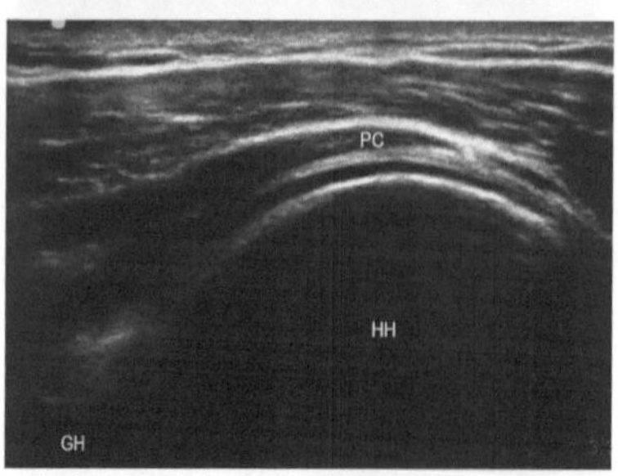

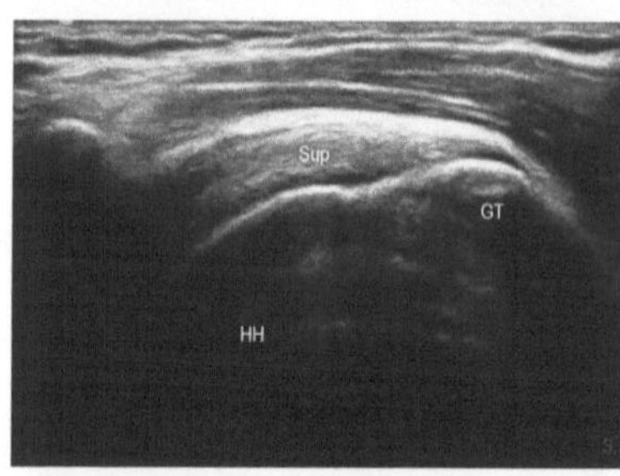

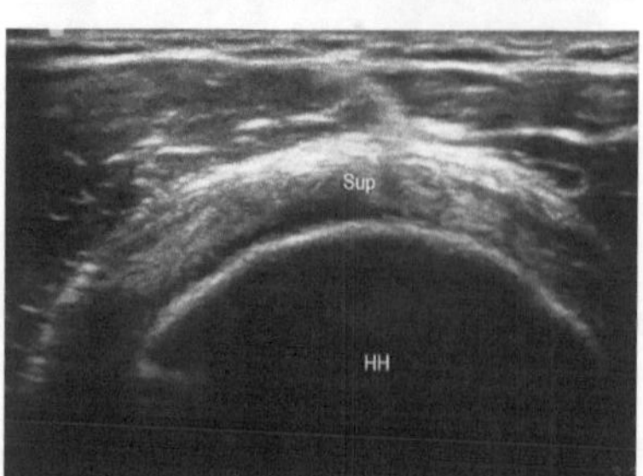

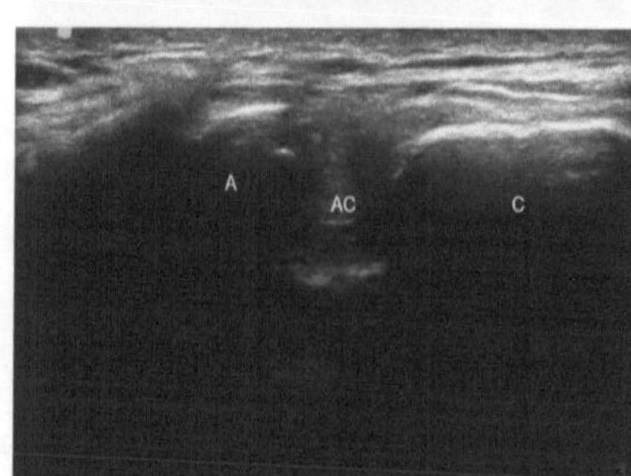

Figure 2-3.1: Example of normal biceps tendon, B, within bicipital groove.

Figure 2-3.2: Longitudinal view of subscapularis (Sub) inserting into the lessor tuberosity (LT). The thickness of the tendon can be measured and recorded.

Figure 2-3.3: Longitudinal image of the biceps tendon (B) in the bicipital groove.

Figure 2-3.4: Transverse view of subscapularis tendon (Sub) and the lesser tuberosity, LT.

Figure 2-3.5: Longitudinal view of the posterior shoulder including infraspinatus tendon and posterior capsule (PC), muscle belly and transverse view of glenohumeral joint (GH).

Figure 2-3.6: Longitudinal view of Supraspinatus (Sup) tendon attaching to the greater tuberosity (GT) with tendon pulled out to length by positioning the patient with their arm internally rotated and extended.

Figure 2-3.7: Transverse (short axis) view of the supraspinatus tendon (Sup) forming concentric circle over the humeral head (HH) articular surface.

Figure 2-3.8: Transverse view of acromioclavicular joint (AC) between medial clavicle (C) and lateral acromion (A).

About 50% of shoulders have a supraspinatus aponeurotic extension, SAE, which is a portion of the anterior supraspinatus tendon that inserts down the bicipital groove. A large SAE may make the biceps long head appear to be split (Figure 4).

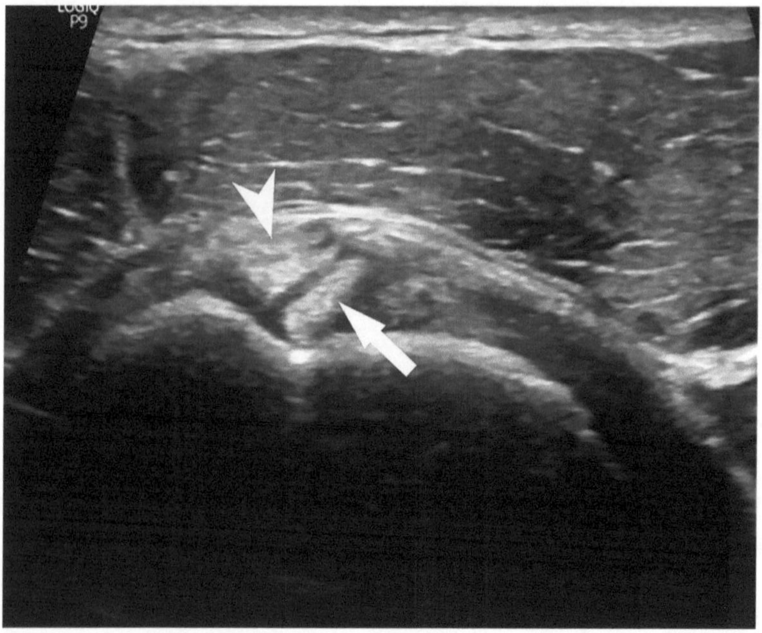

Figure 2-4: Example of supraspinatus aponeurotic extension (arrowhead) extending down into the bicipital groove adjacent to the biceps tendon (arrow). This might be misinterpreted as a split tendon.

Medial displacement of the tendon out of the groove implies subscapularis tearing, usually the superior border. Dynamic stability of the tendon in the groove can be assessed by observing the tendon while internally and externally rotating the shoulder. The probe should be moved along with shoulder rotation to maintain the bicipital groove and tendon in the center of the visual field. Stability versus instability of the tendon in the groove should be documented. Just as in arthroscopy, this position can be returned to as a point of reference throughout the exam if there is ever any confusion as to what is being visualized.

2) Subscapularis tendon (long axis)

With the elbow and forearm in the same position, rotate the shoulder to approximately 40-50 degrees of external rotation. Orient the probe in the long axis of the subscapularis tendon on the anterior shoulder. Locate the biceps tendon and lesser tuberosity and then translate the probe slightly more medial to locate the subscapularis tendon inserting on the lesser tuberosity (Figure 3.2). Upper border tears are commonly seen on this view especially if the biceps tendon is subluxated medially. The probe can be moved superior and inferior to fully visualize the supraspinatus tendon insertion. Further external rotation of the shoulder and medial translation of the probe can allow for visualization of the musculotendinous junction of the subscapularis as well as the movement of the subscapularis under the coracoid process. Evaluate the integrity of the tendon by translating the probe from superior to inferior and back during both static and dynamic imaging. Measure and record the thickness of the tendon. Evaluate the integrity of the tendon during an isometric internal rotation contraction. Evaluate for sub coracoid roughness during passive and active shoulder rotation. Any tenderness or discomfort experienced by the patient during imaging due to pressure of the probe, contraction of the subscapularis or during sub coracoid clearance should be noted.

3) Biceps tendon (long axis)

Keeping the elbow at 90 degrees of flexion with full forearm supination, and neutral shoulder rotation, orient the probe longitudinally to the biceps tendon and arm to obtain the long axis view of the tendon. Locate the tendon in the groove just lateral to the lesser tuberosity (Figure 3.3). Moving the probe more distally will reveal the biceps muscle belly. If this is difficult to visualize, find the biceps tendon in the groove on the transverse view, center the tendon in the field of view, and then rotate the probe 90 degrees. Toggle the probe as needed to obtain the best image an eliminate anisotropy. Note any disruption of the tendon, thickening of the tendon, absence of the tendon or effusion as well as any tenderness or lack thereof when imaging over the tendon.

4) Subscapularis tendon (short axis)

From the position of the biceps tendon longitudinal view, translate the probe slightly medial and/or rotate the shoulder slightly externally. Toggle slightly or rotate to best orient the probe transverse to the subscapularis tendon (Figure 3.4). Concentric hyperechoic circles representing the superficial border of the subscapularis tendon and humeral head articular surface should be visualized. Translate the probe superior to inferior as well as medial to lateral to make sure the tendon is intact. Absence or thinning of the tendon superior implies a tear. Thinning of the tendon as the probe is translated lateral over the lessor tuberosity is normal.

5) Posterior rotator cuff (Infraspinatus and Teres Minor)

Adduct the arm and internally rotate the shoulder to place the patient's hand on the contralateral thigh. This will bring the infraspinatus, teres minor, and posterior glenohumeral joint into view. However, if this amount of internal rotation pulls the tendon insertions too far anterior, simply place the patient's hand on their ipsilateral thigh. Orient the probe medially-laterally by placing it parallel and just inferior to the scapular spine to obtain the long view of the infraspinatus and more inferior the teres minor. These two muscles can be difficult to delineate. Move the probe more laterally to view their insertions on the greater tuberosity. Move the probe medially to view the posterior glenohumeral joint. This view is often used for ultrasound-guided glenohumeral joint injection or aspiration. Figure 3.5 depicts an image showing the posterior cuff and glenohumeral joint. Move the probe further medial and the muscle belly of the infraspinatus superior and teres minor inferior can be visualized. Thickness can be measured and recorded, and the quality of the muscle can be assessed at rest and during an isometric external rotation contraction. The quality of these muscle bellies should be similar to the overlying deltoid muscle. Rotation of the probe 90 degrees allows evaluation of the muscles in a short-axis or transverse view. From this position translating the probe laterally provides short-axis visualization of the infraspinatus and teres minor tendon insertions. In the short-axis view the inferior neck of the glenoid marks the border between the infraspinatus and teres minor. This is particularly helpful if the intervening fascia between the infraspinatus and teres minor is not visualized as that fascia lies parallel to the ultrasound beam and is frequently not seen. Otherwise, one can differentiate the two by using the fact that the infraspinatus is bipinnate while the teres minor is purely muscular, lacking a central tendon.

6) Supraspinatus (long axis)

The supraspinatus can be imaged longitudinally, positioning the probe superior just off the anterior/lateral acromion. From this position a static image of the supraspinatus tendon attachment can be viewed from anterior to posterior. Also, dynamic imaging can be performed by moving the arm passively into slight extension and flexion as well as external and internal rotation to evaluate movement of the tendon with the humeral head. Lack of movement of the overlying tissue as the humeral head is rotated implies a tear. However, this view is limited by the overlying acromion. Therefore, to enhance supraspinatus imaging, have the patient internally rotate and extend the shoulder by positioning their hand as if they were putting it in their back pants pocket with the palm facing the patient. This will bring the anterior portion and insertion of the supraspinatus out from underneath the acromion, closest to the skin and therefore closest to the ultrasound probe. If there is rotator cuff pathology, this positioning may cause discomfort to the patient, but it is necessary to obtain quality images. The orientation of the probe is slightly different in this position due to the shoulder position – the probe is oriented toward the patient's ipsilateral ear to obtain the long view of the supraspinatus, and the probe is oriented toward the patient's umbilicus to obtain the short axis of the supraspinatus. It is easiest to get a good long (coronal) view of the supraspinatus inserting on the greater tuberosity on the long view – find this first and then orient yourself to the most anterior portion of the supraspinatus insertion (Figure 3.6). The anterior border can be seen just posterior to the biceps tendon which longitudinally courses over the humeral head as the probe is translated anterior. Tears are often seen here. In this view, move the probe anterior to posterior along the shoulder, traveling from the supraspinatus insertion to the infraspinatus insertion. This dynamic imaging can be recorded moving from anterior to posterior and back again. During static imaging, the probe should be slightly toggled and rotated to obtain the best image and make sure that any abnormalities appreciated are not artifacts due to anisotropy. Improper toggling can make a good tendon appear bad, but it never makes a bad tendon look good. Evaluate the integrity of the supraspinatus and infraspinatus tendon. Tears are implied by complete absence of the tendon, a loss of integrity of the tendon, a hypo-echoic focus within the normal tendon tissue or an adjacent hyper-echoic focus (implying a partial-thickness tear), and a loss in the normal convexity of the superior border of the supraspinatus tendon attachment (often appreciated when dynamically imaging from posterior to anterior as the superior supraspinatus border flips from a smooth convexity to concavity indicating a tear). Any tenderness experienced by the patient when imaging over these abnormalities should be recorded.

7) Supraspinatus (short axis)

Keeping the arm in the same position, orient the probe orthogonally to the long axis (sagittal) view. Sweep the probe anterior to posterior and slightly medial to lateral. The concentric circles created by the superior border of the supraspinatus and the humeral head indicate an intact tendon. In the normal tendon there may be a slight thickening of the tendon going from posterior to anterior as well as symmetric thinning of the tendon as the probe is translated lateral over the greater tuberosity. Asymmetric anterior thinning indicates a tear. Tendon thickness should be measured and recorded, as should any asymmetric thinning (recording both the thickest and thinnest portions of the tendon). During static imaging, the probe should be slightly toggled and rotated to obtain the best image and make sure that any abnormalities appreciated are not artifacts due to anisotropy. Any reported tenderness when imaging over areas of abnormality should be recorded. Figure 3.7 depicts a normal superior rotator cuff on this view.

The supraspinatus tendon can also be evaluated on its short axis with the arm at the side. The probe should be held parallel and just off the lateral edge of the acromion. The concentric circles of the superior border of the supraspinatus and the humeral head should be imaged. Slight rotation and toggle of the probe should be performed to confirm the best image. The thickness of the tendon and any asymmetry within it should be recorded. As with the long axis view with the arm at the side, this view is limited by the overlying acromion.

8) Acromioclavicular joint (long axis)

Though not always routine, the acromioclavicular (AC) joint can be examined with ultrasound to evaluate for arthritis, effusion, or trauma. With the shoulder held neutral and the arm at the patient's side, orient the probe longitudinal to the clavicle directly over the AC joint. In a normal AC joint, there is a wide-open joint space on this view (Figure 3.8). Irregularity of the joint, effusion within the joint and extending the joint capsule, and tenderness when imaging directly over the joint implies pathology. This view is often used for AC joint injection or aspiration.

9) Dynamic/Functional ultrasound Imaging

Dynamic imaging with ultrasound is one of its greatest advantages over other, static modes of imaging. In the shoulder, all the rotator cuff tendons can be imaged dynamically to better define integrity and pathology. Having the patient actively move the shoulder while imaging can also bring functionality to the exam, as can imaging with isometric muscle contraction. Tissue that does not move with the humeral head during either passive or active motion is not attached to the humeral head. This either represents torn tendon tissue or non-functional bursal tissue.

The subscapularis can be evaluated dynamically by rotating the shoulder while imaging the subscapularis longitudinally as well as transversely. Moving the probe slightly medial while externally rotating the shoulder allows evaluation of the musculotendinous junction. It also allows for evaluation of the subscapularis as it dynamically moves under the coracoid process. This provides a good way to evaluate "sub-coracoid impingement" or roughness. Moving the probe slightly inferior/distal allows evaluation of the subscapularis moving under the short head of the biceps (Figure 5).

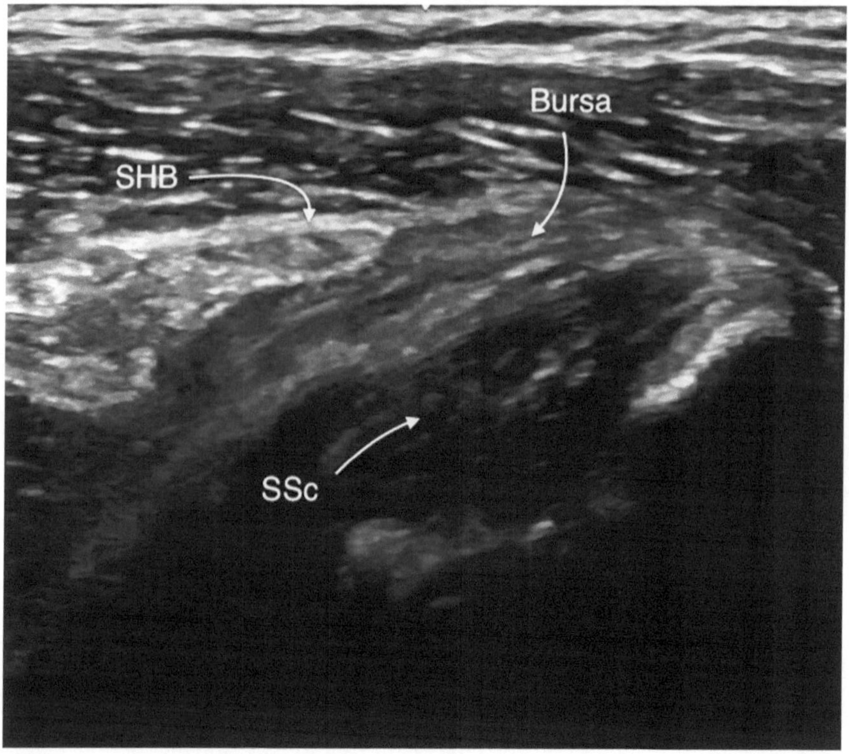

Figure 2-5: Subscapularis (SSc) in the long axis imaged deep to short head of biceps (SHB) including interposed thickened bursa. Usually there is no tissue seen between these two tendons.

Continuing to image the tendon longitudinally during an isometric internal rotation contraction evaluates the functional integrity of the tendon. Movement of tendon tissue medially during contraction without movement of the humeral head implies loss of integrity of the tendon attachment/tearing.

The infraspinatus and teres minor tendons can be imaged dynamically in a similar fashion, rotating the shoulder with the arm at the side and the probe positioned to image the infraspinatus/teres minor muscle bellies and tendons longitudinally. Smooth movement of the tendons and accompanying muscle bellies can be assessed as can their integrities during an isometric external rotation contraction.

The supraspinatus tendon can be imaged dynamically with the arm at the side and the probe positioned longitudinally just off the anterolateral edge of the acromion, parallel to the supraspinatus fossa. Moving the shoulder into extension and back to flexion, allows for a dynamic evaluation of the tendon attachment to the greater tuberosity. Slight rotation can also be incorporated in this evaluation. Lack of movement of the tendon tissue with the tuberosity implies a tear. This evaluation is somewhat limited by the overlying acromion which can be improved by moving the arm into internal rotation and extension.

Functional evaluation of the supraspinatus can be performed while imaging the movement of the tendon, its attachment, and the greater tuberosity as they rotate under the acromion during passive and active elevation of the shoulder in the scapular plane. With the probe positioned longitudinally just off the anterolateral border of the acromion the greater tuberosity is imaged clearing under the acromion as the examiner passively elevates the patient's shoulder. The patient is then asked to actively elevate the arm in a similar manner while the examiner continues to image the shoulder. The clearance of the greater tuberosity under the acromion is classified as: smooth, painful, rough or abutment (the tuberosity hitting the acromion and not being able to clear underneath). The patient should report subjective feelings of pain and/or roughness. Anything other than smooth clearance implies some pathology in the supraspinatus tendon. An inability to actively have the tuberosity even approach the acromion implies either a massive rotator cuff tear or neurologic injury and should be further evaluated accordingly.

Ultrasound for Massive Rotator Cuff Tear

It has been well-documented that ultrasound can be used to diagnose full-thickness rotator cuff tears. Multiple studies have shown that orthopaedic surgeons can obtain the same level of sensitivity and specificity as a musculoskeletal radiologist reading MRIs in the diagnosis of full-thickness rotator cuff tears [29, 30, 31, 32, 33, 34, 35] becoming facile with ultrasound in a fairly short time, roughly fifty exams.[33]

A concern some clinicians have regarding diagnostic ultrasound is with its ability to quantify tendon retraction, muscle atrophy and fatty infiltration, and of using the Goutallier classification when assessing massive tears. This is important, especially for the shoulder surgeon who is comfortable using MRI to determine whether a rotator cuff tear has a high failure rate with repairing, or if it is even repairable at all. This information strongly influences the decision-making process of the surgeon as to whether they can undergo a primary repair versus an augmented reconstruction, tendon transfer or even reverse shoulder arthroplasty.

However, all this information and more can be obtained from ultrasound. Multiple papers have shown the atrophy quantified on ultrasound can equal that of the modified Goutallier classification on MRI with the same levels of inter- and intra-observable reliability.[36] When assessing repairability of a tear, the key is the ability to visualize the lateral edge of the torn tendon lateral to the acromion on long axis supraspinatus and infraspinatus tendon views. If the torn edge of the tendon can be visualized lateral to the acromion, then that is a repairable tear 100% of the time.[37]

If the supraspinatus and/or infraspinatus torn tendon has retracted medial to the lateral edge of the acromion and therefore cannot be visualized on ultrasound, then there is legitimate concern regarding the repairability of the tendon. However, there are many tears that are retracted medial to the lateral border of the acromion and therefore cannot be visualized on ultrasound that are repairable tears. The ability to discern that subset of repairable versus irreparable tears when the tendon edge is medial to the acromion using ultrasound, is by looking at the clues that have been previously looked at on MRI.

Initially, evaluate the short axis of the teres minor and infraspinatus posteriorly, especially in the setting of a chronic retracted tear. Typically, the teres minor will hypertrophy as the infraspinatus atrophies and so you get this dual effect of the muscle belly that is dramatically larger than the other side. Next evaluate the quality of the muscle. Muscles with fatty infiltration will be hyperechoic because they have fat, which has less water than muscle. Water tends to be hypoechoic and dark on ultrasound. High quality, elastic muscle will be hypoechoic while poor quality muscle will be more hyperechoic due to the loss of water that occurs with fat infiltration. Quality muscle has standard architecture with the pennate structure intact. A fatty infiltrated muscle will lose its pennate structure. These qualities can be easily evaluated using ultrasound (Figure 6).

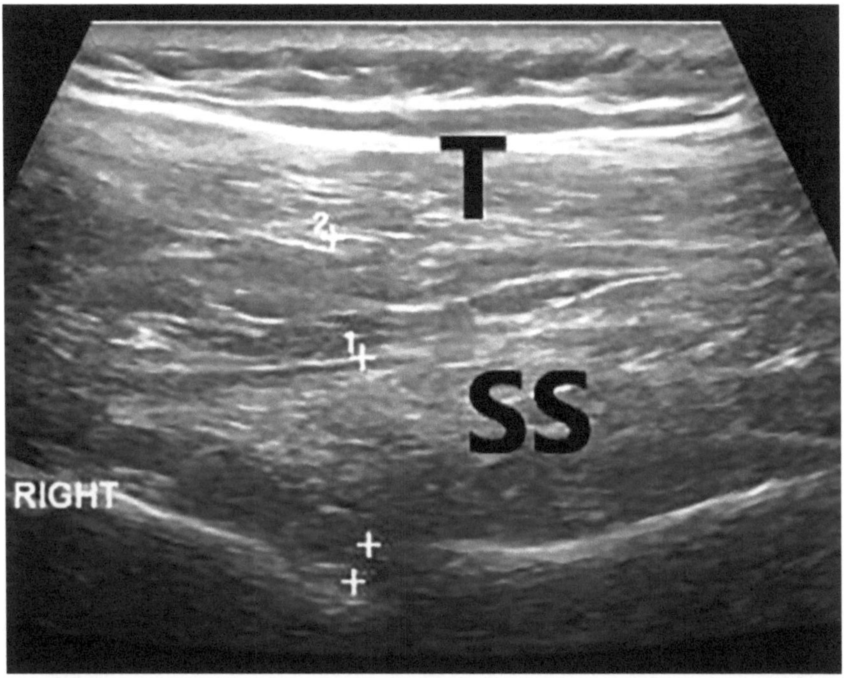

Figure 2-6: Longitudinal image of the supraspinatus muscle belly (SS) with fatty infiltration, including increased echogenicity and loss of normal pennate architecture and a hyperechoic appearance compared to normal trapezius muscle (T).

The sagittal or "Y" view of the supraspinatus muscle belly on ultrasound can be imaged, just as with MRI, by positioning the probe just medial to the medial border of the acromion, imaging the short axis of the supraspinatus. The probe can then be translated medial, over the supraspinatus fossa, slightly toggled and rotated to obtain an excellent transverse image of the supraspinatus muscle belly. Rotating the probe 90 degrees provides a longitudinal view of the supraspinatus muscle belly. In this case the probe is parallel and just anterior to the scapular spine. Slight toggle and rotation provide enhancement of the image. The quality of the supraspinatus muscle belly on both views can be compared to the overlying trapezius muscle, whose quality normally does not change with age. The quality of the infraspinatus and teres minor muscle bellies can be evaluated in a similar fashion, comparing them to the overlying deltoid muscle.

A second ultrasonic method of assessing muscle quality is utilizing dynamic contraction during isometric resistance. This is typically done with the supraspinatus, but occasionally the infraspinatus will be evaluated as well. Place the probe parallel and just anterior to the scapular spine obtaining a longitudinal image of the supraspinatus muscle belly with the arm relaxed at the side. Either have the patient gently elevate the arm against a small amount of force or have the patient perform an isometric abduction contraction while ultrasonically visualizing the supraspinatus muscle. Muscle tissue contracting dynamically implies that the muscle still has elasticity and that is very commonly a repairable tear. This can be quantitated by initially observing the portion the tissue within the supraspinatus fossa that is actively contracting. With the muscle at rest, measure the width of the contractile tissue and the overall width of the space available at its thickest location (from the deep border of the trapezius to the scapula). This quantifies potential atrophy of the muscle belly. Then have the patient activate the supraspinatus as described above. Freeze the image at maximum thickness of contraction, measure this thickness in the same spot and then compare it to the thickness of the muscle at rest (Figure 7).

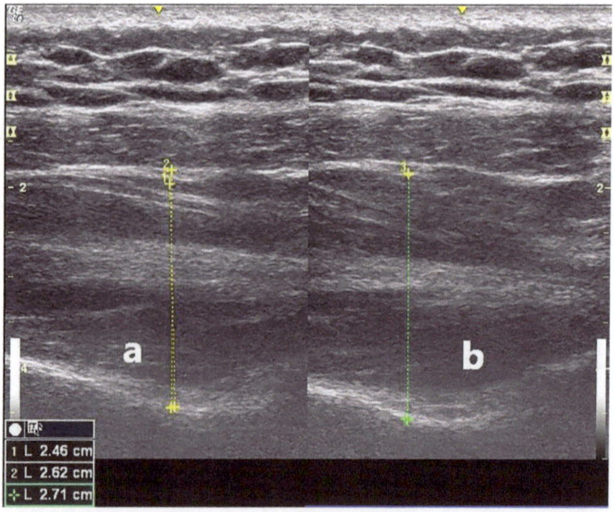

Figure 2-7: Longitudinal image of supraspinatus muscle belly at rest on the left (a) measuring contractile tissue (2.46 cm) and total space (2.62 cm), compared to thickness of supraspinatus muscle belly during contraction (2.71 cm) on the right (b).

This can be done easily by splitting the screen (a feature present on many ultrasounds machines) and recording the image. Comparing thickening of the muscle belly during isometric contraction to that of the contralateral shoulder can be extremely helpful because while the contractility is variable between patients, it is very consistent within the same patient. Significant atrophy and loss of contractility is an indication of a chronic and oftentimes irreparable tear (Figure 8).

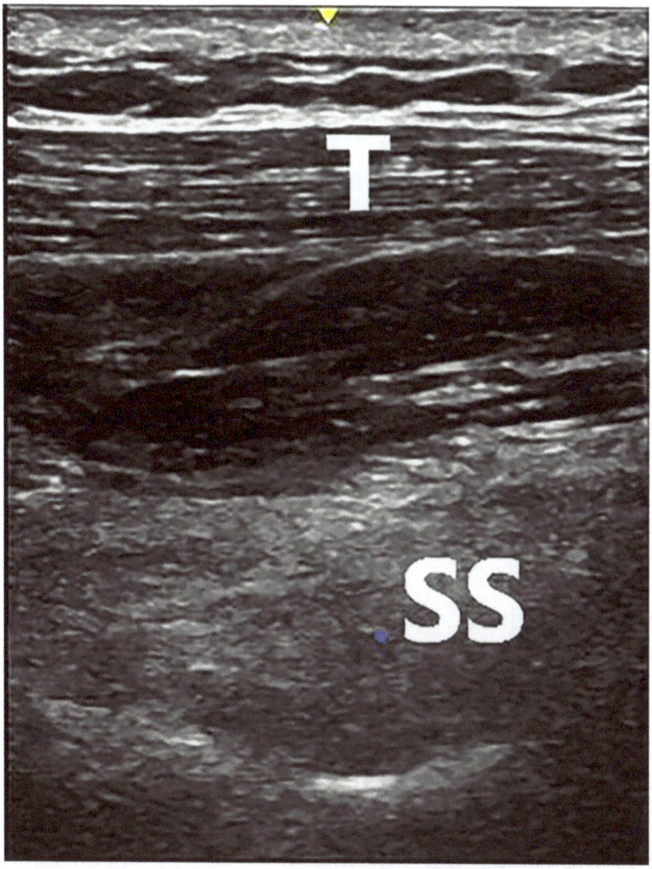

Figure 2-8: Atrophied, hyper echogenic supraspinatus muscle belly (SS) with loss of normal architecture in shoulder with irreparable tear compared to normal muscle belly of overlying trapezius (T).

This information is helpful when determining management of patients, especially those presenting with an acute injury. Non-operative management should certainly be initially tried when there is evidence of a chronic tear that was exacerbated by an acute injury. Similar assessment can be made of the infraspinatus and teres minor muscle bellies utilizing isometric external rotation contraction to activate the muscles. This information can be used to not only assess reparability of the rotator cuff but also potential neurologic dysfunction.

Information gained from the above two methods should be incorporated into the surgeon's individual decision-making process regarding potential irreparable rotator cuff tears. The subscapularis is more difficult to assess in this fashion on ultrasound given the location of its muscle belly. Image the entire lessor tuberosity attachment of the tendon as there is often some tissue still attached inferior. Moving the probe medial while fully externally rotating the shoulder may move some retracted tendon tissue into the field of view.

Post-Operative Shoulder

One of the most valuable uses of diagnostic ultrasound for orthopaedic surgeons is the evaluation of patients following surgery. Potentially even more significant than with pre-operative patients, is the convenience of in-office ultrasound for both patients and surgeons. The utilization of MRI is also limited in the post-operative setting due to artifacts, whether the patient is status post shoulder arthroplasty with substantial implants; tendon repair, tenodesis or shoulder stabilization utilizing suture anchors; or even debridement with micro-metallic shaver or burr fragments present. Artifacts do exist with sonographic imaging; however, given real-time imaging these artifacts can be avoided and at times even manipulated to enhance the image and interpretation of post-operative pathology (Figure 9).

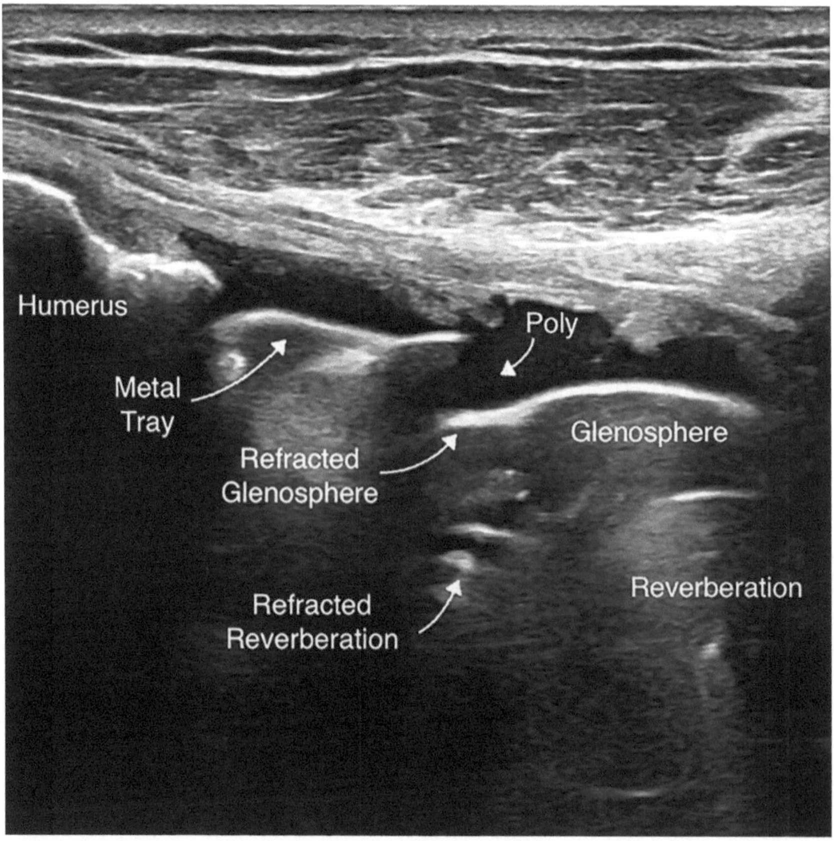

Figure 2-9: Example of post-operative artifact in shoulder of patient following Reverse Total Shoulder Arthroplasty. Note how the little triangle of UHMWPE, Poly, causes the surface of that portion of the glenosphere to appear flattened.

By utilizing dynamic and functional imaging of both tendon and muscle, passive and active movement can be evaluated including functional motion and muscle contractility. This along with the added benefit of immediate patient feedback helps to eliminate significance of potential artifacts.

Just as in patients prior to surgery, care must be taken when utilization the imaging of the post-operative shoulder. While there may be temptation to image the shoulder of any patient having problems following surgery, indications should be like those for pre-operative patients. If there has been an acute traumatic injury with dramatic change in motion, function or comfort, immediate sonographic imaging may be indicated following appropriate history, physical exam, and plain radiographs. Imaging should be delayed in a patient who has discomfort explained by post-operative stiffness and who has not adequately rehabilitated their shoulder. If the patient has failed appropriate post-operative management, thorough pre-operative, intra-operative and post-operative history should be obtained including presumed diagnosis and management. Particular attention should be focused on the fact that pre-operative diagnosis may have been either inaccurate or incomplete.

Post-Rotator Cuff Repair

Following rotator cuff repair in patients, history should include whether the procedure was arthroscopic, open or combined; what tendons were torn/repaired and was it a single or double row repair; were anchors utilized and how many; and was there a biceps tenodesis or tenotomy performed? Including a complete exam, particular attention should focus on dynamic and functional imaging. Tendons are best imaged under full tension (internal rotation for infraspinatus and teres minor, external rotation for subscapularis, and internal rotation and extension for supraspinatus). These movements can also be utilized dynamically while following the movement of tendon tissue with the humeral head to determine the integrity of the repair. Movement of tendon tissue without humeral head rotation during isometric contraction is another useful strategy for evaluation of the post-operative shoulder (isometric external rotation for infraspinatus/teres minor, internal rotation for subscapularis and abduction for supraspinatus). Functional maneuvers can also be performed including active elevation, imaging the greater tuberosity clearing under the acromion.

Shoulder Arthroplasty

The importance of history following shoulder arthroplasty includes type of procedure: anatomic, reverse, hemiarthroplasty, or Ream & Run with a non-prosthetic arthroplasty of the glenoid. Also important is the management of the subscapularis: tenotomy, peel, osteotomy and whether there was a repair in the case of a reverse shoulder arthroplasty. Plain radiographs help defining placement of the prosthesis which helps explain findings on ultrasonic imaging. A complete standard exam is necessary to avoid misdiagnosis with particular attention to the integrity of the subscapularis (Figure 10) on static, dynamic and functional imaging (including isometric internal rotation contraction).

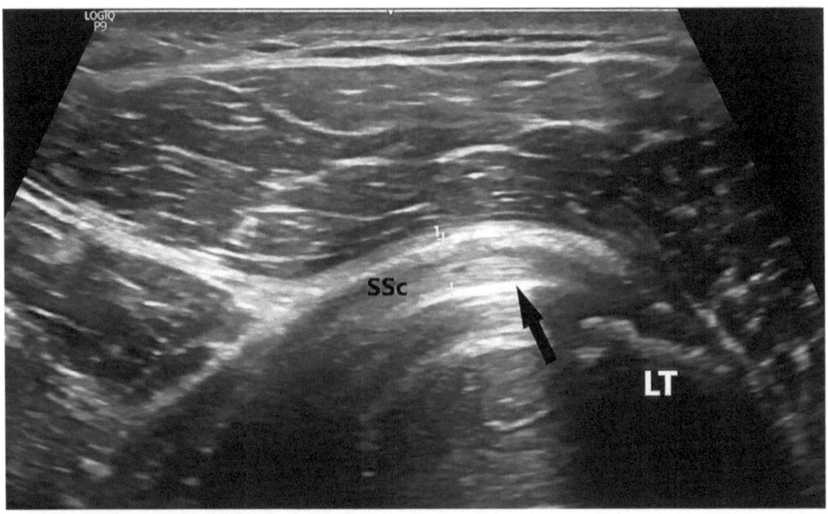

Figure 2-10: Imaging of the subscapularis (SSc) overlying the hyperechoic prosthetic humeral head (arrow) in a shoulder following Total Shoulder Arthroplasty. The lessor tuberosity (LT) is on the right.

However, a complete exam is important especially for the patient who does not appear to have other evidence for post-arthroplasty pain or dysfunction (Figure11).

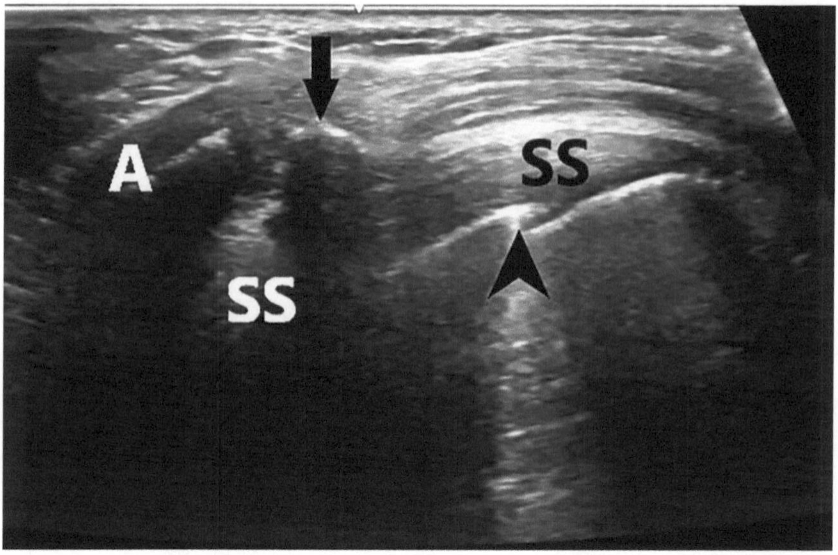

Figure 2-11: Image of avulsed fragment (arrow) of an otherwise intact acromion (A) in a patient with pain following anatomic total shoulder arthroplasty with intact supraspinatus tendon (SS) overlying prosthetic humeral head (arrowhead).

Other Pathology

Calcific Tendonitis

Calcific tendonitis in the shoulder can present acutely with severe shoulder pain or with mild to moderate chronic shoulder pain that may be intermittent. Acute calcific tendonitis can be a real symptomatic emergency for the patient and is best treated almost emergently. Patients present with severe shoulder pain even at rest, significantly worse with any movement, with no history of significant trauma and with symptoms out of proportion to clinical findings. Plain radiographs are extremely helpful in making the diagnosis including a True AP of the glenohumeral joint, an Axillary Lateral and a Scapular Y or Outlet view. The radiologic opaque calcium nodule can be identified and its location 3-dimensionally determined, appearing somewhat fluffy in the acute setting and sharper and more demarcated in the chronic state (Figure 12).

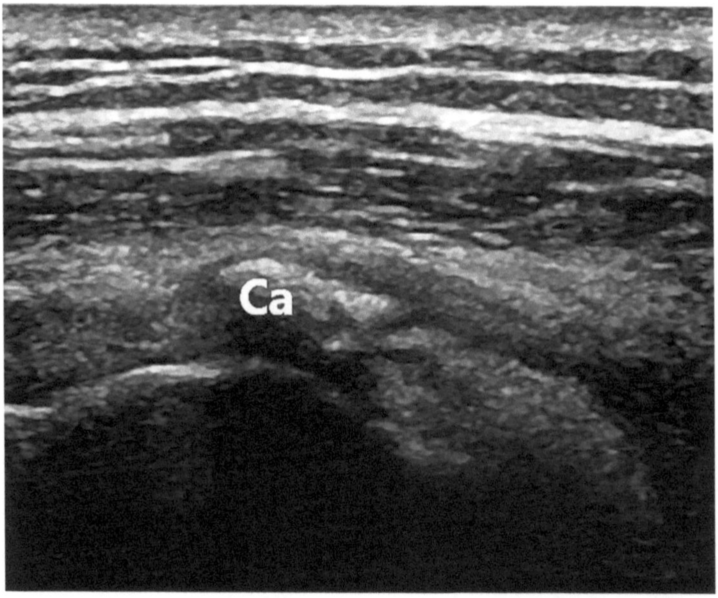

Figure 2-12 a

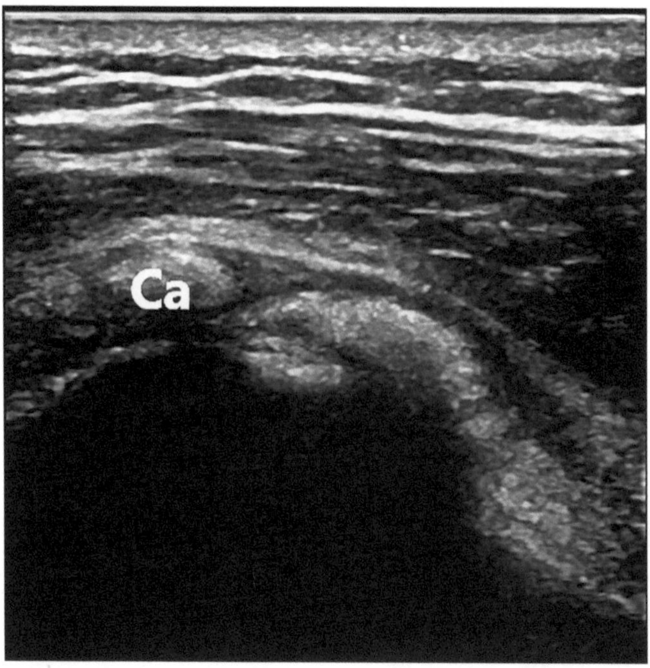

Figure 2-12 b

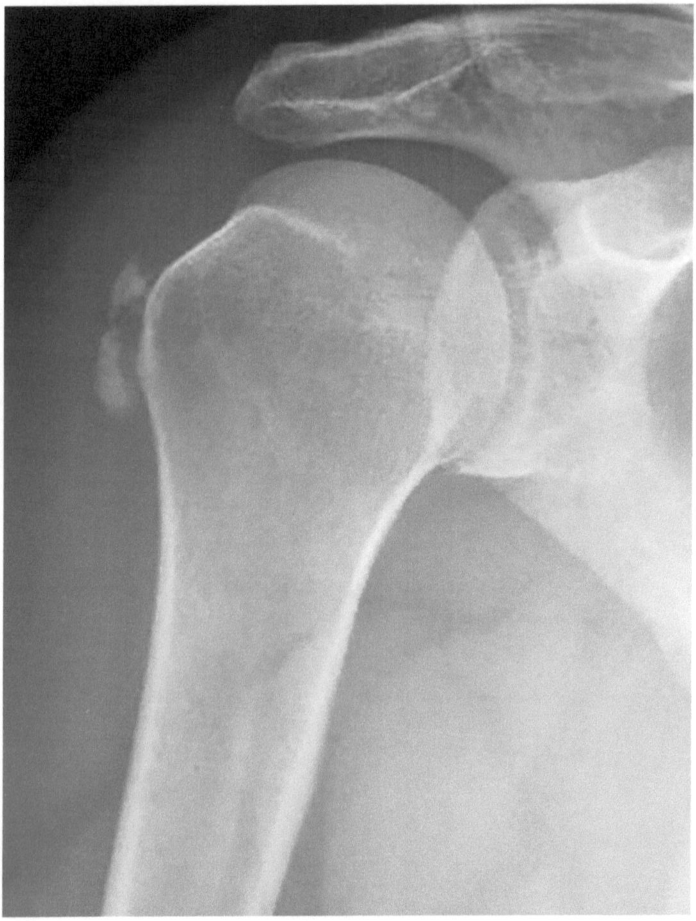

Figure 2-12 c

Figure 12: Calcific nodule (Ca) present within the infraspinatus tendon on longitudinal (a) and transverse (b) views which can be compared with nodule seen on AP radiograph of the shoulder (c).

This is an example of when plain radiographs are extremely helpful if not imperative both in all patients presenting with shoulder pain but certainly prior to ultrasound evaluation. In the very acute setting there may also be instances in which the calcification is not visualized on plain radiographs and only picked up on ultrasound.

A complete standard ultrasound exam of the shoulder should be performed to evaluate for other pathology with particular attention paid to the location of the calcific nodule as seen on plain radiographs. On ultrasound, the calcific nodule appears as a hyperechoic focus within the tendon and anechoic shadow deep to the nodule with a break in the underlying bony contour (Figure 13). Patients may complain of increased tenderness when imaging over the nodule.

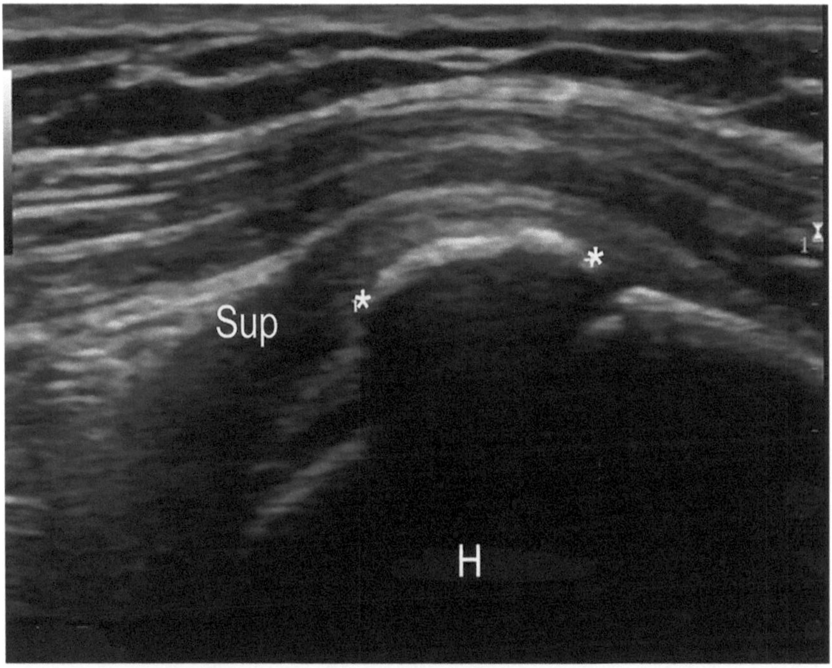

Figure 2-13: Calcific nodule within supraspinatus tendon (Sup) creating anechoic shadow and break in underlying humeral head (H) articular surface.

Management of calcific tendonitis, whether acute or chronic, can be performed under ultrasound guidance. This management could be as simple as an ultrasound guided subacromial injection. However, given the ability of ultrasound to definitively localize the nodule, the needle can be guided directly into it (Figure 14).

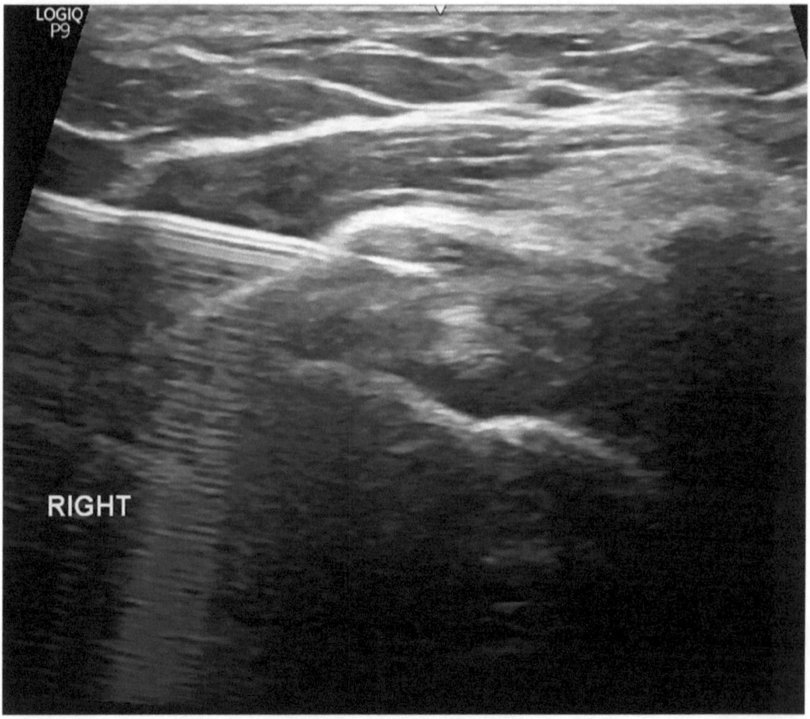

Figure 2-14: Needle guided with ultrasound directly into the calcific nodule.

In the true acute phase, aspiration can yield the typical thick, white calcific paste. Usually this is done with an 18- or 16-gauge needle after local anesthetic has been placed in the area under ultrasonic guidance. In the subacute or chronic setting, even if nothing can by aspirated, barbotage can be performed with the needle and injection with corticosteroid, NSAIDs or both placed directly at the nodule and in the subacromial space.

Pectoralis Major Tear

Evaluation of the pectoralis major is usually performed as a directed, focused exam based on the patient's presenting history and clinical presentation. Pectoralis major tendon rupture occurs secondary to an eccentric load and may present acutely, though often subacute or secondary to chronic dysfunction. Patients complain of weakness and pain with presses and resisted internal rotation from an externally rotated position. Exam findings include weakness with those maneuvers, chest wall deformity and absence of pectoralis tendon on palpation in the axilla.

Ultrasound exam of the pectoralis major begins from the already described starting position with the arm in neutral rotation, the probe transverse over the anterior shoulder, obtaining an image of the bicep's tendon proximally in the bicipital groove. Slight medial translation of the probe identifies the subscapularis tendon attachment. As the probe is moved distal past the inferior border of the subscapularis, the pectoralis major tendon is visualized as it traverses over the long head of the biceps tendon, attaching to the humerus lateral to the bicipital groove. Slight lateral translation of the probe allows imaging of the attachment. The probe is moved distal and back proximal, visualizing the entire length of the tendon attachment and then medial to the musculotendinous junction obtaining both longitudinal and transverse images. In the acute setting hematoma may be visualized in the longitudinal plane at the musculocutaneous junction as the sternal head rotates beneath the clavicular head and in the transverse plane medial to the fused tendon superficial to the short head of the biceps muscle. The exam is maximized with passive and active dynamic rotation as well as resisted internal rotation. Tendon tears are represented by hypoechoic and anechoic disruption of the tendon attachment, lack of movement of the tendon with dynamic rotation of the humerus or medial retraction of the tendon on resisted, isometric internal rotation. Most tears are partial-thickness involving the sternal head of the pectoralis major. In this case a patient presented with obvious clinical evidence of pectoralis major tendon rupture but an MRI reported as negative for a tear. Proximal imaging of the pectoralis major tendon demonstrates an intact clavicular head tendon (Figure 15).

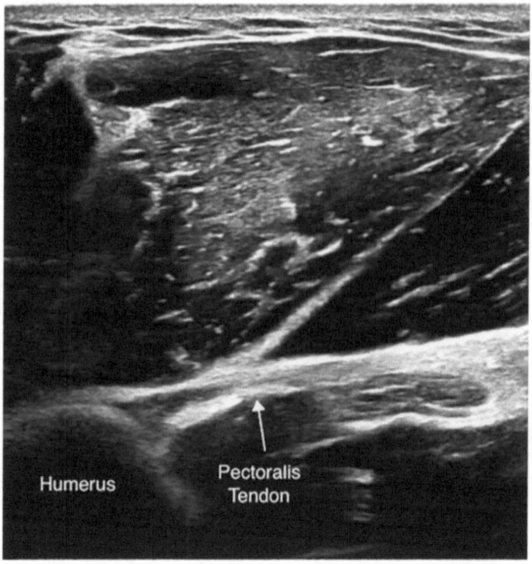

Figure 2-15: Intact clavicular head of the pectoralis major tendon.

Slightly more distal demonstrates a torn and retracted sternal head tendon (Figure 16) , with edematous sternal head muscle belly imaged by moving the probe medial (Figure 17).

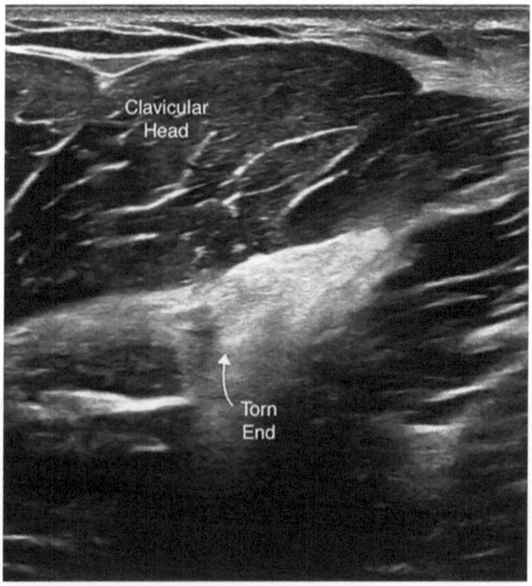

Figure 2-16: Probe moved distally to image the retracted torn edge of the sternal head tendon.

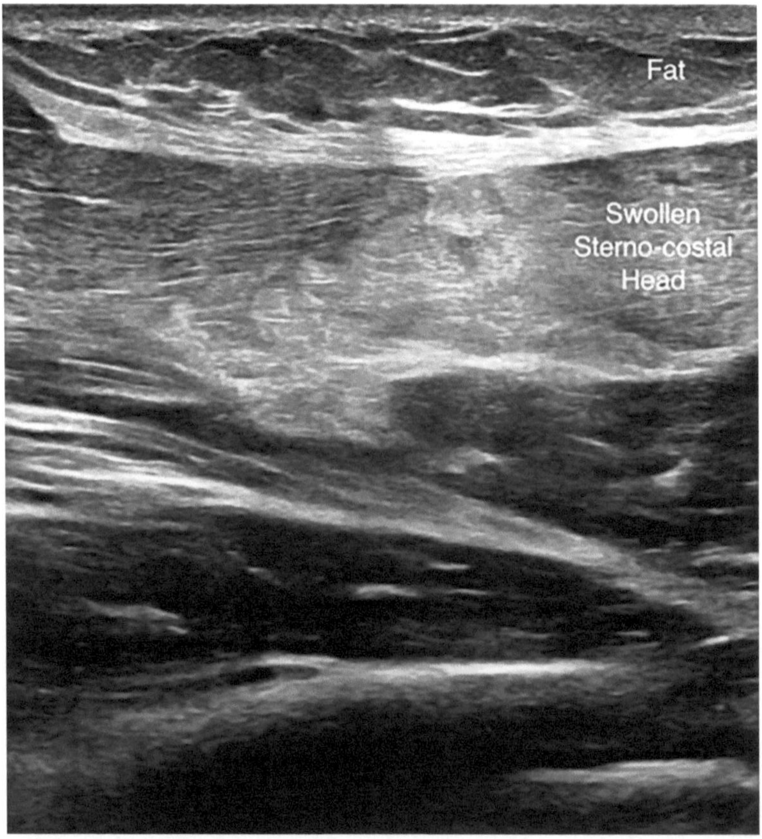

Figure 2-17: Medial translation of the probe imaging swollen, hyperechoic, sternal head muscle belly.

Snapping Scapular Bursitis

Ultrasound can be very helpful in the evaluation of a symptomatic snapping scapula. Position the probe longitudinally over the superior-medial corner of the acromion, centering it on the tip of the acromion. Translation of the probe superior and inferior around the contour of the scapula allows for evaluation of any hypertrophic bursa initially in the static state. Imaging with static and dynamic movement confirms any pathology in the scapulothoracic articulation. Having the patient attempt to reproduce their symptoms can be very beneficial. Diagnostic injection can be performed, as described below, to further aid in evaluation of pathology.

Post-Operative Rotator Cuff Imaging:

Ultrasound provides an excellent means of evaluating patients who are struggling following previous rotator cuff surgery. Not only does it allow for the convenience of immediate documentation of the status of the rotator cuff, but it also avoids artifacts that may obscure other modes of advanced imaging. In this case a 50-year-old female presented with pain and weakness following previous rotator cuff repair and appropriate post-operative rehabilitation. In-office ultrasound (Figures 18, 19) documented a full-thickness tear of the supraspinatus tendon with slight retraction of the tendon confirmed at surgery.

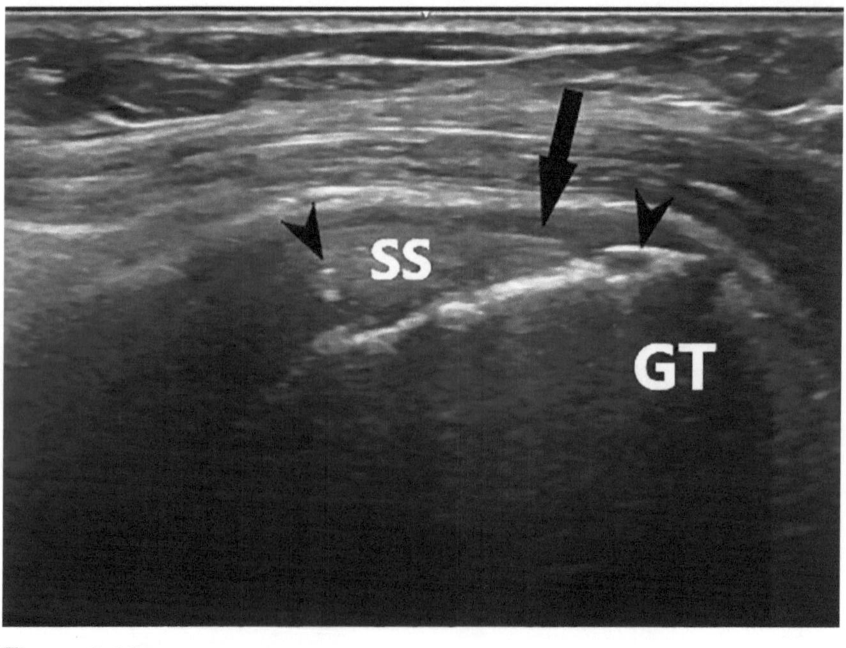

Figure 2-18a

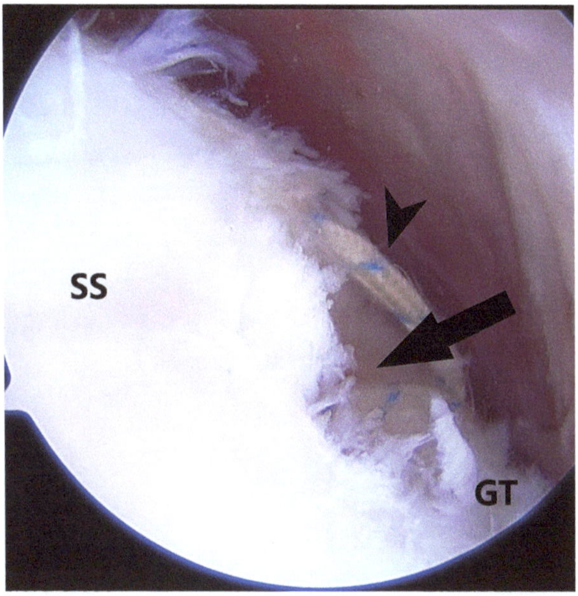

Figure 2-18b

Figure 18: Long axis post-operative ultrasound image (a) of the supraspinatus (SS) tendon with slight retraction from the greater tuberosity (GT). The defect in the tendon can be seen as hypoechoic discontinuity (arrow) along with hyperechoic dots representing suture (arrowhead). Similar view at the time of revision arthroscopy (b) confirms the ultrasound findings.

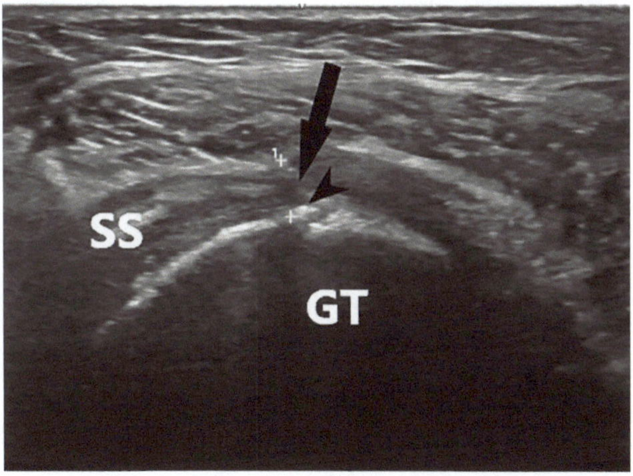

Figure 2-19a

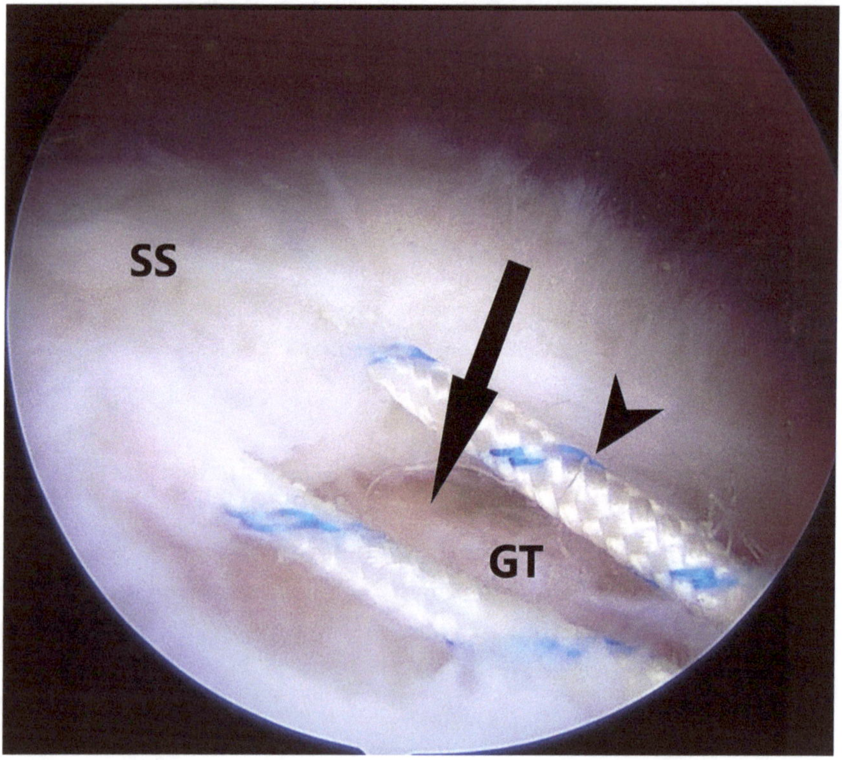

Figure 2-19b

Figure 19: Short axis ultrasound image (a) demonstrating supraspinatus tendon (SS) posterior with thinning anterior indicating a tearing (arrow) of the tendon as it attaches to the greater tuberosity (GT). Hyperechoic sutures are again visualized (arrowhead) and the tear is confirmed on similar arthroscopic image from the lateral portal (b).

Also documented on ultrasound was the quality of the supraspinatus muscle belly (Figure 20).

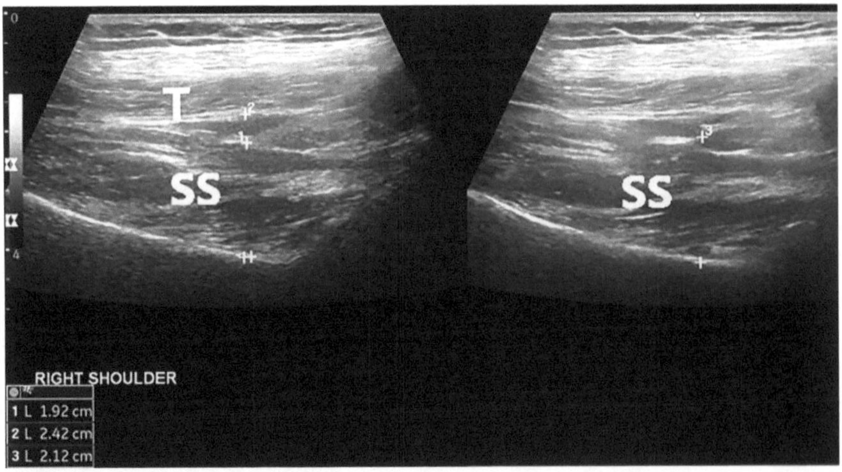

Figure 2-20: Ultrasound image of supraspinatus muscle belly (SS) demonstrating normal echogenicity and architecture compared to the overlying trapezius (T). Good quality of the muscle is also demonstrated by the thickening of the muscle with contraction (right image) compared to the resting state (left image).

While there was slight atrophy, the muscle showed normal echogenicity, architecture, and contractility.

Evaluation of Glenohumeral Roughness

Diagnostic ultrasound can at times be very helpful in not only the management of but also the evaluation of glenohumeral roughness in the form of osteoarthritis, rheumatoid arthritis or rotator cuff tear arthropathy. Radiographs may hint at cartilage loss in the shoulder with inferior osteophytes (Fig. 21) or slightly asymmetric joint line narrowing (Fig. 22).

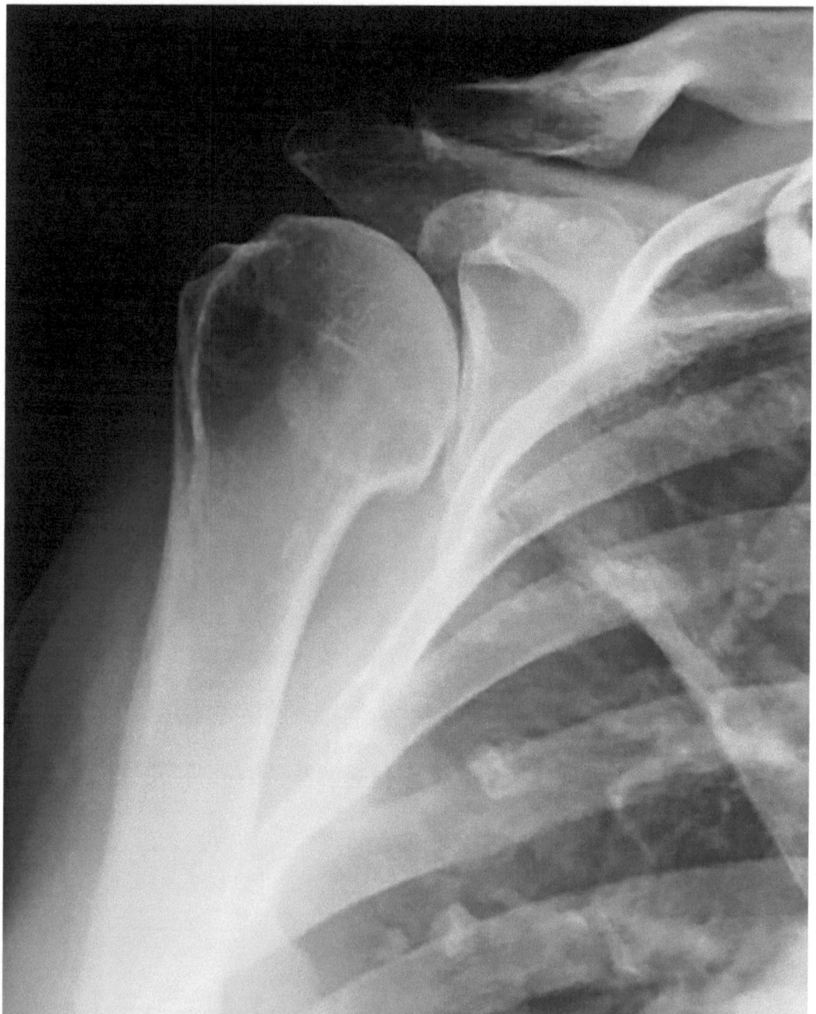

Figure 2-21: AP radiograph of the shoulder demonstrating an inferior humeral head osteophyte and slight joint space narrowing.

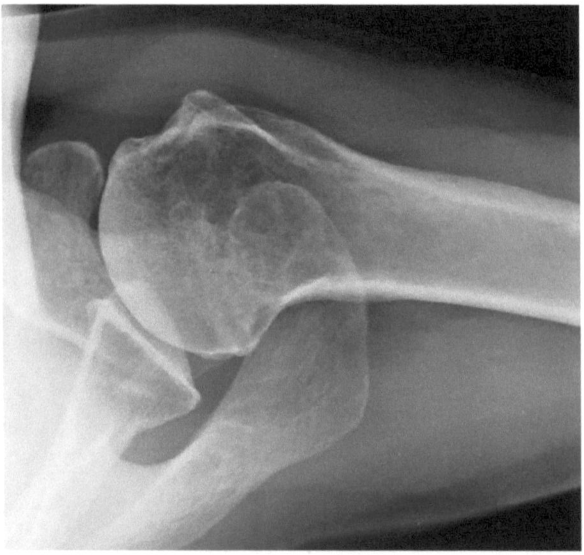

Figure 2-22: Axillary lateral view of the glenohumeral joint demonstrating slight anterior joint narrowing.

Ultrasound can be even more demonstrative visualizing peripheral osteophytes (Fig. 23), humeral head collapse (Fig. 24) and articular surface irregularity (Fig. 25).

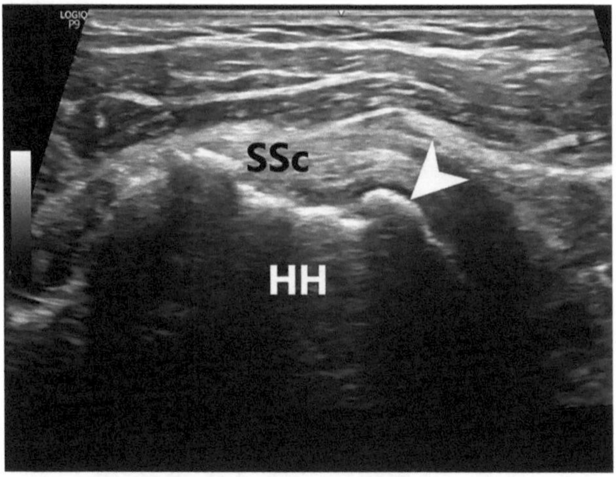

Figure 2-23: Peripheral humeral head (HH) osteophyte (arrowhead) imaged with ultrasound from anterior including the overlying subscapularis tendon (SSc).

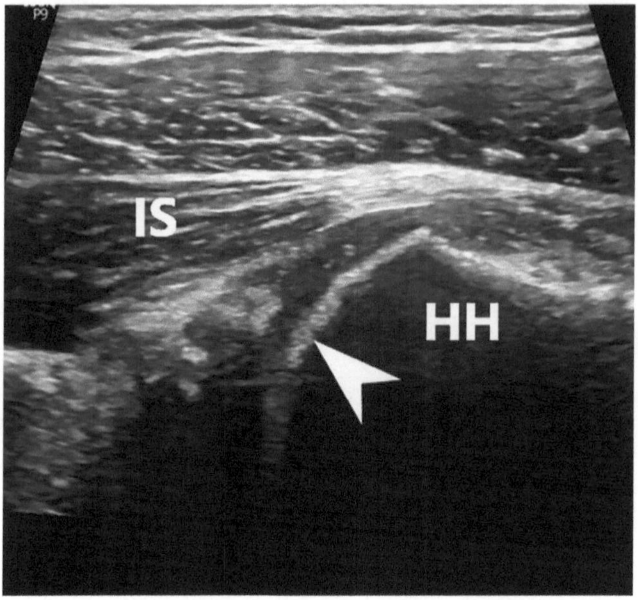

Figure 2-24: Ultrasound visualization of humeral head (HH) flattening (arrowhead) imaged from posterior including the overlying infraspinatus (IS).

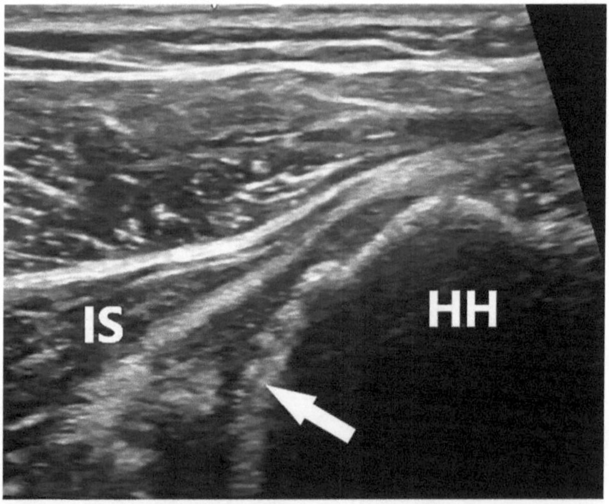

Figure 2-25: View of the glenohumeral joint from posterior in the long axis of the infraspinatus imaging the humeral head (HH), infraspinatus (IS) and demonstrating irregularity of the articular cartilage (arrow).

In this 60-year-old female there was significant degenerative changes confirmed at the time of anatomic shoulder arthroplasty (Fig. 26).

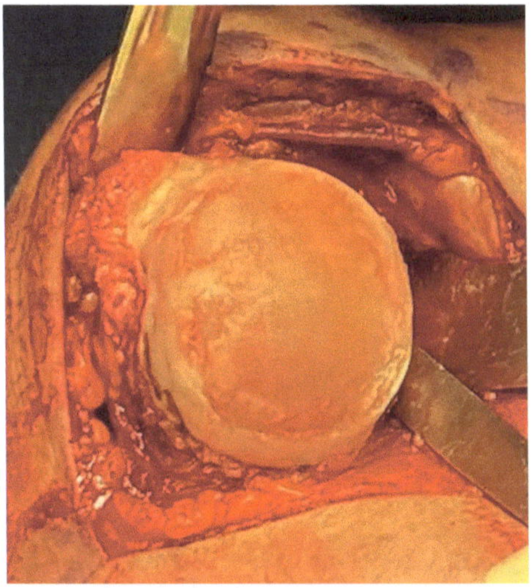

Figure 2-26a

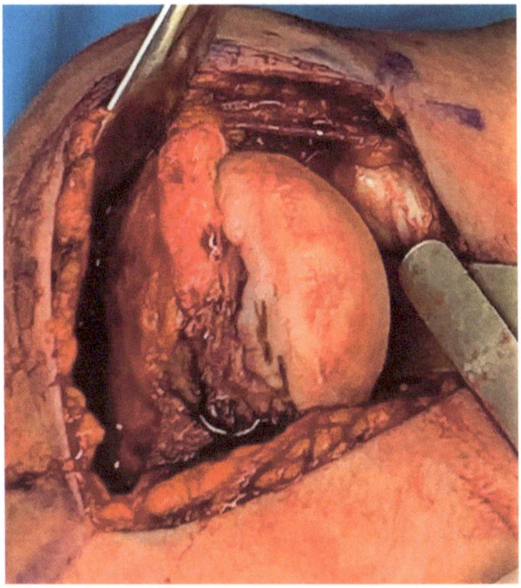

Figure 2-26b

Figure 26: Intra-operative image of the humeral head with significant cartilage loss (a) and peripheral osteophytes (b).

Interventional Ultrasound

Injection: As with all ultrasound guided injections, the proper technique including patient positioning, orientation of the probe relative to the anatomic structure being managed, and position of the needle relative to the probe is what works best in the hands of the surgeon performing the intervention. Most important is that both the patient and surgeon feel safe and comfortable throughout the procedure. While many of these injections can be performed with the patient seated upright, there are times in which the patient may be safer and more comfortable supine, prone, or lateral decubitus. You need to find what works best for you and your patients. You can certainly change your approach as you get more experience.

Subacromial

The subacromial injection is one that may be best done with the patient sitting upright so that gravity helps to open up the subacromial space. If the patient needs to sit in a chair with arms for better support, make sure that the arm of the shoulder being injected is resting comfortably in the patient's lap, not on the arm of the chair. After performing your brief diagnostic exam, position the probe just off the antero-lateral corner of the acromion. Position the probe so that the acromion is on the far side of the screen with the superior border of the supraspinatus (if intact) in the center and the greater tuberosity on the other side. Perform a Heel-Toe maneuver with the probe to position it so that it would be parallel with the needle coming in from lateral. The ruler on the lateral side of the screen will allow you to estimate how far down from the probe you need to insert the needle. After proper prepping, insert the needle, attempting to advance it parallel to the probe, until it reaches the bursa superficial to the supraspinatus tendon. Slowly inject and adjust the position of the probe until you meet minimal resistance and can see the bursa expand. Then continue to advance the probe while injecting as the bursa further expands (Figure 27).

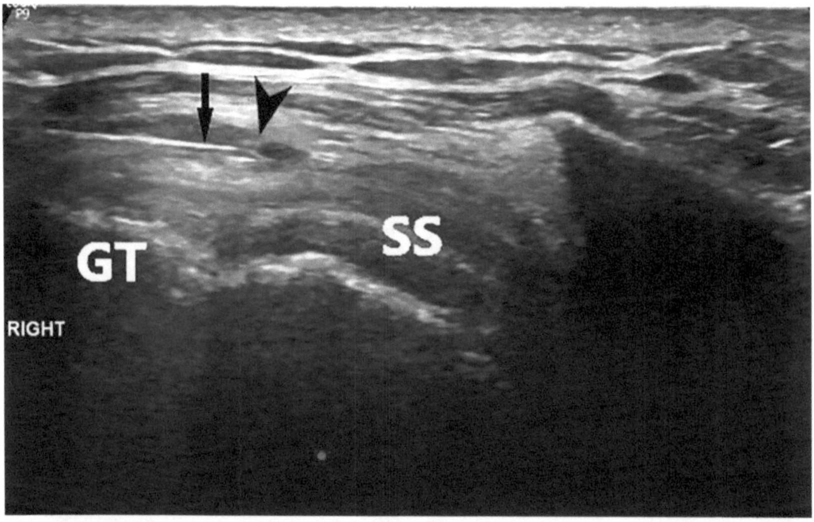

Figure 2-27a

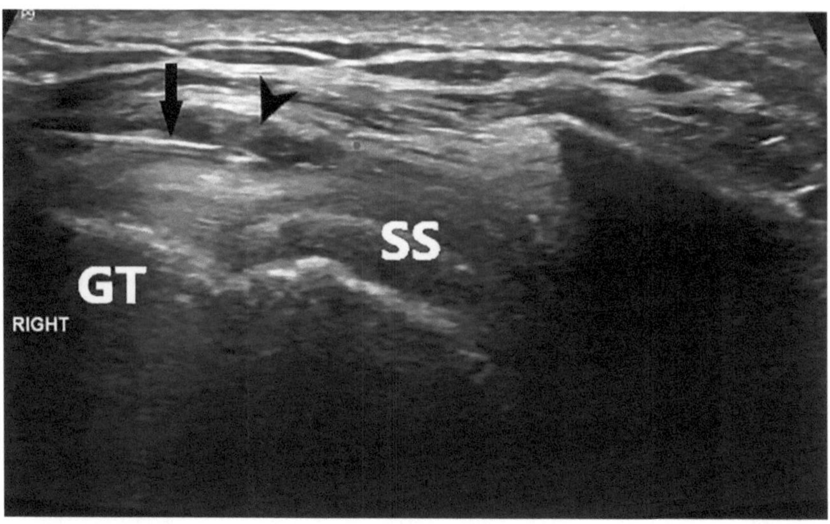

Figure 2-27b

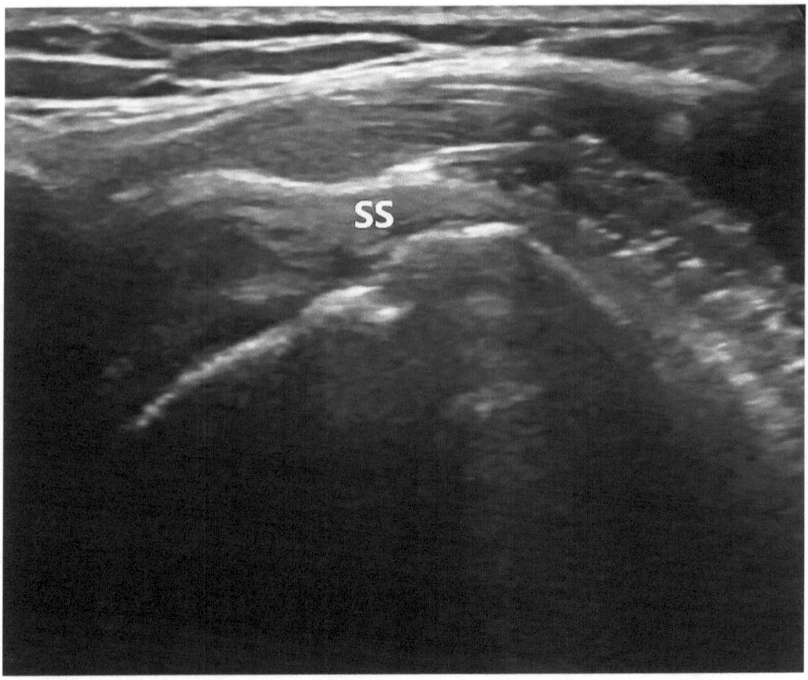

Figure 2-27c

Figure 27: Needle (arrow) advanced into subdeltoid bursa (arrowhead) between deep surface of deltoid and superficial surface of supraspinatus (SS) (a). Bursa expands, elevating the deltoid as fluid is injected (b) with intact supraspinatus tendon (SS) thickness maintained. In the case of a tear the supraspinatus (SS) is compressed with the injection of fluid (c).

In the case of an intact rotator cuff, the tendon tissue will remain intact and the bursa will expand superiorly into the deltoid. However, if there is a tear, the fluid will advance unimpeded to the humeral head and into the joint, thus further confirming the diagnosis of a tear. Confirmatory images of the needle in the subdeltoid bursa should be recorded.

Biceps

Biceps tendon injections can be performed upright or supine. Usually, the injection is done while imaging the tendon transversely. Position the probe so that the tendon is in the center of the screen. After proper prepping, the needle can be advanced either transverse or longitudinal to the probe until it enters the tendon sheath. The injection should then be performed watching for fluid flowing into the tendon sheath, expanding it somewhat (Figure 28).

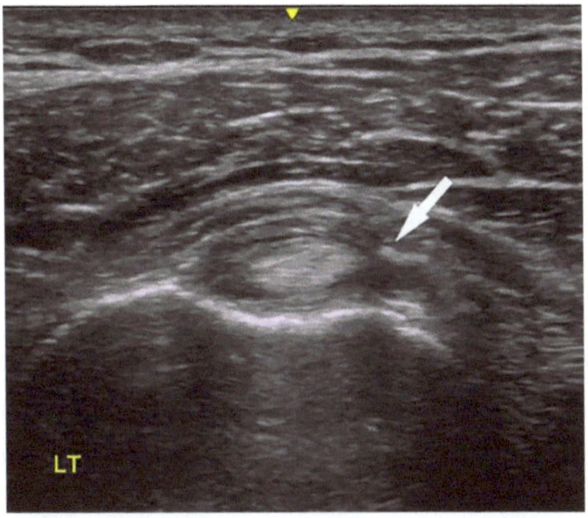

Figure 2-28a

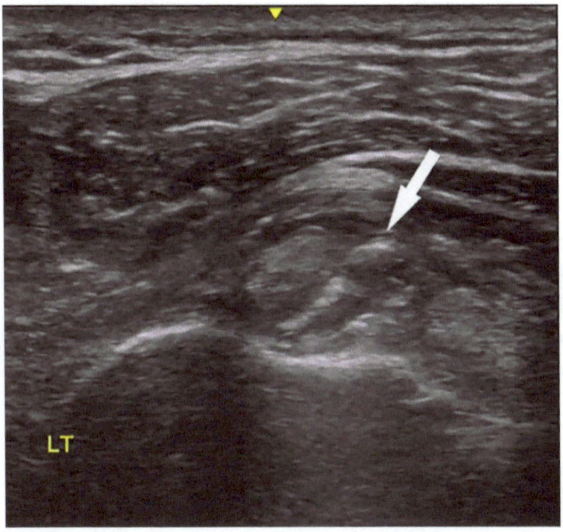

Figure 2-28b

Figure 28: Biceps tendon sheath injection imaging the tendon transverse with the needle advanced in transverse to the probe (a) seen as a hyperechoic dot (N) within the sheath. As fluid is injected the sheath it can be seen to expand confirming proper placement of the needle (b).

If this is not seen and there is a fair amount of resistance, it may be because the needle is in the tendon. This can be avoided by always visualizing the tip. However, if it is the case, adjust the position of the needle outside the tendon but still within the sheath and perform the injection. Record images of the needle in the tendon sheath.

Glenohumeral

Glenohumeral joint injections can be performed either anterior or posterior with the patient sitting upright, supine or prone. Whatever the position, the probe should be imaging the glenohumeral joint in the short axis (transverse), centering the probe just lateral to the glenoid edge. The needle can then be inserted either longitudinal or transverse to the probe until it enters the joint. If longitudinal, the needle enters from posterolateral approaching the joint space tangentially. In this case the needle can be visualized during the entire injection and adjusted accordingly. Using a curvilinear probe may be helpful with resolution providing more of a panoramic view (Figure 29).

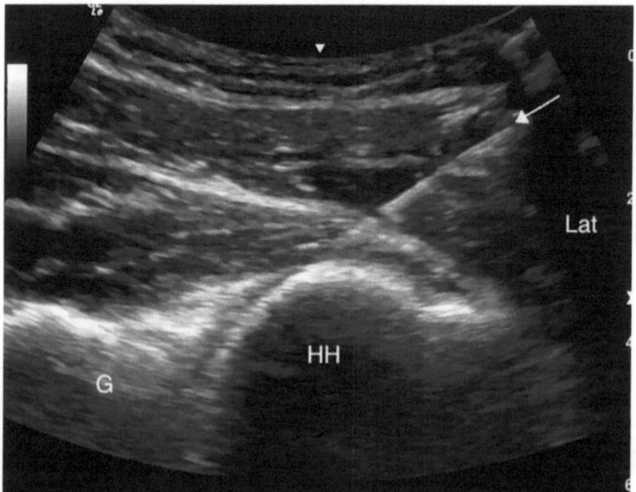

Figure 2-29: Some prefer to inject in the long axis of the infraspinatus. In this case the needle (arrow) enters from posterolateral approaching the joint space tangentially. The use of the curvilinear probe allows for some resolution to gain a panoramic view.

If transverse, you will just see a disturbance in the soft tissues as the needle advances and the tip of the needle as a bright dot as it enters the plane of the probe. If positioned and advanced correctly, this will be as the needle enters through the joint capsule (Figure 30).

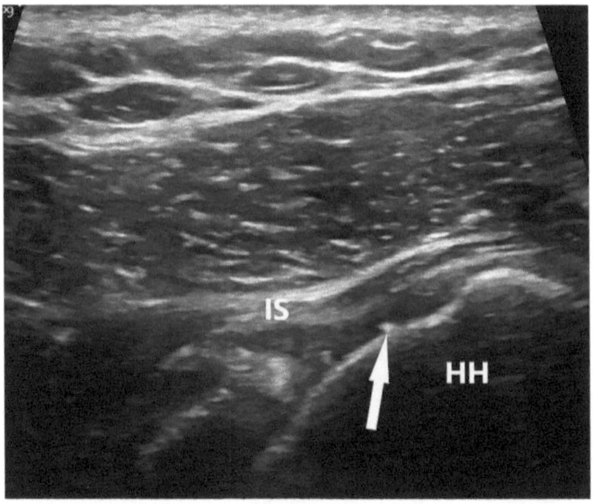

Figure 2-30a

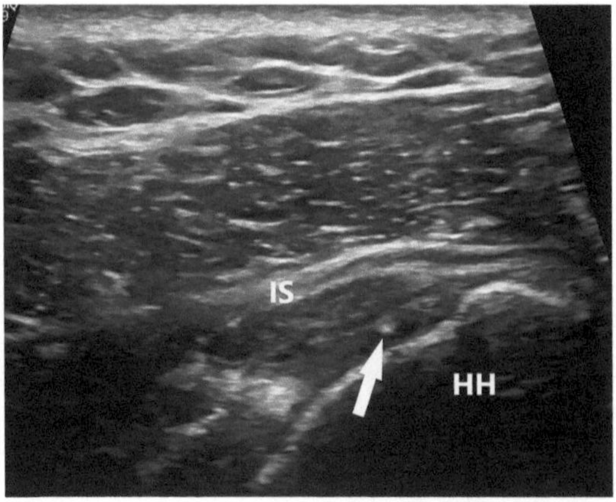

Figure 2-30b

Figure 30: Glenohumeral joint injection with the probe posterior, imaging the humeral head (HH) in the short axis with the needle advanced transverse to the probe, seen as a hyperechoic dot (arrow) entering deep to the infraspinatus (IS) into the joint (a). The capsule expands with injection of fluid (b).

It is helpful to tell the patient that they will feel a slight poke as the needle goes through the skin and a sharper one as it enters the joint penetrating the capsule. The image of the needle entering the joint should be recorded.

Acromioclavicular

The acromioclavicular joint can be injected with the probe transversely imaging the joint, adjusting the probe so that joint is centered on the screen. Osteophytes on the clavicular and/or acromial side should be noted, as should any effusion which usually expands the capsule superior. Tenderness while imaging the joint should be noted. After proper prepping, the needle can be inserted and advanced either longitudinal or transverse to the probe until it enters the joint (Figure 31).

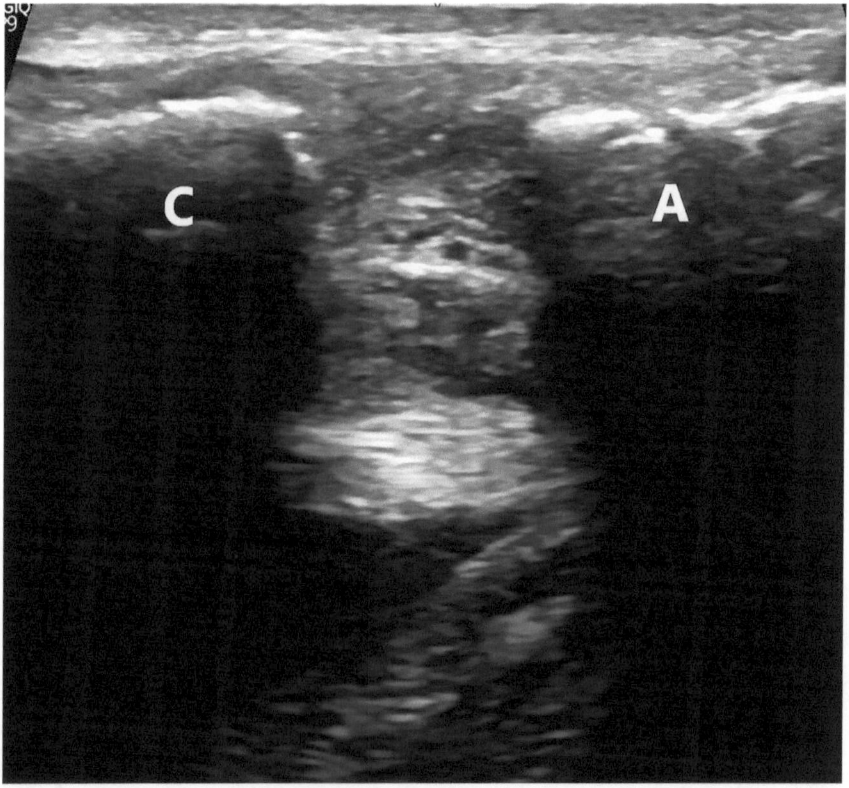

Figure 2-31a

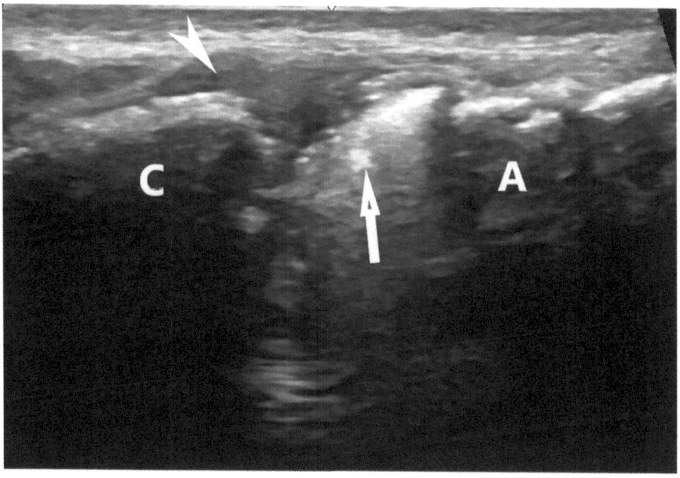

Figure 2-31b

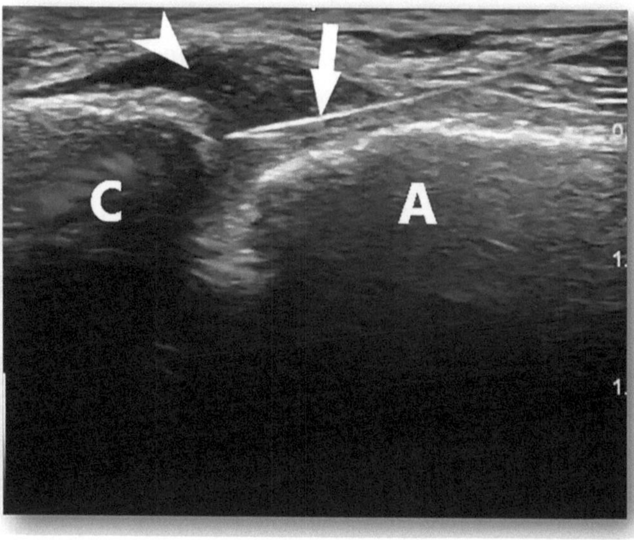

Figure 2-31c

Figure 31: Acromioclavicular joint injection imaging the joint transverse (a) with the clavicle (C) medial and acromion (A) lateral, with the needle advanced transverse to the probe (b) and seen as a hyperechoic dot (arrow) entering the AC joint with overlying effusion (arrowhead). Example of longitudinal injection (c) visualizing the entire length of the needle (arrow).

If properly in the joint the injection will meet minimal resistance. If this is not the case, adjust the position of the probe and attempt to visualize better to confirm that it is in the joint. If inserting the needle transverse to the probe, the needle can be advanced all the way into the subacromial space. Since the acromioclavicular joint is substantially smaller than the glenohumeral joint, not nearly as much fluid can be injected and there will be slightly more resistance when in the joint. Also, at times patients may react to the pressure within the joint in a vaso-vagal fashion, even to the point of passing out. As always, document the image of the needle in the joint.

Scapulo-thoracic

Scapulo-thoracic injections are usually performed at the posterior superior pole of the scapula, into the bursa between the undersurface of the scapula and the rib cage. This injection can be performed with the patient sitting upright or prone if necessary. The superior pole of the scapula should be visualized and the needle advanced longitudinal to the probe as it enters just deep to the scapula but superficial to the ribs. The injection should then be performed, meeting minimal resistance, recording the position of the needle tip (Figure 32).

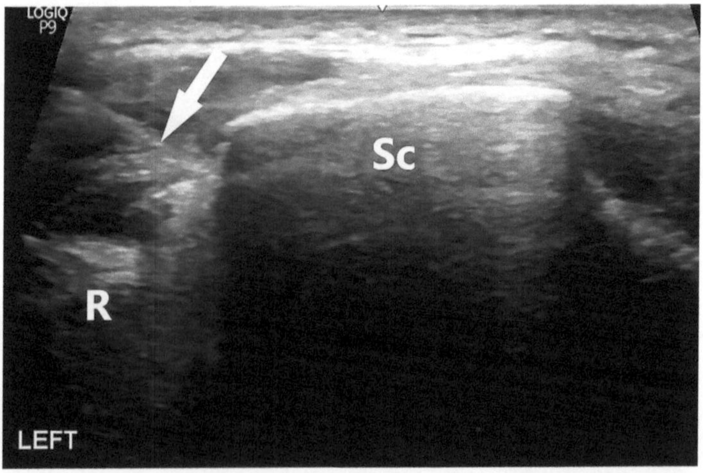

Figure 2-32: Scapulo-thoracic joint injection imaging edge of the scapula (Sc), underlying rib (R) with the needle advanced longitudinal (arrow).

The ST bursa can also be injected with the patient seated and the shoulders protracted. The needle is advanced deep to the rhomboid to the outer surface of the rib under direct ultrasound visualization. In this way the hydro-dissection can be observed in real time (Figure 33).

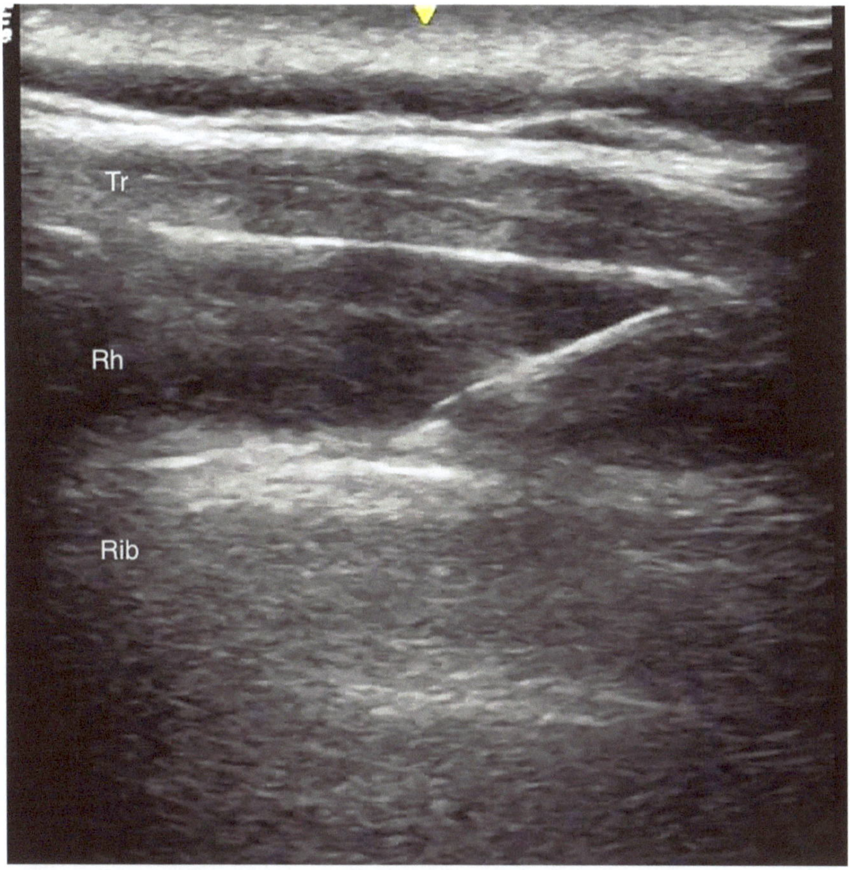

Figure 2-33: Needle advanced longitudinally through the trapezius (Tr), deep to the rhomboid (Rh) and superficial to the rib (Rib). The scapula has been protracted to allow full visualization of the needle and subsequent hydro-dissection.

References:

1. Katthagen BD. *Ultrasonography of the Shoulder*. New York: Thieme, 1990.

2. Farrar EL, Matsen FA, Rogers JV et al. Dynamic sonographic study of lesion of the rotator cuff [abstract]. Presented at the American Academy of Orthopedic Surgeons 50th Annual Meeting. 10–15 March 1983; 49.

3. Middleton WD, Edelstein G, Reinus WR et al. Ultrasonography of the rotator cuff: technique and normal anatomy. *J Ultrasound Med* 1984; 3:549–51.

4. Middleton WD, Edelstein G, Reinus WR et al. Sonographic detection of rotator cuff tears. *AJR* 1985; 144:349–53.

5. Middleton WD, Reinus WR, Melson CL et al. Pitfalls of rotator cuff sonography. *AJR* 1986; 146:555–60.

6. Mack LA, Matsen FA, Kilcoyne RF et al. US evaluation of the rotator cuff. *Radiology* 1985; 157:205–9.

7. Drakeford MK, Quinn MJ, Simpson SL et al. A comparative study of ultrasonography and arthrography in evaluation of the rotator cuff. *Clin Orthop* 1990; 253:118–22.

8. Alasaarela E, Leppilahti J, Hakala M. Ultrasound and operative evaluation of arthritic shoulder joints. *Ann Rheum Dis* 1998; 57:357–60.

9. Brandt TD, Cardone BW, Grant TH et al. Rotator cuff sonography: a reassessment. *Radiology* 1989; 173:323–327.

10. Burk DL, Karasick D, Kurtz AB et al. Rotator cuff tears: prospective comparison of MR imaging with arthrography, sonography, and surgery. *AJR* 1989; 153:87–92.

11. Chiou HJ, Hsu CC, Chou YH et al. Sonographic signs of complete rotator cuff tears. *Chung Hua I Hsueh Tsa Chih* (Taipei) 1996; 58:428–34.

12. Fabis J, Synder M. The sensitivity and specificity of sonographic examination in detection of rotator cuff. *Chir Narzadow Ruchu Ortop Pol* 1999; 64:19–23.

13. Hedtmann A, Fett H. Sonography of the shoulder in subacromial syndromes with diseases and injuries of the rotator cuff. *Orthopade* 1995; 24:498–508.

14. Kurol M, Rahme H, Jilding S. Sonography for diagnosis of rotator cuff tear. *Acta Orthop Scand* 1991; 62:465–7.

15. Middleton WD, Reinus WR, Totty WG et al. Ultrasonic evaluation of the rotator cuff and biceps tendon. *J Bone Joint Surg* 1986; 68A: 440–50.

16. Miller CL, Karasick D, Kurtz AB et al. Limited sensitivity of ultrasound for the detection of rotator cuff tears. *Skeletal Radiol* 1989; 18:179–83.

17. Read JW, Perko M. Shoulder ultrasound: diagnostic accuracy for impingement syndrome, rotator cuff tear, and biceps tendon pathology. *J Shoulder Elbow Surg* 1998; 7:264–71.

18. Soble MG, Kaye AD, Guay RC. Rotator cuff tear: clinical experience with sonographic detection. *Radiology* 1989; 173:319–21.

19. van Holsbeeck MT, Kolowich PA, Eyler WR et al. US depiction of partial-thickness tear of the rotator cuff. *Radiology* 1995; 197:443–6.

20. van Moppes FI, Veldkamp O, Roorda J. Role of shoulder ultrasonography in the evaluation of the painful shoulder. *Eur J Radiol* 1995; 19:142–6.

21. Vick CW, Bell SA. Rotator cuff tears: diagnosis with sonography. *AJR* 1990; 154:121–3.

22. Wiener SN, Seitz WH. Sonography of the shoulder in patients with tears of the rotator cuff: accuracy and value for selecting surgical options. *AJR* 1993; 160:103–7.

23. Hedtmann A, Fett H. Atlas und Lehrbuch der Schultersonografie, 2nd ed. Stuttgart: Enke, 1991.

24. Helweg G, Moriggl B, Sperner G et al. Ultrasound diagnosis of the shoulder. *Radiologe* 1996; 36:971–80.

25. Mellerowicz H, Kefenbaum A, Stelling E. Soft tissue diagnosis of the shoulder joint using sonography, computerized tomography and magnetic resonance tomography (MRT). *Zentralbl Chir* 1989; 114:209–21.

26. Sonnabend DH, Hughes JS, Giuffre BM et al. The clinical role of shoulder ultrasound. *Aust NZ J Surg* 1997; 67:630–633.

27. Tallroth K. Shoulder imaging. A review. *Ann Chir Gynaecol* 1996; 85:95–103.

28. Balogh B, Fruhwald F, Neuhold A et al. Sonoanatomy of the shoulder. *Acta Anat* (Basel) 1986; 126:132–5.

29. Iannotti JP, Ciccone J, Buss DD, Visotsky JL, Mascha E, Cotman K. Accuracy of office-based ultrasonography of the shoulder for the diagnosis of rotator cuff tears. *J Bone Joint Surg Am.* 2005;87:1305–1311. doi: 10.2106/JBJS.D.02100.

30. Jeyam M, Funk L, Harris J. Are shoulder surgeons any good at diagnosing rotator cuff tears using ultrasound?: a comparative analysis of surgeon vs radiologist. *Int J Shoulder Surg.* 2008;2:4–6. doi: 10.4103/0973-6042.39580. - DOI - PMC – PubMed

31. Moosmayer S, Heir S, Smith HJ. Sonography of the rotator cuff in painful shoulders performed without knowledge of clinical information: results from 58 sonographic examinations with surgical correlation. *J Clin Ultrasound* 2007;35:20–26. doi: 10.1002/jcu.20286.

32. Moosmayer S, Smith HJ. Diagnostic ultrasound of the shoulder—a method for experts only? Results from an orthopedic surgeon with relative inexpensive compared to operative findings. *Acta Orthop.* 2005;76:503–508. https://doi.org/J82K536U54N24054 - PubMed

33. Murphy RJ, Daines MT, Carr AJ, Rees JL. An independent learning method for orthopaedic surgeons performing shoulder ultrasound to identify full-thickness tears of the rotator cuff. *J Bone Joint Surg Am.* 2013;95:266–272. doi: 10.2106/JBJS.K.00706.

34. Ok JH, Kim YS, Kim JM, Yoo TW. Learning curve of office-based ultrasonography for rotator cuff tendons tears. *Knee Surg Sports Traumatol Arthrosc.* 2013;21:1593–1597. doi: 10.1007/s00167-012-2105-4.

35. Strobel K, Hodler J, Meyer DC et al. Fatty atrophy of the supraspinatus and infraspinatus muscles: diagnostic performance of ultrasound. *Radiology* 2005;237:584–9.

36. Khoury 1 V, Cardinal E, Brassard P. Atrophy and fatty infiltration of the supraspinatus muscle: sonography versus MRI. *AJR Am J Roentgenol.* 2008 Apr;190(4):1105-11. doi: 10.2214/AJR.07.2835.

37. Cox JL, Laughlin MS, Elkousy HA, Baker HM, Badman BL, Buford DA, Ziegler DW, Kruse KK. Determination of rotator cuff tear reparability: an ultrasound-based investigation. *Journal of Shoulder and Elbow Surgery International* [Accepted pending publication]

Chapter 3 Ultrasound of the Elbow and Forearm

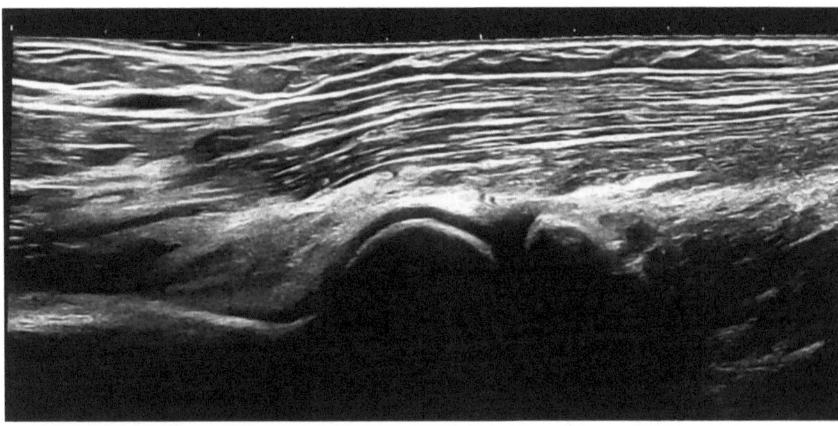

- Ethan W. Dean, MD
- Joseph J. King III, MD

1. Introduction

The elbow and forearm are frequently injured in sports and occupational activities in all age groups. Ultrasound is increasingly utilized in the evaluation and management of patients presenting with elbow and forearm pathology as it provides a low-cost, noninvasive, dynamic, and high-resolution image of both the elbow joint and its periarticular structures. Both acute and chronic conditions can be assessed including overuse syndromes, traumatic tendon or ligament tears, fractures, inflammatory diseases, soft tissue masses, and neuropathies. Ultrasound can aid in needle placement during aspiration procedures or therapeutic injections. Additionally, ultrasound can assist in the localization and evaluation of neurovascular structures in the elbow and forearm. Several factors lend to the suitability of this region to sonographic evaluation: the elbow is a relatively small joint which is easily manipulated by the examiner to facilitate dynamic evaluation; the upper extremity is accessible around its entire circumference which allows for a comprehensive examination; the contralateral extremity is readily accessible for comparison imaging; and the structures of interest are relatively superficial and frequently linear in nature which improves the reliability of identification and evaluation. Familiarity with the techniques of elbow and forearm ultrasound imaging along with knowledge of both the normal and pathologic appearance of the associated anatomic structures increases the diagnostic effectiveness of the provider and facilitates the appropriate treatment.[1] In contrast to the shoulder which has a standard scanning protocol, the elbow ultrasound exam is performed by placing the transducer at the site of clinical interest. However, to facilitate an organized anatomic approach, this chapter divides the elbow into four quadrants (anterior, lateral, posterior, and medial) and the forearm into two halves (anterior and posterior) while recognizing that there is considerable overlap between the elbow and proximal forearm anatomy.

2. Diagnostic Exam of the Elbow and Forearm

a. Anterior Elbow

For sonographic evaluation of the anterior elbow, the patient should be seated with the elbow comfortably extended (Figure 1). The supine or semi-supine position may also be utilized (Figure 2) to facilitate patient comfort or if there is concern for a syncopal episode in response to an interventional procedure such as an aspiration or injection. The examiner is seated facing the patient on the same side as the extremity of interest. The monitor should be easily visible and is generally placed on the contralateral side of the patient. A linear high-frequency transducer is utilized.

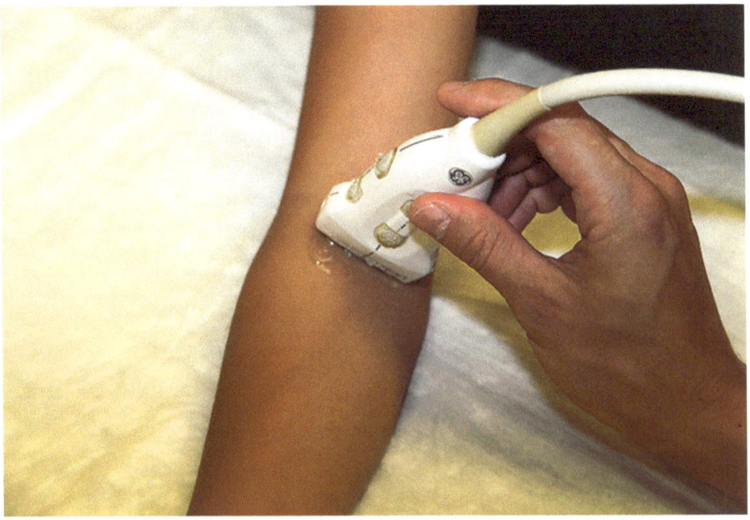

Figure 3-1: Access to the anterior elbow with the patient in the seated position is facilitated by shoulder external rotation and supination of the forearm.

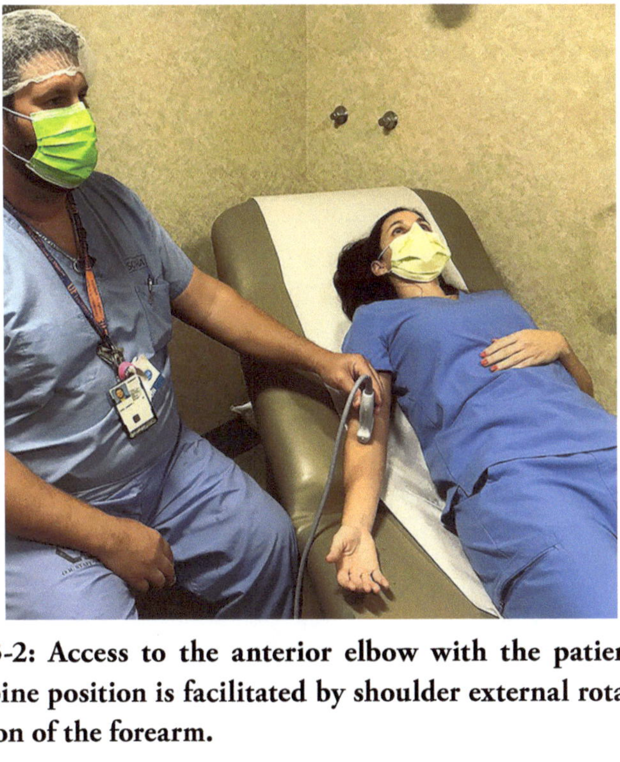

Figure 3-2: Access to the anterior elbow with the patient in the semi-supine position is facilitated by shoulder external rotation and supination of the forearm.

The primary structures of interest in the anterior quadrant include the biceps muscle and tendon, the median nerve, and the anterior aspects of the humeroulnar and radiocapitellar joints (Figure 3). The transducer is placed transversely over the anterior aspect of the distal arm and is slid distally until the curvilinear anterior surface of the distal humerus, composed of the capitellum and trochlea, is visualized. The distal humeral articular surfaces are covered by a thin anechoic layer of articular cartilage. The brachialis muscle is immediately anterior to the distal humerus and appears as a large pyramid-shaped hypoechoic structure. The pulsating brachial artery is superficial to the brachialis and is a helpful landmark as it is midline and generally easily visualized. The biceps brachii tendon lies immediately lateral to the brachial artery and superficial to the brachialis. The hyperechoic median nerve is identified medial to the artery. The pronator teres muscle belly is seen medial to the median nerve. The biceps aponeurosis, also referred to as the lacertus fibrosus, is a fascial structure that extends from the flexor pronator muscle group to the biceps tendon and is visualized superficial to the brachial artery and median nerve. The brachioradialis muscle belly lies lateral to the brachialis, and the radial nerve is located within the oblique fascial plane separating these two muscles (Figure 3). The lateral antebrachial cutaneous nerve is located immediately lateral and superficial to the biceps tendon. This nerve is a continuation of the musculocutaneous nerve which can be imaged more proximally as it courses between the biceps brachii and brachialis muscle bellies in the arm.[2]

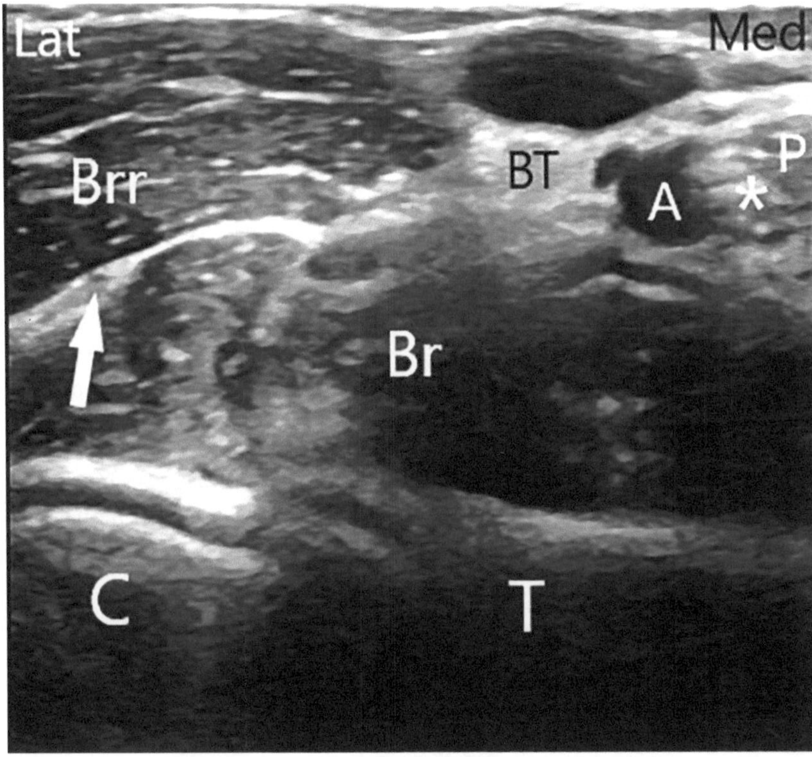

Figure 3-3: Transverse ultrasound image of the antecubital fossa. The biceps tendon (BT) lies lateral to the brachial artery (A) and the median nerve (asterisk). The brachialis muscle (Br) lies anterior to the capitellum (C) and trochlea (T) of the distal humerus. The radial nerve (white arrow) passes between the brachialis and the brachioradialis (Brr). P = pronator teres.

The median nerve arises from the medial and lateral cords of the brachial plexus receiving contributions from the ventral rami from C6-8 and T1 spinal levels. It courses distally adjacent to the brachial artery within the anterior compartment and passes through the antecubital fossa deep to the biceps aponeurosis and anterior to the brachialis. At the level of the elbow joint, the nerve lies between the superficial (humeral) and deep (ulnar) heads of the pronator teres muscle (Figure 4). The median nerve enters the anterior compartment of the forearm by passing deep to the proximal fibrous arch of the flexor digitorum superficialis (FDS) muscle and continuing distally between the FDS and flexor digitorum profundus (FDP) (Figure 5). The nerve supplies the pronator teres, flexor carpi radialis (FCR), palmaris longus, and FDS at the elbow and proximal forearm. The anterior interosseous nerve (AIN) arises from the median nerve in the proximal forearm at the level of the humeral head of the pronator teres (discussed further in the anterior forearm section).

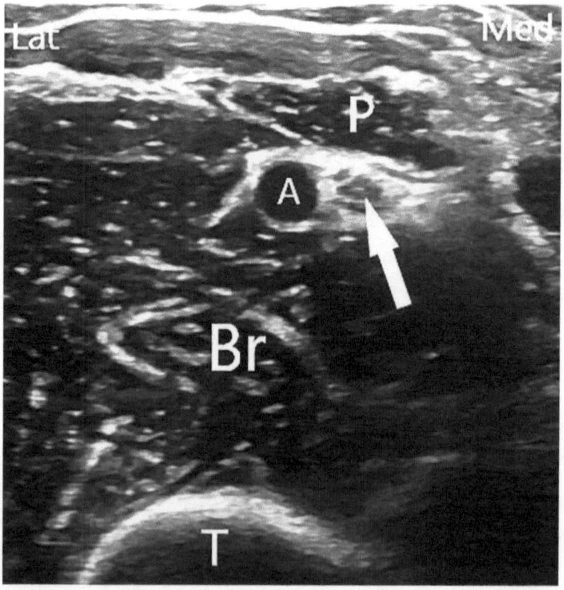

Figure 3-4: Transverse ultrasound image of the anteromedial elbow. The median nerve (white arrow) passes under the superficial head of the pronator teres muscle (P) medial to the brachial artery (A). The hypoechoic brachialis muscle (Br) is seen anterior to the trochlea (T).

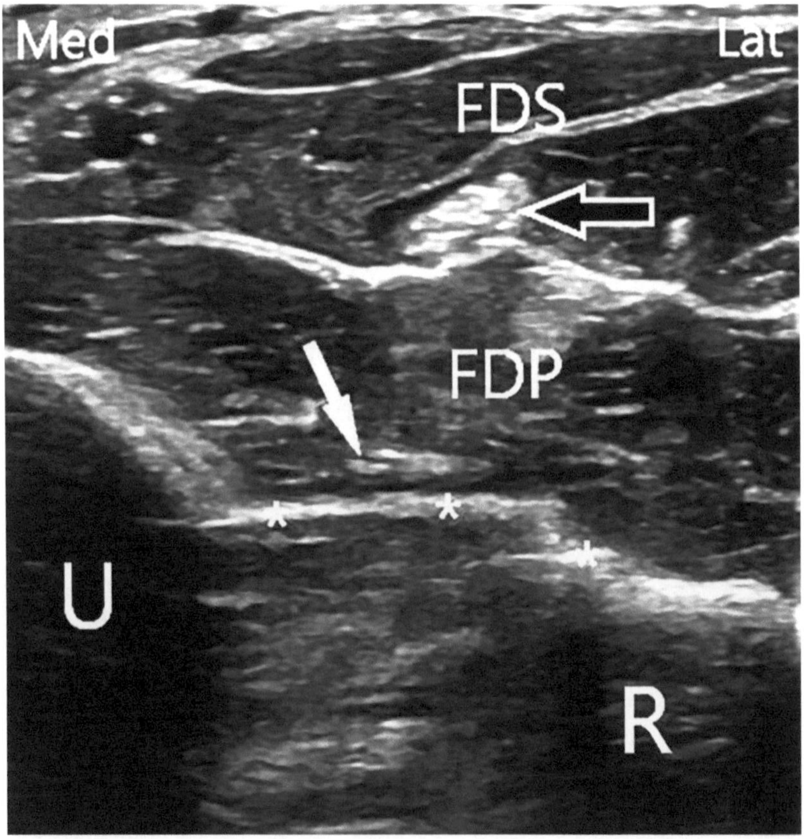

Figure 3-5: Transverse ultrasound image of the proximal anterior forearm. The median nerve (black arrow) lies between the flexor digitorum superficialis (FDS) and the flexor digitorum profundus (FDP). The anterior interosseous nerve (white arrow) is seen anterior to the echogenic interosseous membrane (asterisks). R = radius. U = ulna.

Evaluation of the biceps tendon in the transverse axis over the distal arm may reveal the individual long and short heads, however they are typically sonographically indistinct. Subtle adjustment of the transducer to create anisotropy may aid in differentiation, in which case the long head will be identified laterally and the short head medially.[3] As the biceps tendon passes distally into the antecubital fossa and proximal forearm, the long head rotates into a position deep to the short head and inserts on the proximal aspect of the radial tuberosity, while the short head inserts more distally.[1] When appropriately visualized in the longitudinal axis, the biceps tendon has a uniform caliber with an echogenic, fibrillar appearance typical of tendon (Figure 6). It should appear round and well-defined in the transverse axis, although one can occasionally appreciate a subtle bilobed appearance representing the long and short heads. In contrast to the more proximal aspect of the tendon, the distal biceps tendon can be challenging to image due to its oblique course and deep insertion.

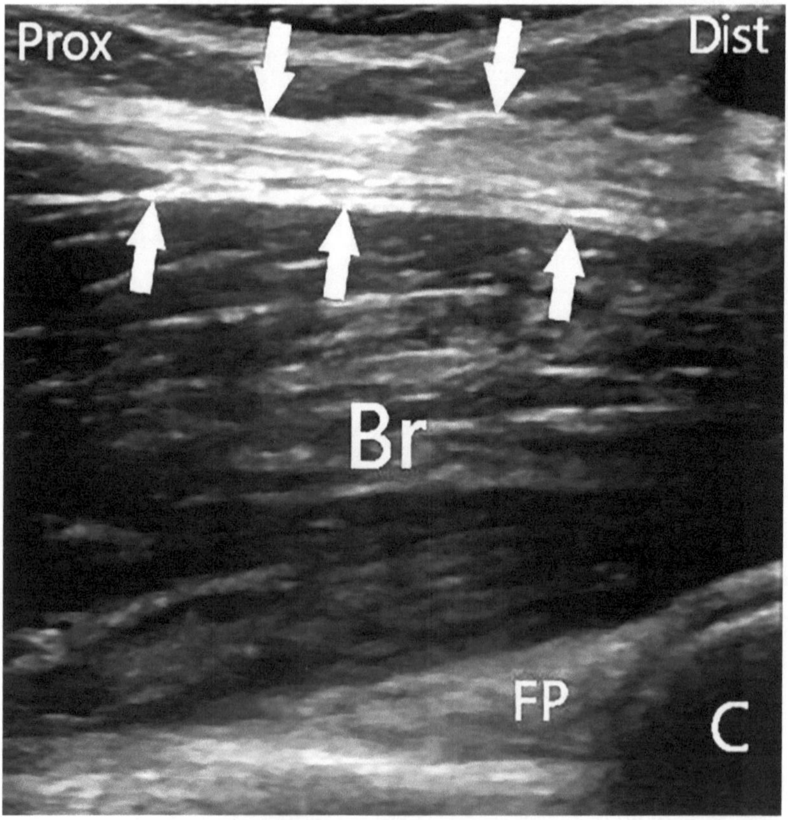

Figure 3-6: Longitudinal ultrasound image of the distal anterior arm. The echogenic biceps tendon (white arrows) lies anterior to the hypoechoic brachialis muscle (Br). FP = fat pad. C = capitellum.

Several approaches may be employed in order to obtain a suitable image:

1. Anterior approach: The elbow is extended and the forearm is maximally supinated. The biceps tendon is visualized in its short axis distal to the elbow crease and the transducer is then rotated 90 degrees into the long axis (Figure 7). Alternatively, the brachial artery can be localized longitudinally in the antecubital fossa and the transducer is then translated just lateral to the artery to reveal the tendon. The "heel-toe" maneuver in which the distal aspect of the transducer is pressed into the forearm while rotating it towards the radius can aid in visualization as the transducer and the tendon become more parallel (Figure 8).

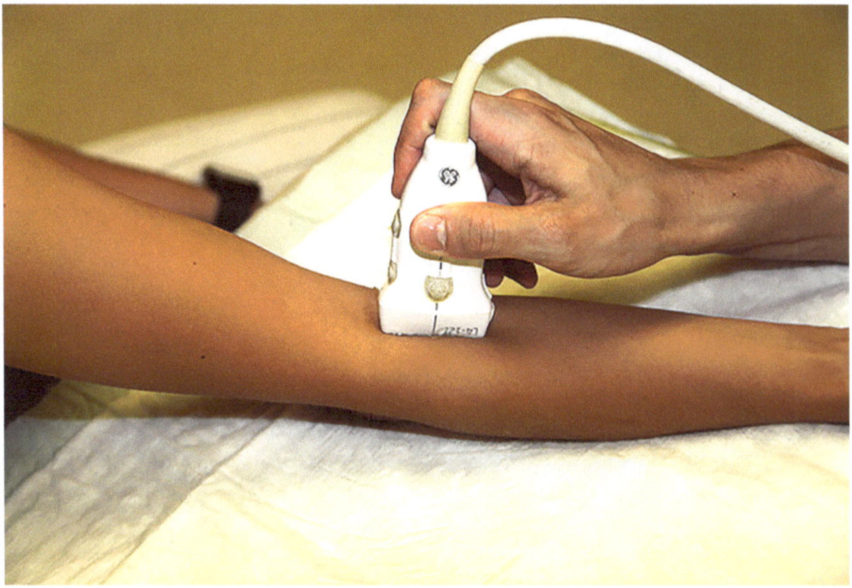

Figure 3-7: Anterior approach to the biceps tendon. The transducer is placed longitudinally in the interosseous space of the maximally supinated forearm. Pressing the distal aspect of the transducer into the forearm ("heel-toe" maneuver) can improve visualization.

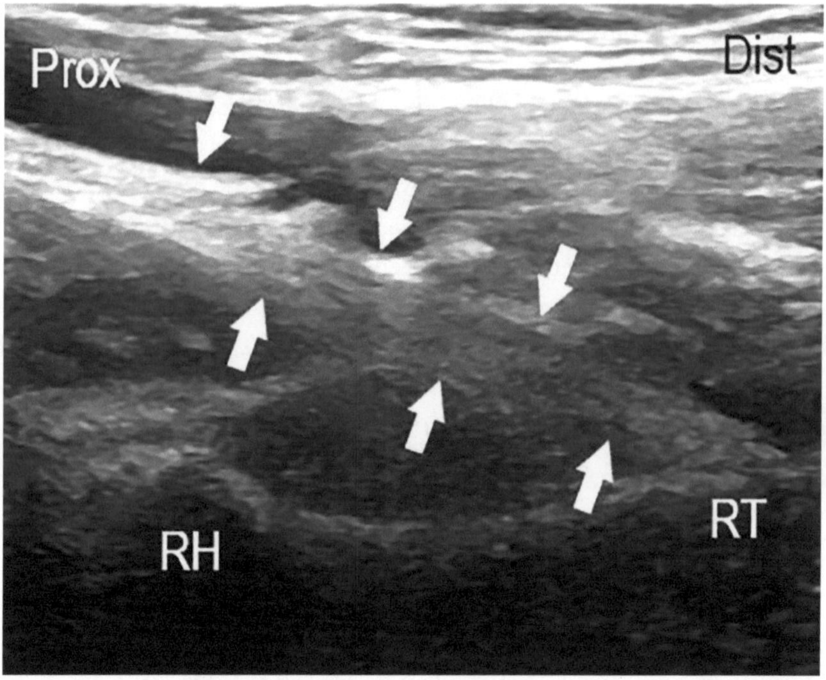

Figure 3-8: Anterior approach ultrasound image of the distal biceps tendon (white arrows) as it inserts on the radial tuberosity (RT). RH = radial head.

2. Medial approach:[4] The elbow is flexed approximately 30 degrees and the forearm is supinated. The transducer is placed longitudinally over the medial aspect of the distal arm (Figure 9). The transducer is first translated anteriorly until the biceps tendon is identified and then distally to reveal its insertion on the radial tuberosity. The flexor pronator mass acts as the acoustic window in this approach and will be visualized more superficially (Figure 10).

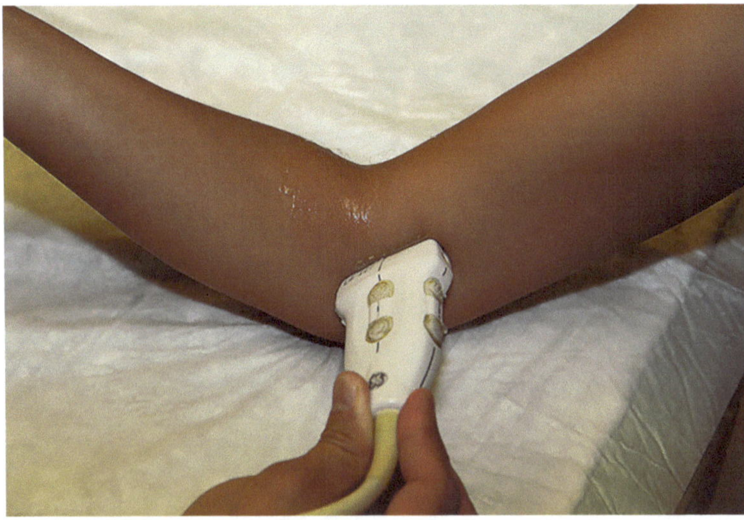

Figure 3-9: Medial approach to the biceps tendon. The elbow is flexed approximately 90 degrees and the transducer is placed parallel to the arm. (For a dynamic view the forearm is supinated and pronated.)

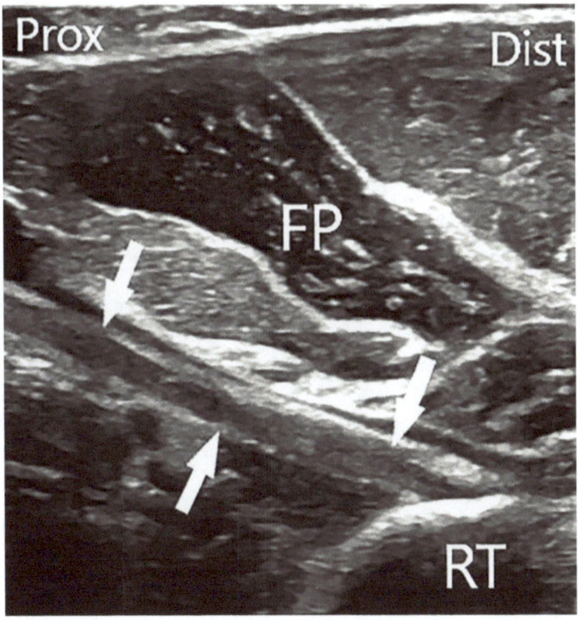

Figure 3-10: Medial approach ultrasound image of the distal biceps tendon (white arrows) as it inserts on the radial tuberosity (RT). FP = flexor pronator mass.

3. Posterior approach:[5] The elbow is maximally flexed and the forearm is fully pronated. The transducer is placed transversely over the dorsal forearm at the level of the radial tuberosity (Figure 11). The patient is instructed to slowly supinate and pronate the forearm until the distal biceps tendon is identified as it inserts on the radial tuberosity (Figure 12).

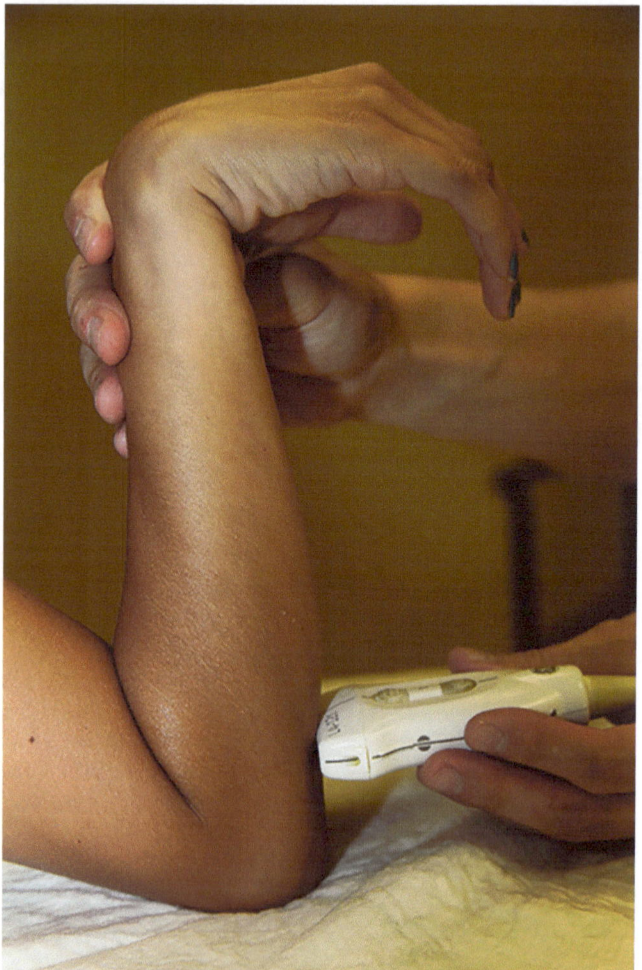

Figure 3-11: Access to the posterior elbow for visualization of the distal biceps tendon in the seated position is facilitated by elbow flexion and full pronation of the forearm with the probe overlying the bicipital tuberosity.

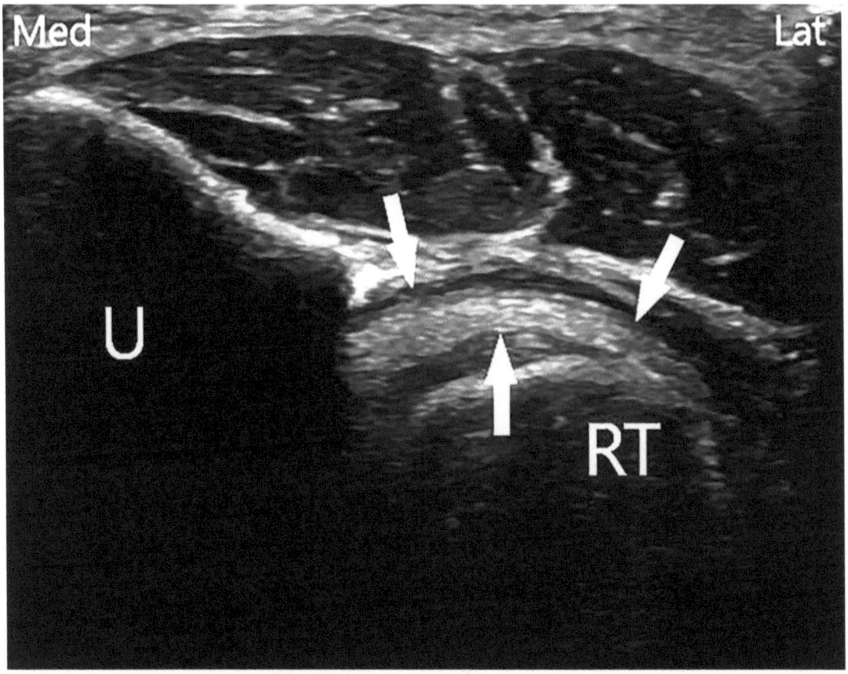

Figure 3-12: Posterior approach ultrasound image of the distal biceps tendon (white arrows) as it inserts on the radial tuberosity (RT). U = ulna.

4. Lateral approach:[6] The elbow is flexed to approximately 90 degrees and the forearm is supinated. The transducer is placed longitudinally over the lateral forearm along the course of the biceps tendon (Figure 13). The tendon will be visible in the long axis while the radial tuberosity will be visualized in the short axis. The brachioradialis acts as the acoustic window in this approach and will be visualized more superficially (Figure 14).

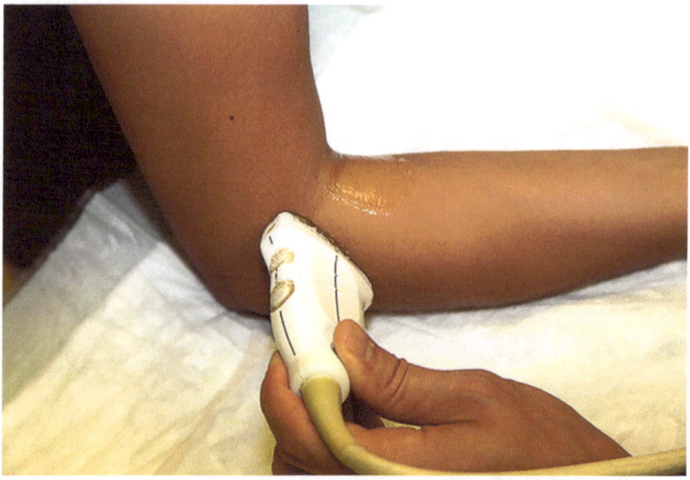

Figure 3-13: Lateral approach to the biceps tendon. The elbow is flexed to approximately 90 degrees with the forearm maximally supinated and the transducer is placed obliquely along the course of the biceps tendon.

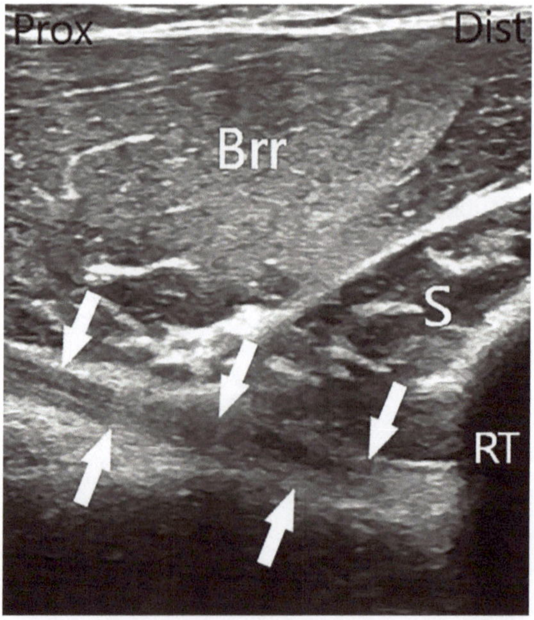

Figure 3-14: Lateral approach ultrasound image of the distal biceps tendon (white arrows) as it inserts on the radial tuberosity (RT). Brr = brachioradialis. S = supinator.

The transducer is placed longitudinally over the distal humerus with the elbow extended to reveal the anterior aspects of the humeroulnar and radiocapitellar articulations. A thin layer of anechoic articular cartilage can be noted over the superficial surfaces of the capitellum and trochlea. The anterior recess of the elbow joint consists of the coronoid fossa medially and the smaller radial fossa laterally, both of which appear as concavities over the distal anterior humerus. Triangular hyperechoic structures are typically seen within these fossae, representing the anterior intracapsular fat pad (Figure 15). The coronoid fossa can be assessed for the presence of intra-articular loose bodies as well as the presence of an effusion.

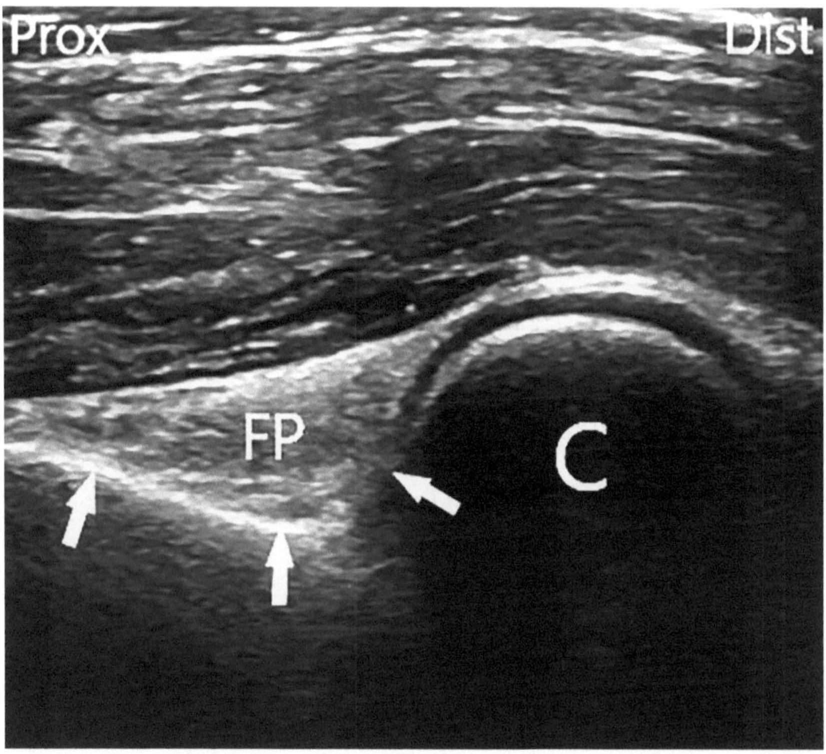

Figure 3-15: Longitudinal ultrasound image of the anterior elbow demonstrating the radial fossa (white arrows) and the echogenic anterior fat pad (FP). C = capitellum.

e. Lateral Elbow

For sonographic evaluation of the lateral elbow, the patient should be seated with the elbow comfortably flexed and resting on the examination table. The shoulder is internally rotated and the forearm is pronated (Figure 16). The supine or semi-supine position may be utilized as needed to facilitate patient comfort. The examiner is seated facing the patient on the side of the ipsilateral extremity. The monitor should be easily visible and is generally placed on the contralateral side. A linear high-frequency transducer is utilized.

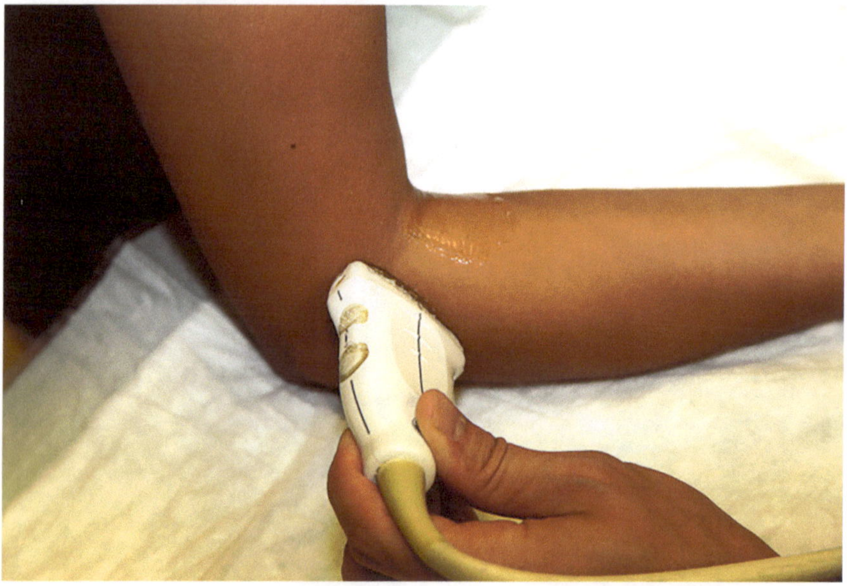

Figure 3-16: Access to the lateral elbow in the seated position can be down with elbow flexion (shown) as well as elbow extension (using a higher table).

The primary structures of interest in the lateral quadrant include the common extensor tendon, the radial tunnel, the lateral aspect of the radiocapitellar joint, and the lateral collateral ligament complex consisting of the annular ligament, radial collateral ligament, and lateral ulnar collateral ligament. Utilizing the lateral epicondyle and the radial head as landmarks, the transducer is placed longitudinally on the lateral elbow at the level of the radiocapitellar joint (Figure 17).

The characteristic contour of the radial head is readily identified and the transducer is slid more proximally to reveal its articulation with the capitellum (Figure 18). The lateral epicondyle is visualized proximal to the radiocapitellar joint and is the site of origin for the common extensor tendon which has a thin, fibrillar, echogenic appearance (Figure 19).[7] Rotating the transducer 90 degrees while centered over the common extensor tendon origin at the lateral epicondyle allows one to visualize the extensor tendon in the transverse plane. From anterior to posterior, the common extensor tendon consists of the extensor carpi radialis brevis (ECRB), extensor digitorum communis (EDC), extensor digiti minimi (EDM), and extensor carpi ulnaris (ECU) although it is frequently difficult to identify these separate components. Care should be taken to ensure that the anterior-most aspect of the tendon is visualized as this is the most common site of tendon abnormalities.

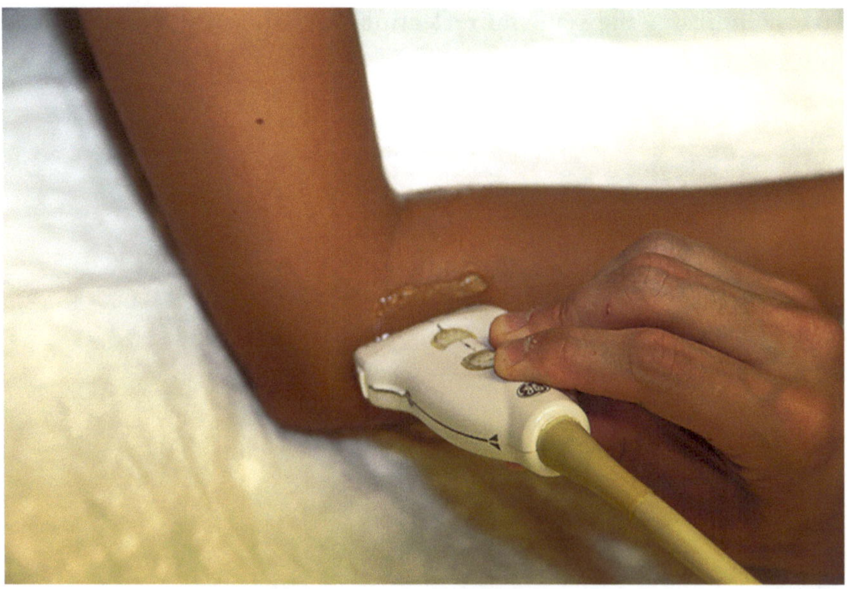

Figure 3-17: Visualization of the radiocapitellar joint is done with the proximal end of the probe centered over the lateral aspect of the elbow at the capitellum and the other end of the probe in line with the forearm. This can easily be done in the seated position as shown.

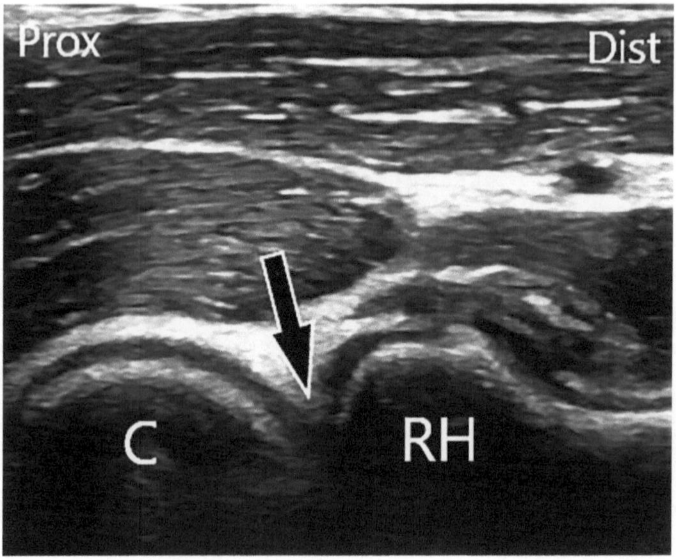

Figure 3-18: Longitudinal ultrasound image of the lateral elbow demonstrating the capitellum (C) and radial head (RH). The black arrow indicates the synovial reflection, known as the posterolateral plica.

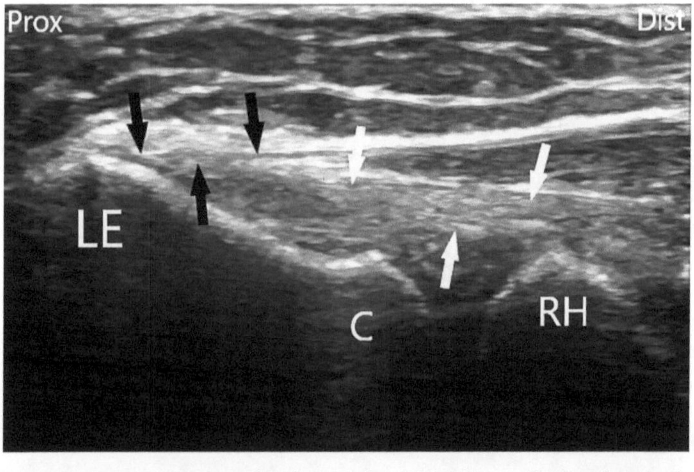

Figure 3-19: Longitudinal ultrasound image of the lateral elbow demonstrates the common extensor- tendon (black arrows) originating from the lateral epicondyle (LE). The underlying echogenic radial collateral ligament (white arrows) extends from the lateral epicondyle to the radial head (RH). C = capitellum.

With the transducer placed longitudinally, the deeper radial collateral ligament can be seen in the long axis as it originates from the distal undersurface of the lateral epicondyle and extends distally to blend with the annular ligament. It is often difficult to distinguish the radial collateral ligament from the overlying common extensor tendon as both appear hyperechoic and fibrillar, however slight rotation of the transducer can demonstrate subtle differences in the fiber orientations between each structure. It has been demonstrated that the common extensor tendon originates from the proximal half of the lateral epicondyle and a subtle bony ridge may occasionally be visualized between the two footprints.[8] As the radial collateral ligament is traced distally to the level of the radiocapitellar joint, a triangular, hyperechoic synovial reflection is visualized extending into the joint from the radial collateral ligament and joint capsule. This appears similar in appearance to the knee meniscus and is termed the posterolateral plica (Figure 18).[9]

To evaluate the capitellum from the lateral approach, the elbow is placed in extension and the transducer is applied to the anterolateral aspect of the elbow in the longitudinal plane. The characteristic hyperechoic contours of the capitellum and radial head are visualized. The thin anechoic layer of articular cartilage over the anterior surface of the capitellum can be evaluated for any irregularities. Sliding the transducer slightly posteriorly at this level may reveal an abrupt change in the contour of the posterolateral margin of the capitellum. This cortical irregularity is a normal anatomic finding referred to as the capitellar pseudo defect and should not be misinterpreted as an osteochondral defect.[10] The elbow is brought into flexion and the transducer is translated even more posteriorly in the longitudinal plane to reveal the central and posterior aspects of the capitellum which can be evaluated in a similar fashion.

The lateral ulnar collateral ligament (LUCL) originates on the posterior surface of the lateral epicondyle and passes posterior to the radial head and neck where it acts as a supportive sling prior to inserting upon the supinator crest of the ulna. The transducer must be angled obliquely to obtain an effective image of the LUCL. This is accomplished by first placing the transducer longitudinally over the radial head in line with the axis of the lateral collateral ligament and then angling it dorsally towards the ulna to reveal the LUCL.[11] Slight rotation of the transducer may be required to bring it into the appropriate longitudinal alignment.

The radial nerve arises from the posterior cord of the brachial plexus with contributions from the ventral rami at the C5-8 and T1 spinal levels. It courses distally in the upper arm posterior to the humerus in the spiral groove and then pierces the lateral intermuscular septum to lie anterior to the lateral condyle of the humerus. The radial nerve supplies the triceps, anconeus, brachioradialis, and the lateral half of the brachialis. At the level of the elbow joint, the radial nerve divides into a superficial sensory branch (radial sensory nerve) and a deep motor branch. The RSN courses into the forearm along the deep surface of the brachioradialis while the deep motor branch enters the radial tunnel. Placing the transducer transversely over the lateral aspect of the antecubital fossa with the elbow extended allows one to identify the radial nerve as it courses along the oblique fascial plane between the brachioradialis and brachialis (Figure 3). By sliding the transducer slowly distally, its division into the deep and superficial branches can be visualized. Turning the probe 90 degrees from the transverse plane while centered over the radial nerve or one of its branches, demonstrates the characteristic hypoechoic, linear, and fibrillar appearance of these structures in the long axis (Figure 20).

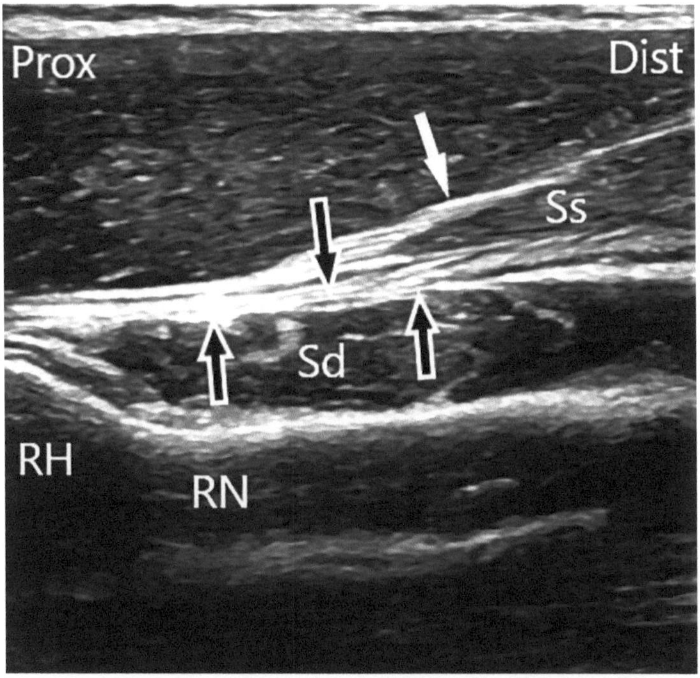

Figure 3-20: Longitudinal ultrasound image of the proximal anterolateral forearm demonstrating the hyperechoic deep branch of the radial nerve (black arrows) passing into the interval between the deep (Sd) and superficial (Ss) heads of the supinator muscle. The proximal aspect of the superficial head (white arrow) is known as the Arcade of Frohse. RH = radial head. RN = radial neck.

The radial tunnel extends from the level of the radiocapitellar joint to the proximal aspect of the supinator muscle. It is bounded posteriorly by the joint capsule, medially by the brachialis muscle and biceps tendon, and laterally by the brachioradialis and the extensor carpi radialis longus and brevis muscles. The deep branch enters the interval between the deep and superficial heads of the supinator anteriorly at the distal aspect of the radial tunnel and exits the posterior aspect of the supinator as the posterior interosseous nerve (PIN) in the dorsal forearm (Figure 21). The proximal aspect of the superficial head of the supinator is termed the Arcade of Frohse and is a common site of radial nerve entrapment.[12] The deep branch supplies the extensor carpi radialis brevis and supinator at the elbow. The PIN supplies the extensor carpi ulnaris, the extensor digitorum communis, the extensor digiti minimi, the abductor pollicis longus, the extensor pollicis longus and brevis, and the extensor indicis proprius in the posterior forearm.

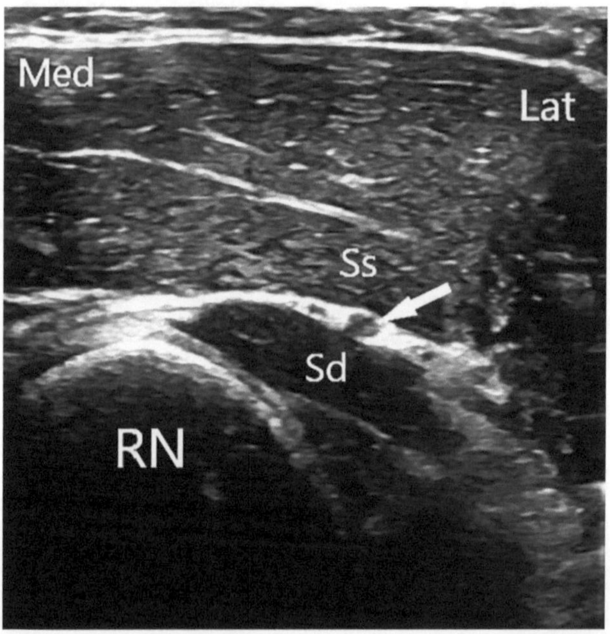

Figure 3-21: Transverse ultrasound image at the radial neck (RN) demonstrating the deep branch of the radial nerve in the interval between the deep (Sd) and superficial (Ss) heads of the supinator muscle.

f. Medial Elbow

For sonographic evaluation of the medial elbow, the patient can be placed in one of several positions. In the seated position facing the examiner, the patient abducts and externally rotates the shoulder while the supinated forearm is placed on the exam table (Figure 22). A second option is the hand-above-head position in which the patient is placed supine or semi-supine with the shoulder abducted and externally rotated with the elbow flexed (Figure 23). Alternatively, the shoulder can be slightly abducted and the flexed elbow allowed to hang over the side of the examining table which effectively applies a passive valgus stress to the elbow (Figure 24). An active valgus stress exam is most easily performed with the patient sitting or standing with the elbow flexed and the supinated forearm placed against the examiner's side while the examiner applies a force to the lateral aspect of the elbow (Figure 25).

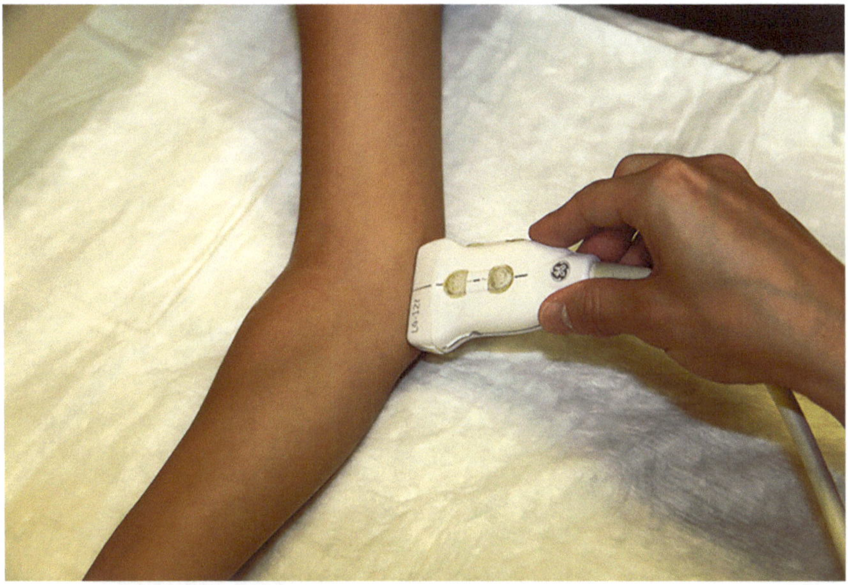

Figure 3-22: Medial elbow access can be achieved in the seated position with the elbow on a table with shoulder abduction and external rotation and the forearm supinated.

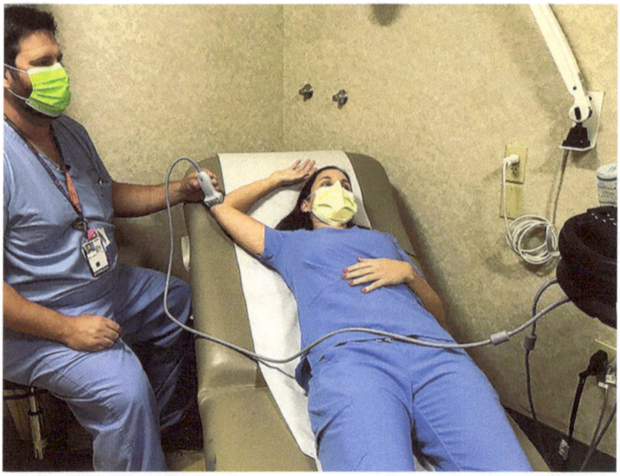

Figure 3-23: Medial elbow access can be achieved by the patient placing their hand over their head with the shoulder abducted and elbow flexed in the semi-supine position. The hand should be free (not behind the patient's head) to allow for dynamic evaluation with elbow flexion and extension if needed.

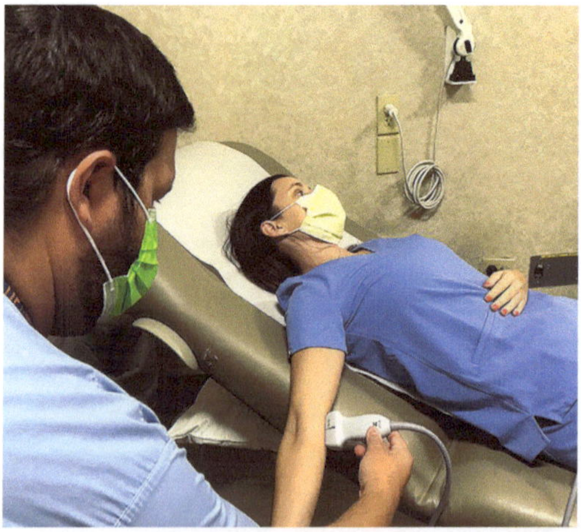

Figure 3-24: Medial elbow access can be achieved in the semi-supine position with the patient's shoulder abducted and externally rotated, the elbow extended, and the forearm supinated. Increased shoulder external rotation allows for gravity to place a valgus stress on the elbow as well (valgus stress in this manner is easier with the patient in the full supine position).

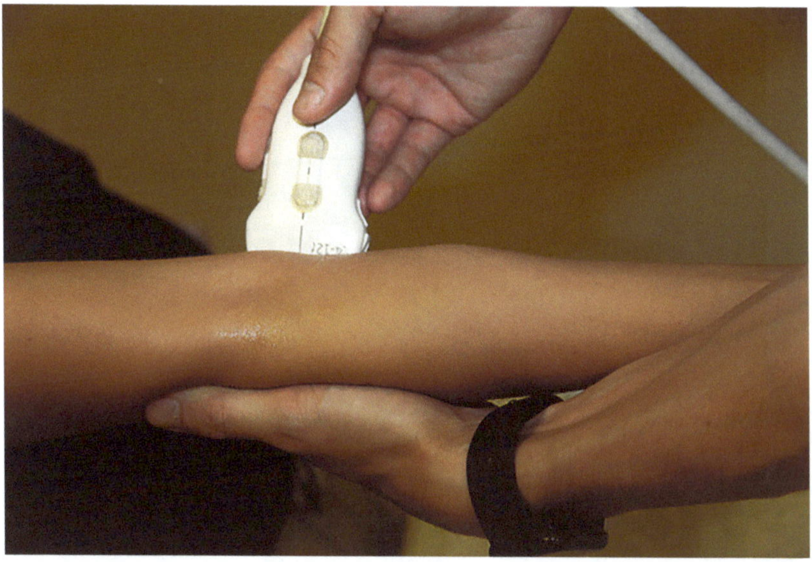

Figure 3-25: Medial elbow access with a valgus stress can be done standing with the examiner's hand that is not holding the probe used to create a valgus force at the elbow.

The primary structures of interest in the medial quadrant include the common flexor tendon, the medial ulnar collateral ligament (UCL), and the ulnar nerve. The common flexor tendon originates on the medial epicondyle of the humerus and is composed of the pronator teres, flexor carpi radialis, palmaris longus, and flexor carpi ulnaris. Sonographic images are obtained by first palpating the medial epicondyle with the elbow slightly flexed. The transducer is then placed with its proximal aspect over the medial epicondyle and its distal aspect angled towards the longitudinal axis of the forearm. The characteristic hyperechoic contour of the medial epicondyle is visualized proximally and the trochlea and proximal ulna are visualized distally. Both the common flexor origin and the anterior bundle of the UCL can be identified in this longitudinal axis. The common flexor tendon origin is visualized at the superficial aspect of the medial epicondyle and appears hyperechoic and fibrillar with a gradual transition to hypoechoic muscle distally (Figure 26). This transition occurs more proximally as compared to the common extensor tendon which results in a relatively shorter and broader appearance.

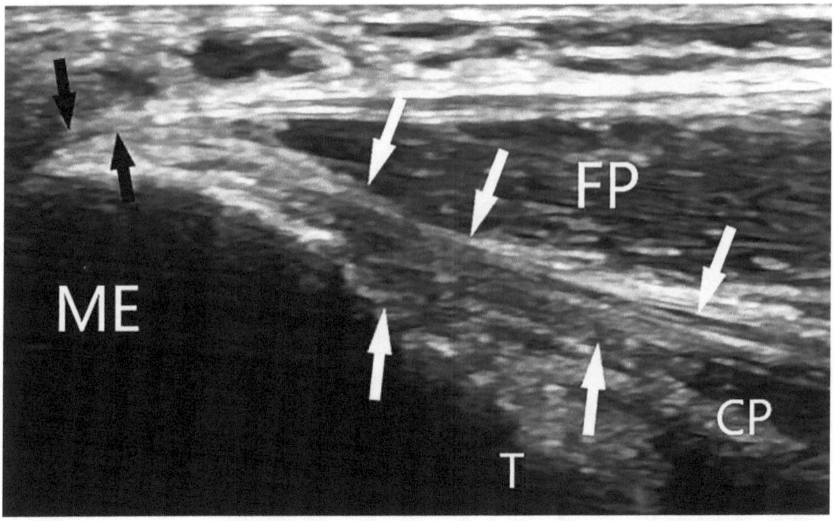

Figure 3-26: Longitudinal ultrasound image of the medial elbow demonstrating the echogenic common flexor tendon (black arrows) originating from the medial epicondyle (ME). The anterior bundle of the UCL (white arrows) is seen originating from the medial condyle and inserting on the sublime tubercle of the coronoid process (CP) distally. T = trochlea.

The anterior bundle of the UCL is visualized deep to the common flexor tendon. It has a comparatively thicker appearance than the radial collateral ligament and may appear somewhat hypoechoic due to its oblique course distally (Figure 27).[13] Pressing the distal aspect of the transducer into the forearm may improve visualization. The UCL also consists of posterior and transverse bundles, however the anterior bundle is most readily visualized via sonography. Additionally, it is a primary restraint to valgus stress and is generally the bundle of primary clinical concern. The anterior bundle has a broad, fan-shaped origin on the underside of the medial epicondyle and a thinner insertion distally on the sublime tubercle of the coronoid process of the ulna. Its proximal attachment may appear as a discrete bundle or alternatively as a less well-defined structure with interspersed hyperechoic regions.[14] Regardless, it should demonstrate a relatively consistent thickness throughout its course. If there is clinical concern for medial ulnar collateral ligament insufficiency, a valgus stress maneuver may be informative. This may be performed by having the patient lie supine with the flexed elbow hanging over the edge of the examining table or, alternatively, by having the sitting or standing patient place the supinated forearm against the examiner's side while the examiner applies a valgus stress to the lateral aspect of the elbow (Figure 25). The elbow should be flexed at least 30 degrees in order to eliminate the osseous stability afforded by the olecranon process within the olecranon fossa. The medial humeroulnar joint line is observed as the valgus stress is applied and the amount of widening is noted.[15] The exam can be repeated on the contralateral uninjured elbow to provide a comparison.

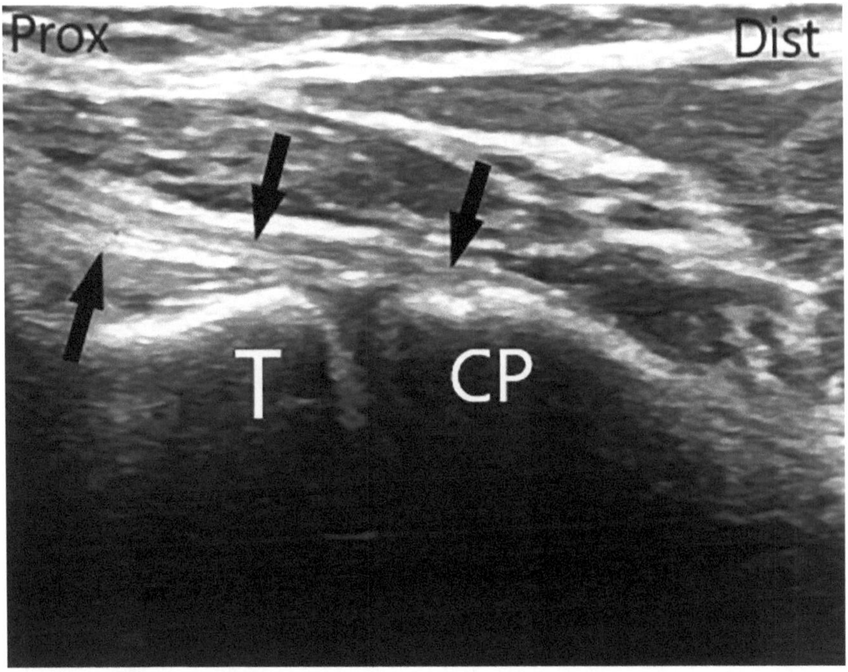

Figure 3-27: Longitudinal ultrasound image of the medial elbow demonstrating the insertion of the anterior bundle of the UCL (black arrows) on the sublime tubercle of the coronoid process (CP). T = trochlea.

The ulnar nerve arises from the posterior cord of the brachial plexus with contributions from the ventral rami at the C8 and T1 spinal levels. It travels distally medial to the brachial artery in the anterior compartment of the upper arm. It subsequently pierces the medial intermuscular septum 8 cm proximal to the medial epicondyle and descends on the anterior surface of the medial head of the triceps muscle. The ulnar nerve courses into the anterior compartment of the forearm through the fibrosseous cubital tunnel which is bordered by the olecranon process laterally, the posterior cortex of the medial epicondyle medially, the posterior bundle of the UCL and the joint capsule anteriorly, and the cubital retinaculum (also referred to as Osborne's ligament) posteriorly. The nerve exits the cubital tunnel and enters the medial forearm between the humeral and ulnar heads of the flexor carpi ulnaris muscle. At the level of the elbow, the ulnar nerve supplies the flexor carpi ulnaris and the medial half of the flexor digitorum superficialis.

Sonographic identification of the ulnar nerve should first be performed with the elbow in extension. Elbow flexion can sometimes result in anterior subluxation of the nerve from the cubital tunnel which can confound identification. The transducer is placed in the transverse plane centered just posterior to the medial epicondyle. The characteristic hyperechoic contours of the medial epicondyle and the olecranon are visualized. The nerve appears round and hypoechoic with a surrounding layer of echogenic fat (Figure 28). The nerve should remain consistent in caliber as the probe is slid proximally and distally. The cubital retinaculum is visualized as a thin structure connecting the olecranon and medial epicondyle superficial to the nerve. The posterior bundle of the UCL is visualized deep to the nerve. As the probe is translated distally, the ulnar nerve is seen coursing between the humeral and ulnar heads of the flexor carpi ulnaris (Figure 29). Rotating the transducer 90 degrees allows for longitudinal visualization in which the nerve should appear linear, fibrillar, and hypoechoic.

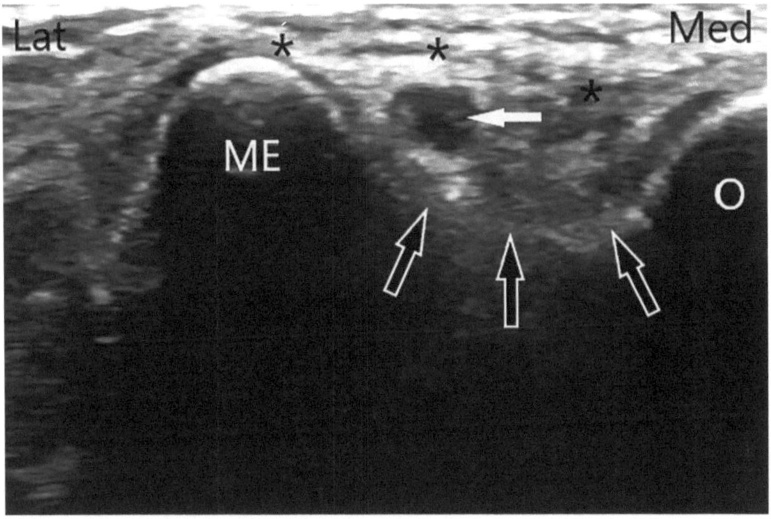

Figure 3-28: Transverse ultrasound image of the cubital tunnel demonstrating the ulnar nerve (white arrow) bounded by the medial epicondyle (ME), posterior bundle of the UCL (black arrows), olecranon (O), and the cubital retinaculum (asterisks).

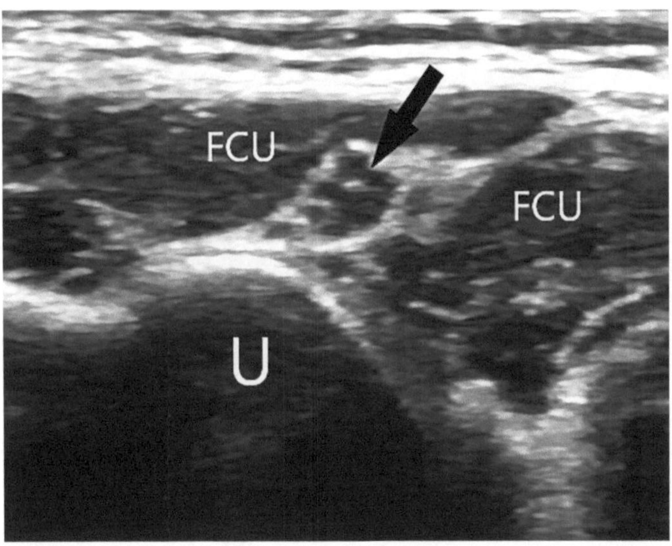

Figure 3-29: Transverse ultrasound image of the medial elbow demonstrating the ulnar nerve (black arrow) passing between the two heads of the flexor carpi ulnaris muscle (FCU) after exiting the cubital tunnel. U = ulna.

A dynamic exam of the cubital tunnel involves placement of the transducer in transverse fashion between the medial epicondyle and the olecranon process (Figure 30). The elbow is passively flexed which moves the olecranon out of the imaging plane and brings the hypoechoic medial head of the triceps brachii muscle into view. The normal contour of the medial epicondyle should be kept in view during the entire maneuver, which may require slight adjustment of the transducer. As the elbow is flexed, the ulnar nerve is noted to shift towards the apex of the medial epicondyle, however it should not translate anteriorly over the epicondyle (Figure 31).[14] Care should be taken not to apply excessive pressure to the transducer as this may affect nerve translation.

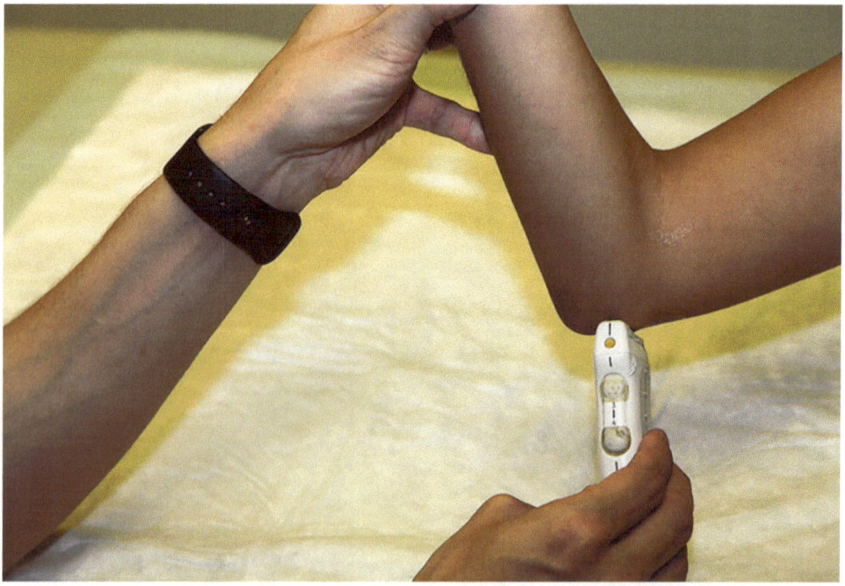

Figure 3-30: Ulnar nerve dynamic exam can be performed by holding the ultrasound probe transversely over the medial elbow cubital tunnel with the other examiners hand on the patient's wrist to allow ultrasound visualization during passive elbow flexion and extension.

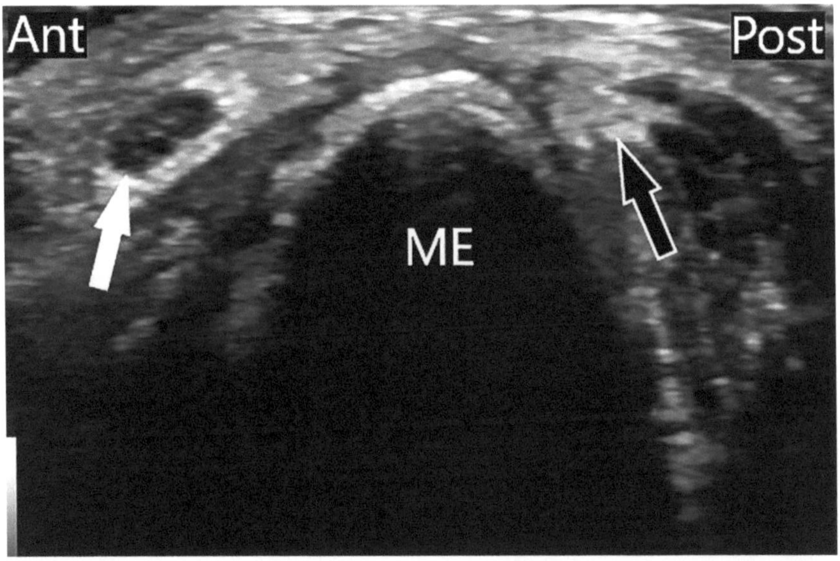

Figure 3-31: Transverse ultrasound image of the cubital tunnel demonstrating subluxation of the ulnar nerve (white arrow) anterior to the medial epicondyle (ME) with elbow flexion. The tendinous portion of the medial head of the triceps is indicated by the black arrow.

g. Posterior Elbow

For sonographic evaluation of the posterior elbow, the patient can be placed in one of several positions. In the seated position facing the examiner, the patient internally rotates the shoulder and pronates the forearm. It may be helpful to have the patient lean away from the examiner, and the elbow can be flexed or extended as necessary (Figure 32). A bump can also be placed under the upper arm to improve posterior access to the elbow (Figure 33). A second option is the so-called "crab" position in which the patient's shoulder is internally abducted and the elbow flexed while the palm of the hand is placed on the exam table (Figure 34). Patients with limited range of motion of the upper extremity may find this position challenging. A third variant is the hand-above-head position in which the patient is placed supine or semi-supine with the shoulder abducted and externally rotated with the elbow flexed (Figure 35). This position is effective for examination of the medial elbow as well. Finally, the patient can be placed supine or semi-supine with the shoulder internally rotated and the forearm allowed to rest across the abdomen (Figure 36).

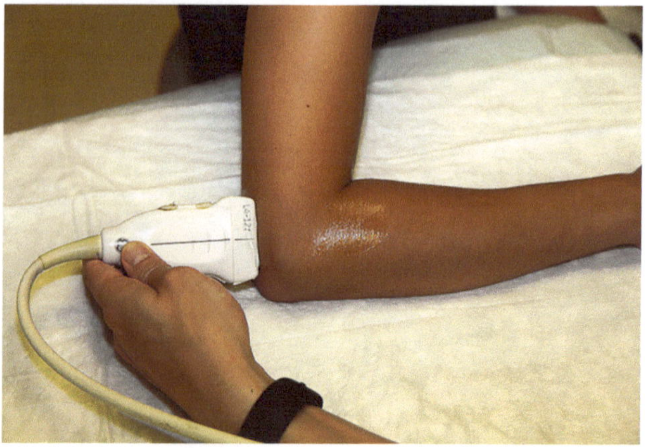

Figure 3-32: Posterior access to the elbow in the seated position can be performed with the patient's elbow flexed to 90 degrees and the forearm laying on a table.

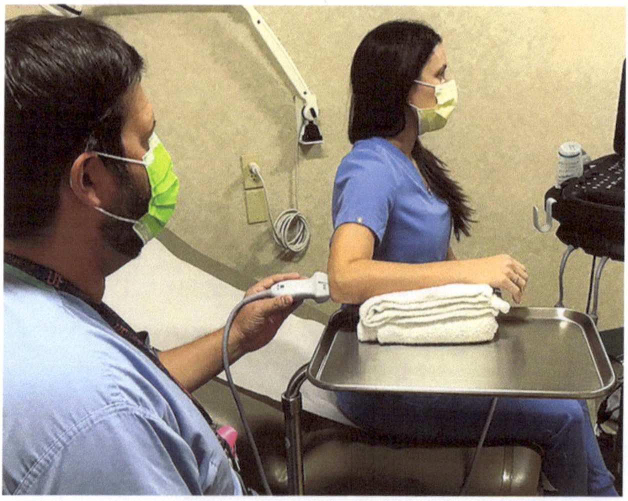

Figure 3-33: Posterior elbow access is facilitated in the seated position by placing the forearm on a bump (towels in this case), but can also be done by allowing the posterior elbow to hang over the edge of a table. The forearm should be well-supported to allow for a comfortable position for the patient, especially if attempting a procedure.

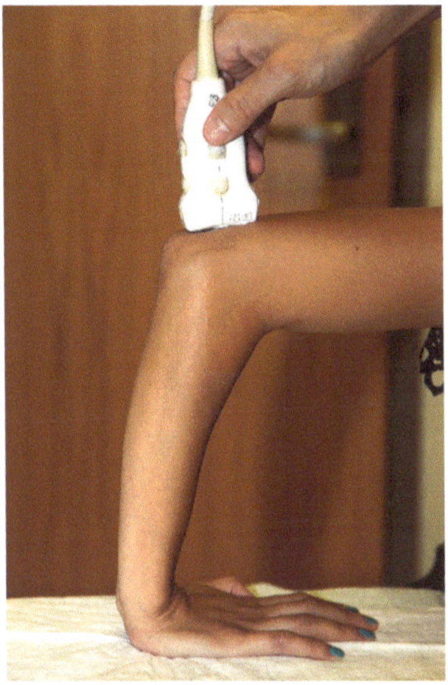

Figure 3-34: Improved posterior elbow access can be achieved with the "crab position" where the patient is standing with their palm flat on the table, wrist extended, elbow flexed, and the shoulder internally rotated. This position allows full access of the posterior elbow to the examiner without the table being in the way.

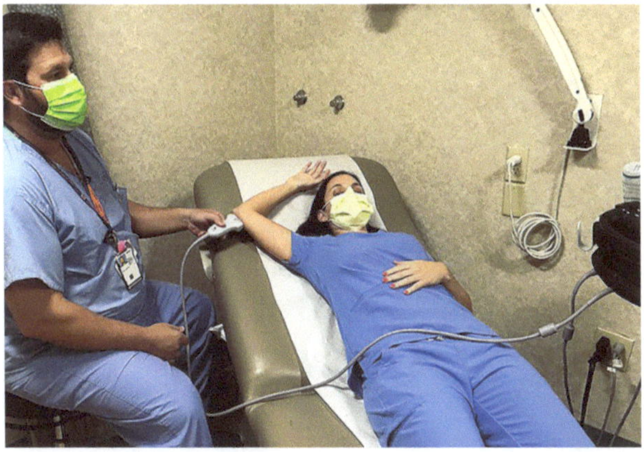

Figure 3-35: Posterior elbow access can be achieved by the patient placing their hand over their head with the shoulder abducted and elbow flexed in the semi-supine position. The hand should be free (not behind the patient's head) to allow for dynamic evaluation with elbow flexion and extension if needed.

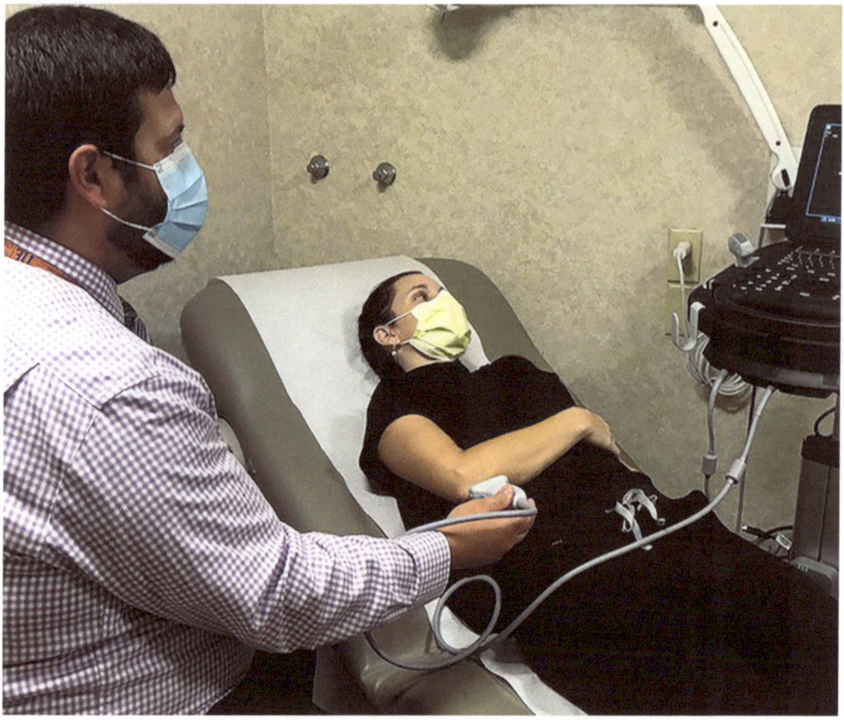

Figure 3-36: Posterior elbow access in the semi-supine position can be achieved by placing the patient's forearm across their abdomen with the elbow flexed and the hand holding their contralateral side.

The primary structures of interest in the posterior quadrant include the proximal olecranon, the olecranon fossa, the olecranon bursa, the triceps tendon, and the posterior joint capsule. The transducer is first placed longitudinally over posterior aspect of the distal arm. The characteristic hyperechoic contour of the humeral diaphysis is visualized. Distal translation of the transducer reveals the concavity of the olecranon fossa which is normally filled with the hyperechoic posterior elbow fat pad (Figure 37). The fossa can be inspected for the presence of an effusion and intra-articular loose bodies. The hyperechoic triceps brachii muscle belly and its more distal hyperechoic tendon are visualized superficial to the olecranon fossa. The triceps tendon is short, broad, and echogenic with a fibrillar appearance characteristic of tendon. Its insertion on the superficial aspect of the olecranon process represents the confluence of the lateral and long heads of the triceps while the medial head has a separate shorter insertion deep (anterior) to the tendon (Figure 37). The elbow is brought into extension to reveal the olecranon process and the overlying olecranon bursa which can be evaluated. Abundant gel should be used in order to float the transducer to avoid excessive compression of the bursa and displacement of fluid out of the image plane. Although the posterior elbow structures are generally best evaluated in the longitudinal plane, they can also be evaluated in the transverse axis.

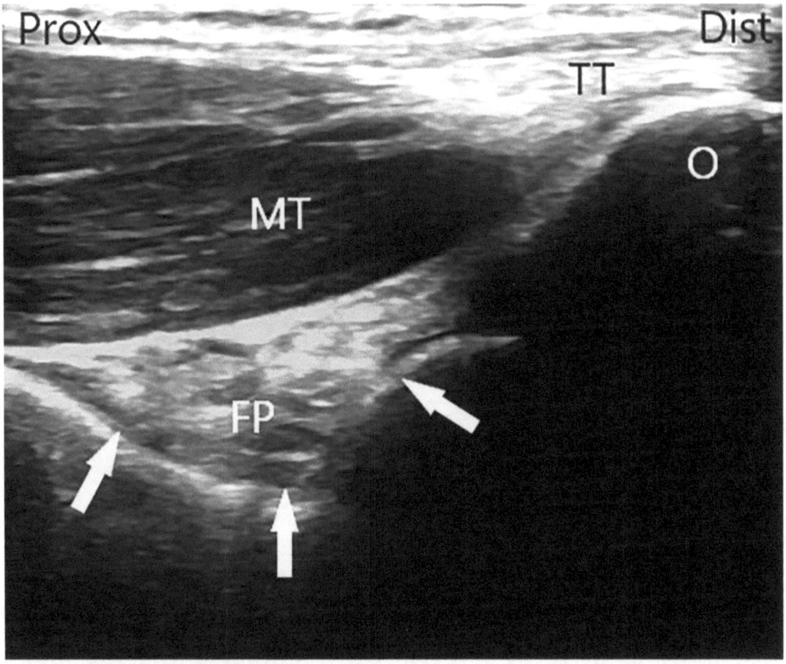

Figure 3-37: Longitudinal ultrasound image of the posterior elbow demonstrating the triceps tendon (TT) inserting on the olecranon (O). The posterior fat pad (FP) is visualized within the olecranon fossa (white arrows) deep to the medial head of the triceps (MT).

h. Anterior Forearm

For sonographic evaluation of the anterior forearm, the patient should be seated with the supinated forearm resting comfortably on the examination table (Figure 38). The supine or semi-supine position may also be utilized. The examiner is seated facing the patient on the ipsilateral side. The monitor should be easily visible and is generally placed at the head of the patient facing the examiner. A linear high-frequency transducer is utilized.

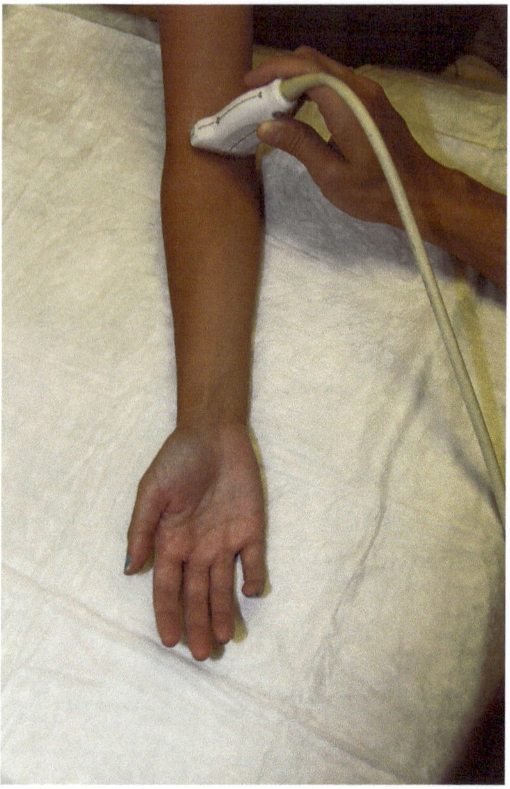

Figure 3-38: Access to the anterior forearm can be achieved in the seated position with the forearm fully supinated and the shoulder externally rotated.

The primary structures of interest in the anterior forearm include the flexor muscles of the wrist and hand, the median nerve, the anterior interosseous nerve, the ulnar nerve, the ulnar artery, and the radial artery. The flexor muscles can be divided into a deep group and a superficial group. The deep flexors include the flexor digitorum profundus and the flexor pollicis longus, while the superficial flexors include the flexor carpi radialis, the palmaris longus, the flexor digitorum superficialis, and the flexor carpi ulnaris. Placement of the transducer transversely over the volar aspect of the mid forearm demonstrates the characteristic profiles of the volar radius and ulna with the hypoechoic interosseous membrane visualized running transversely in the interosseous space (Figure 5). The broad hypoechoic flexor digitorum profundus muscle belly is visualized anterior to the interosseous membrane and the flexor digitorum superficialis lies more superficially.

The hyperechoic median nerve is visualized in cross section as is courses in the interval between the flexor digitorum profundus and flexor digitorum superficialis (Figure 5). In the most superficial layer, from radial to ulnar, the flexor carpi radialis, palmaris longus, and flexor carpi ulnaris muscle bellies are visualized, however they are often difficult to differentiate proximally. The ulnar nerve enters the forearm between the two heads of the flexor carpi ulnaris and subsequently courses superficial to the flexor digitorum profundus, deep to the flexor carpi ulnaris, and medial to the ulnar artery (Figure 39). The ulnar nerve and artery lie lateral to the flexor carpi ulnaris tendon at the wrist.

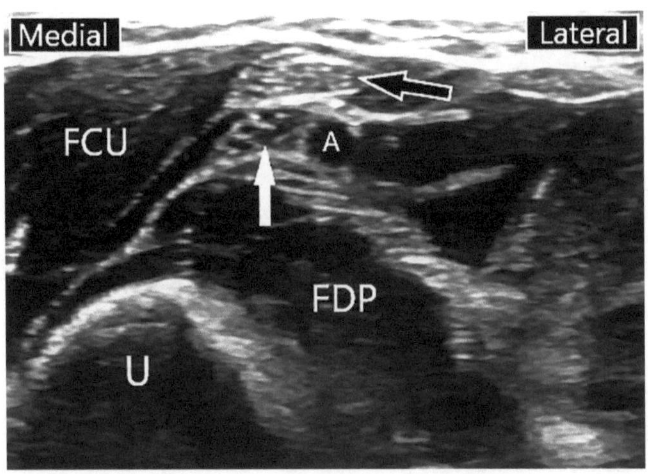

Figure 3-39: Transverse ultrasound image of the distal anterior forearm, demonstrating the relationship between the ulnar nerve (white arrow) and ulnar artery (A). The flexor carpi ulnaris muscle (FCU) and tendon (black arrow) are visualized. FDP = flexor digitorum profundus. U = ulna.

As the transducer is slid distally, the anterior interosseous nerve branches off the median nerve and courses with the anterior interosseous artery along the anterior surface of the interosseous membrane (Figure 5). The flexor pollicis longus muscle belly is identified over the anterior surface of the radius at this level. The median nerve continues to course distally and emerges from the interval between the flexor digitorum superficialis and flexor carpi radialis approximately 5 cm proximal to the flexor retinaculum of the wrist. The radial artery is identified over the anterior radial aspect of the forearm coursing deep to the brachioradialis muscle belly and lateral to the flexor carpi radialis tendon (Figure 40). Turning the probe 90 degrees to any of the previously described nerves, vessels, or muscles will allow for assessment in their longitudinal axis which can aid in visualization and diagnosis.

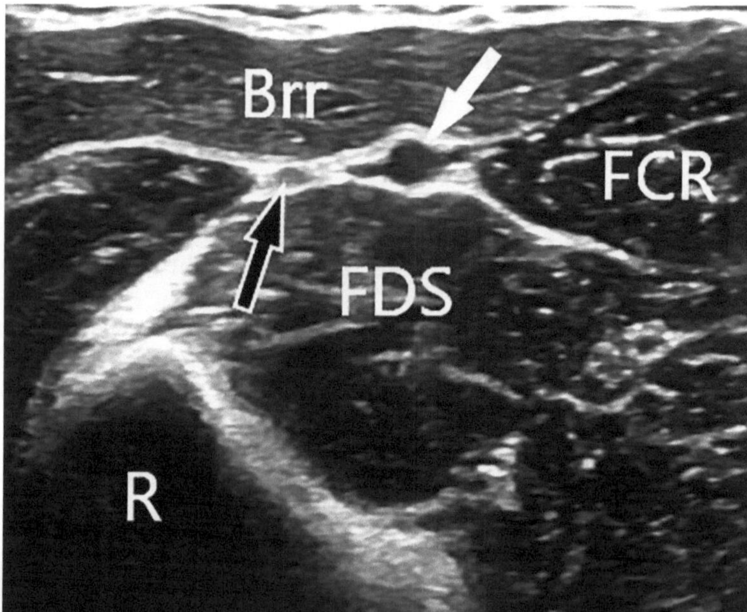

Figure 3-40: Transverse ultrasound image of the volar radial forearm demonstrating the superficial branch of the radial nerve (black arrow) and the radial artery (white arrow) deep to the brachioradialis muscle (Brr). FDS = flexor digitorum superficialis. FCR = flexor carpi ulnaris. R = radius.

i. Posterior Forearm

For sonographic evaluation of the posterior forearm, the patient should be seated with the pronated forearm resting comfortably on the examination table (Figure 41). Another option for the supine or semi-supine patient is that they can place the hand of the affected extremity on the contralateral abdomen (Figure 36). The examiner is seated facing the patient on the ipsilateral side. The monitor should be easily visible and is generally placed at the head of the patient facing the examiner. A linear high-frequency transducer is utilized.

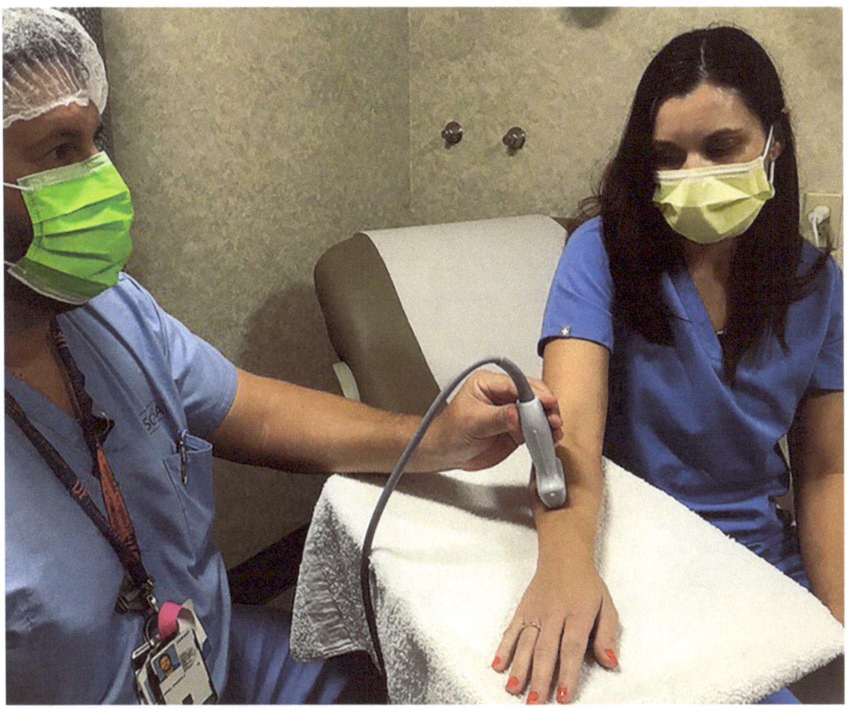

Figure 3-41: Access to the posterior forearm can be achieved in the seated position with the forearm fully pronated.

The primary structures of interest in the posterior forearm include the extensor muscles, the posterior interosseous nerve, and the superficial radial nerve. The extensor muscles can be divided into a deep group and a superficial group. The deep extensors include the abductor pollicis longus, extensor pollicis brevis, extensor pollicis longus, and extensor indicis proprius; the superficial extensors include extensor carpi radialis longus, extensor carpi radialis brevis, extensor digitorum communis, extensor digiti minimi, and extensor carpi ulnaris. Placement of the transducer transversely over the dorsal aspect of the mid forearm demonstrates the characteristic profiles of the dorsal radius and ulna with the hyperechoic interosseous membrane visualized running transversely in the interosseous space (Figure 42). The broad hypoechoic abductor pollicis longus muscle belly is visualized originating from the posterior surfaces of the ulna, interosseous membrane, and radius. The extensor pollicis longus muscle is visualized ulnarly originating from the posterior surface of the ulna. More superficially and from radial to ulnar, the extensor digitorum communis, extensor digiti minimi, and the extensor carpi ulnaris are visualized, however they are frequently indistinct proximally (Figure 43 Dorsal). More distally, the extensor pollicis brevis originates from the posterior surfaces of the interosseous membrane and radius, while the extensor indicis proprius originates from the posterior surface of the ulna. Sliding the probe more distally will bring these latter two muscles into view.

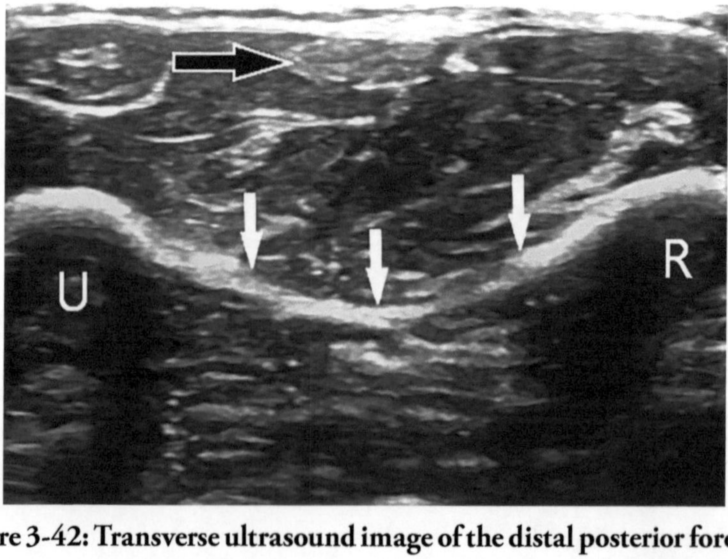

Figure 3-42: Transverse ultrasound image of the distal posterior forearm demonstrating the echogenic interosseous membrane (white arrows) between the radius (R) and ulna (U). The tendons of the extensor digitorum communis (black arrow) are visualized more superficially.

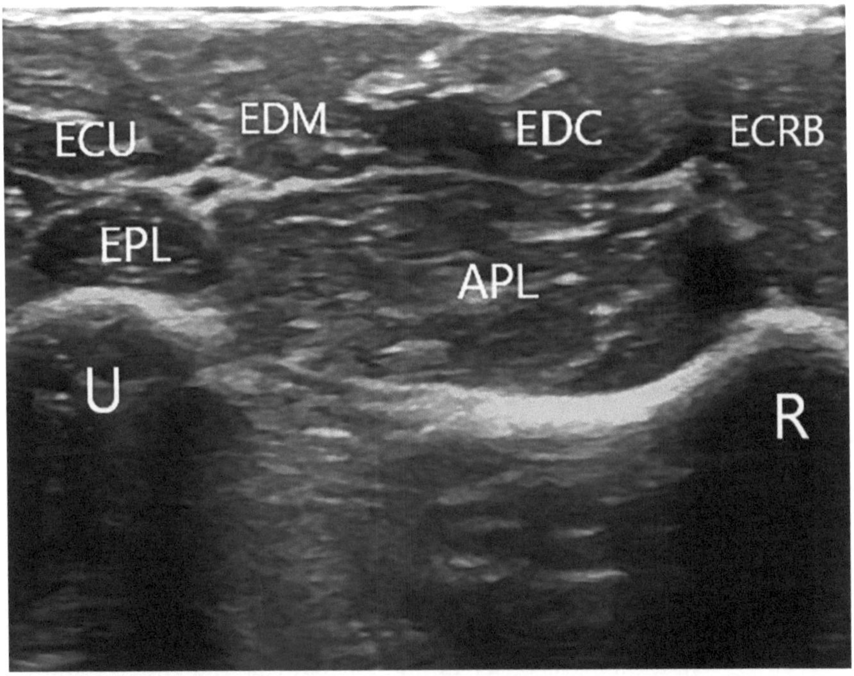

Figure 3-43: Transverse ultrasound image of the posterior forearm. Extensor pollicis longus (EPL) and abductor pollicis longus (APL) constitute the deep layer, while extensor carpi ulnaris (ECU), extensor digitorum minimi (EDM), extensor digitorum communis (EDC) and extensor carpi radialis brevis (ECRB) are visualized more superficially.

The posterior interosseous nerve (PIN) exits the distal aspect of the supinator muscle to enter the posterior forearm. It can be visualized as a hyperechoic structure coursing in the fascial plane between the superficial and deep extensor muscles. Distally, the PIN courses along the posterior surface of the interosseous membrane to ultimately provide sensory innervation to the dorsal carpus, but is difficult to visualize on ultrasound exiting the supinator. The radial sensory nerve (RSN) can be identified coursing deep to the brachioradialis muscle over the radial aspect of the forearm (Figure 40). Turning the probe 90 degrees to any of the previously described nerves or muscles will allow for assessment in the longitudinal plane which can aid in visualization and diagnosis.

3. Surgical Pathology

a. Tendon Pathology

i. **Distal Biceps Tendon** – Distal biceps tendon pathology presents as a spectrum ranging from tendinosis, to partial-thickness tears, to full-thickness tears with or without retraction. Tendinosis is the result of repetitive microtrauma, while partial or full-thickness tears are generally the result of a single episode, classically the forced extension of a flexed elbow resulting in excessive eccentric tension on the tendon. Distal biceps tendon pathology presents most commonly in men, generally involves the dominant arm, and demonstrates increased prevalence with increasing age. Weightlifting, smoking, and anabolic steroid use are recognized risk factors.[16]

Patients with distal biceps tendon ruptures typically recall the inciting event and may report a popping or snapping sensation with onset of sudden pain at the time of injury. Physical exam may demonstrate one or more findings including the reverse "Popeye" sign (referring to the abnormal anterior and proximal arm prominence secondary to the retracted biceps muscle belly), medial forearm/elbow ecchymosis, loss of elbow flexion and forearm supination strength, and a negative hook test in which the examiner's finger is unable to hook under the lateral edge of the distal biceps tendon.[17] Full-thickness tears of the distal biceps tendon commonly result in significant proximal retraction of the ruptured tendon stump. However, if the biceps aponeurosis (lacertus fibrosus) remains intact, retraction may be limited to the level of the radiocapitellar joint.

Sonographically, distal biceps tendinosis is visualized as abnormal hypoechoic signal within the tendon. The caliber of the tendon should be noted as tendinosis may result in tendon thickening or an irregular contour. Partial-thickness tears demonstrate regions of hypoechoic or anechoic tendon fiber disruption with tendon thinning. Complete ruptures result in tendon discontinuity on imaging as well as varying degrees of retraction.[18] Placement of the transducer over the tendon gap may demonstrate a heterogeneous hypoechoic signal indicative of hematoma. If significant retraction is present, the proximal tendon stump can often be visualized near the level of the elbow joint, directly superficial to the brachialis muscle.

Distal biceps tendon injuries may involve isolated tears of one of the two heads, representing a partial-thickness tear (Figure 44). In cases of an isolated tear of the short head, the retracted tendon stump may create refraction shadowing which obscures the intact long head at its more proximal insertion on the radial tuberosity. In these cases in which the diagnosis of a partial-thickness tear versus a non-retracted full-thickness tear is unclear, a dynamic exam can be informative.[19] This is performed by visualizing the biceps tendon longitudinally through the medial or lateral window with the elbow in flexion, while passively moving the patient's forearm from pronation to neutral. In the setting of a partial-thickness tear, the visualized proximal aspect of the biceps tendon will translate in accordance with the rotation of the radial tuberosity, which indicates the presence of intact fibers. In contrast, forearm rotation in the setting of a full-thickness tear will demonstrate little or no translation of the visualized proximal biceps tendon segment. Utilizing these methods, sonographic evaluation of the distal biceps has demonstrated 95% sensitivity and 91% accuracy in differentiating partial from complete ruptures.[19] It should be noted that while sonography is an effective method of diagnosing distal biceps tears, studies have demonstrated that magnetic resonance imaging may have increased sensitivity and specificity in the detection of these injuries.[20] This is certainly dependent on the experience and expertise of the sonographer.

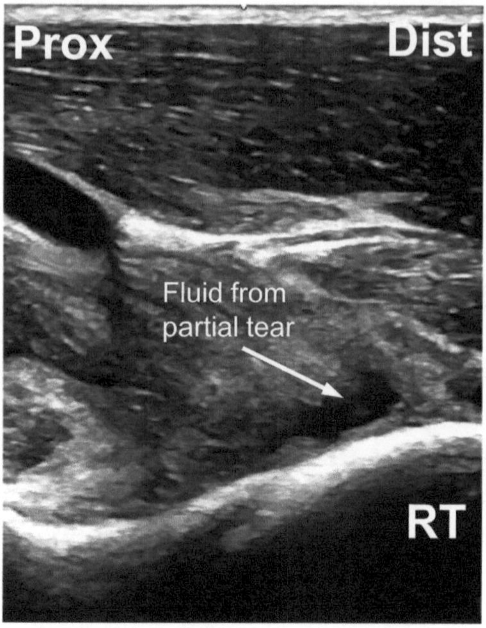

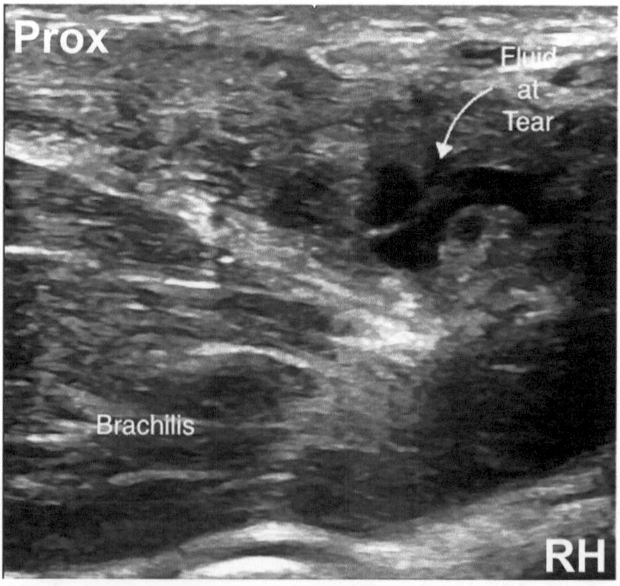

Figure 3-44: Longitudinal ultrasound image of the anterior elbow showing a small fluid collection anterior to the brachialis muscle representing a partial-thickness distal biceps tendon tear. RH is the radial head on the distal aspect of the image.

ii. Distal Triceps Tendon – Distal triceps tendon pathology includes tendinosis, partial-thickness tears, and full-thickness tears. Distal triceps tendinosis is frequently caused by activities that involve repetitive elbow extension such as bench press exercises. Partial or full-thickness tears are typically the result of a forceful eccentric contraction or traumatic event such as a fall onto the outstretched hand. They are uncommon injuries that most typically affect males between the ages of 30 to 50 years. Anabolic steroid use and systemic illnesses such as diabetes, rheumatoid arthritis, and renal failure are recognized risk factors.[21] Patients may recall a painful pop at the time of injury with subsequent ecchymosis and swelling over the posterior elbow. Exam findings include inability or difficulty extending the elbow against resistance, a positive triceps squeeze test (squeezing the triceps fails to elicit passive elbow extension), and a palpable defect proximal to the olecranon.

Sonographically, tendinosis is visualized as abnormal hypoechogenicity and tendon enlargement with intact tendon fibers. Partial-thickness tears appear as areas of anechoic or hypoechoic tendon fiber disruption. Partial-thickness distal triceps tendon tears most commonly involve delamination of the lateral and long head insertions on the olecranon, while the deeper medial head insertion remains intact (Figure 45).[1] Ultrasound can help determine the presence of a triceps tear when overlying olecranon bursitis or swelling makes palpation difficult (Figure 46).

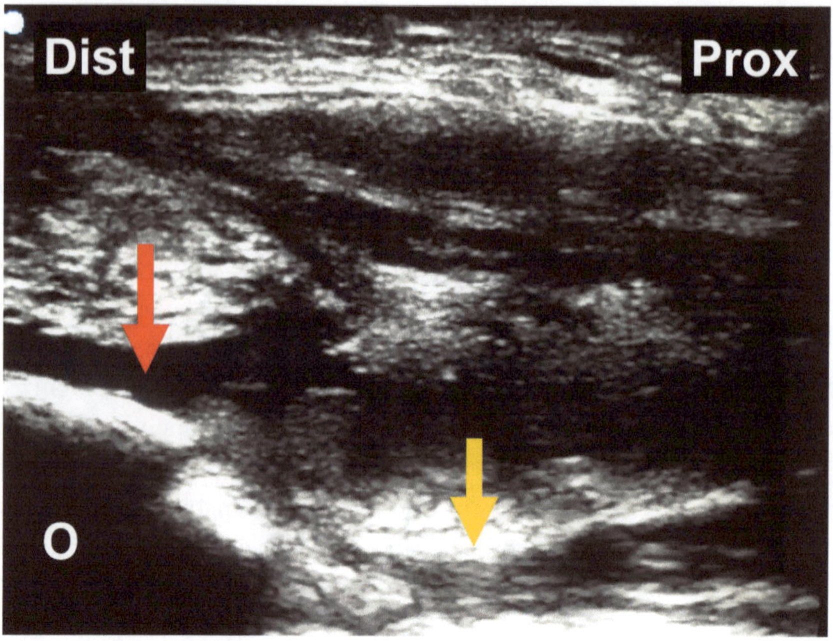

Figure 3-45: Longitudinal ultrasound image of the posterior elbow showing a torn triceps tendon (red arrow) with some of the deep fibers intact (yellow arrow).

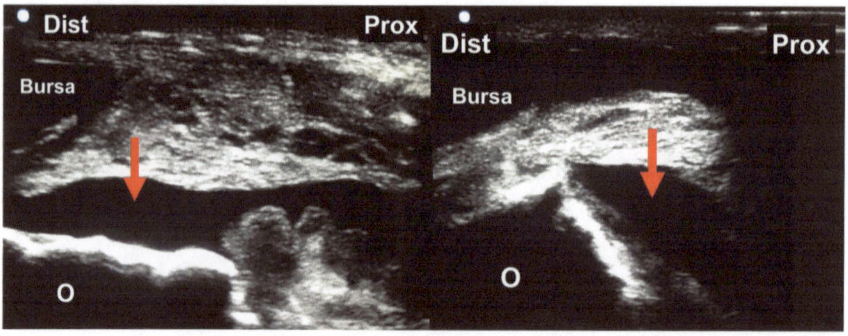

Figure 3-46: Two longitudinal images of the posterior elbow (left image in extension and right image in flexion) showing a torn triceps tendon (red arrow) with an overlying olecranon bursitis. This is a 57 y.o. male presenting 2.5 months after a fall onto the elbow with a large olecranon bursitis and some weakness in elbow extension. No triceps defect could be palpated.

An additional triceps abnormality is referred to as snapping triceps syndrome which is caused by the anterior subluxation of the ulnar nerve and medial head of the triceps over the medial epicondyle with elbow flexion. The patient typically reports the sensation of a single snapping sensation, although occasionally two snaps will be reported with the first representing subluxation of the ulnar nerve and the second representing subluxation of the medial head of the triceps. This is best imaged utilizing the same technique used for dynamic examination of the ulnar nerve in the cubital tunnel .[14] As the elbow is slowly brought into flexion, the ulnar nerve translates anteriorly to the medial epicondyle followed by the hypoechoic medial head of the triceps muscle. This may occur almost simultaneously or as two discrete events. Elbow extension should allow the nerve and medial head of the triceps to return to their anatomic positions.

iii. Common Extensor and Flexor Tendons – Lateral epicondylitis, also known as tennis elbow, refers to pain localized to the common extensor origin over the lateral epicondyle and proximal lateral forearm exacerbated by wrist extension and forearm supination. This is an overuse injury which primarily affects the extensor carpi radialis brevis component of the anterior aspect of the common extensor tendon. While classically associated with poor technique in tennis players, this condition may be encountered in patients who participate in any activity which requires repetitive wrist extension and forearm supination. Lateral epicondylitis has a similar presentation to that of radial tunnel syndrome; consequently, physical examination and imaging can play a valuable role in differentiating these conditions.[22]

Medial epicondylitis, also known as golfer's elbow, refers to pain localized to the common flexor origin over the medial epicondyle with wrist and finger flexion and forearm pronation. This is an overuse injury which primarily affects the flexor carpi radialis and pronator teres components of the common flexor tendon. Classically associated with the trailing arm in golfers with poor swing technique, the condition may be encountered in patients who participate in any activity which involves repetitive wrist flexion and forearm pronation, particularly throwing sports secondary to the valgus stress associated with these activities. Ulnar neuritis is occasionally associated with this condition.[23]

The term epicondylitis is a misnomer as it does not involve a true acute inflammatory process. Epicondylitis is a degenerative process related to repetitive microtrauma of the common extensor or flexor tendons with mucoid degeneration and angiofibroblastic proliferation seen on histology.[24] It is possible for the condition to progress to a frank tendon tear in some cases.

Sonography demonstrates a similar appearance for both lateral and medial epicondylitis.[25-28] The affected tendon may appear hypoechoic with possible thickening. Color or power Doppler imaging may demonstrate hyperemia secondary to angiofibroblastic proliferation (Figure 47). Enthesophytes or calcifications on the epicondyle may be seen in advanced cases as hyperechoic areas superficial to the epicondyle (Figure 48). Partial-thickness tears are visualized as hypoechoic or anechoic clefts with fiber discontinuity. In the rare case of a full-thickness tear, complete discontinuity of the tendon fibers will be noted with distal retraction of the torn stump. Scanning in both the long and short axes is recommended to completely characterize the tendon. Overall ultrasound has a wide range of reported sensitivity (64-100%) and specificity (36-100%) for the diagnosis of lateral epicondylitis suggesting that the diagnostic accuracy is likely largely impacted by technician experience, equipment quality, and disease severity.[29,30]

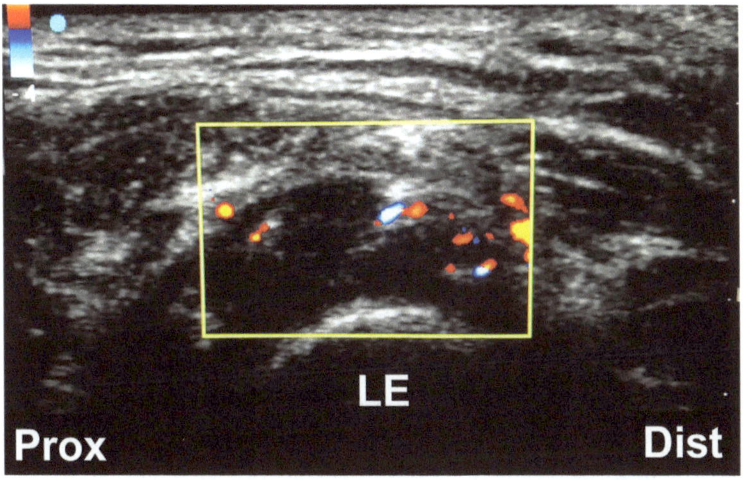

Figure 3-47: Longitudinal ultrasound image of the lateral elbow showing the lateral epicondyle (LE) with surrounding increased vasculature in a case of recalcitrant lateral epicondylitis.

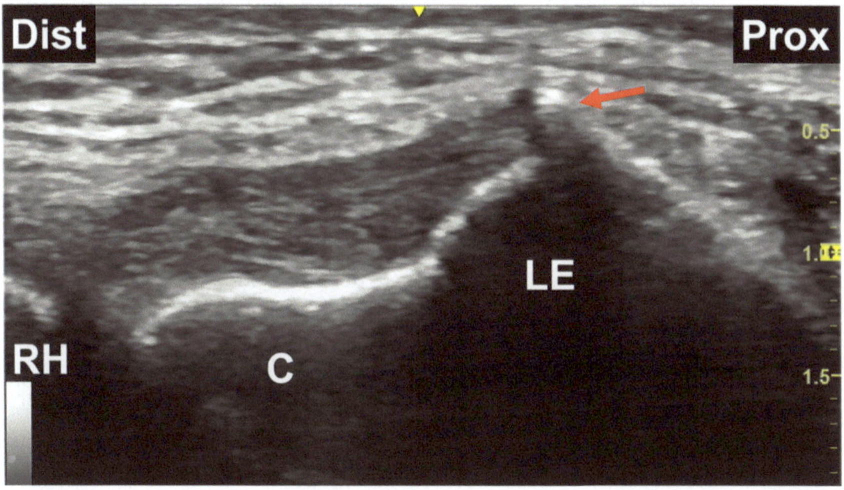

Figure 3-48: Longitudinal ultrasound image of the lateral elbow showing the lateral epicondyle (LE) with a hyperechoic calcium deposit (red arrow) in a case of recalcitrant lateral epicondylitis. RH = radial head. C = capitellum.

b. Ligament Pathology

i. Medial Ulnar Collateral Ligament – The medial ulnar collateral ligament (UCL) is the primary restraint to valgus stress at the elbow. The anterior bundle is biomechanically the most important constituent of this ligament and is generally the focus of sonographic imaging. The posterior bundle forms the floor of the cubital tunnel and acts as a secondary restraint to valgus stress, while the transverse bundle does not provide any significant contribution to elbow stability. Repetitive valgus loading, particularly in throwing sports, increases the risk of injury to the anterior bundle. Traumatic injuries such as a fall onto the elbow or an elbow dislocation may also result in UCL injury.

On imaging, a partial tear of the anterior bundle may appear as a hypoechoic area of thinning or thickening without complete disruption of the tendon fibers.[31] In cases of remote injury, the ligament may be intact on imaging but demonstrates excessive laxity on exam. A full-thickness tear appears as a hypoechoic or anechoic area of fiber discontinuity with surrounding heterogeneous fluid representing hemorrhage.[32] To assist in distinguishing between a partial-thickness and a full-thickness tear, the valgus stress exam can be performed to assess widening at the medial joint line. The applied valgus stress may result in visible separation of the torn tendon ends or abnormal joint space widening. Joint widening greater than 1 mm compared to the contralateral uninjured elbow has been proposed as a threshold for ulnar collateral ligament tears requiring surgery while widening greater than 2.5 mm is commonly used to determine the presence of a full-thickness tear.[33]

It should be noted that the UCL adapts to physiologic forces which may alter its sonographic appearance. Asymptomatic baseball players have demonstrated increased thickness of the ligament and medial joint line widening 1 to 2 mm greater with valgus stress in the dominant arm as compared to the nondominant arm).[34,35] Asymptomatic professional baseball pitchers have also been shown to have abnormal hypoechoic regions and calcifications of the UCL.[36] Correlating the exam findings to the patient's symptoms is therefore particularly important in this region of the elbow. The value of the stress exam is well recognized as its use in combination with MR arthrography in the evaluation of UCL injuries increases the diagnostic accuracy to 98%.[37]

ii. Radial Collateral Ligament Complex – The radial collateral ligament provides the primary restraint to varus stress at the elbow while the lateral ulnar collateral ligament (LUCL) provides the primary restraint to posterolateral stress. The annular ligament stabilizes the proximal radioulnar joint by maintaining the radial head in alignment with the sigmoid notch of the proximal ulna. The radial collateral ligament and LUCL are generally injured during a traumatic event in which the elbow is subjected to an excessive varus load or as a result of a posterior elbow dislocation. The sequence of injury to the stabilizing structures around the elbow during a posterior dislocation is predictable and first involves the radial collateral and lateral ulnar collateral ligaments, followed by the joint capsule, and finally the medial UCL.[38] Notably, atraumatic degeneration of the lateral collateral and radial ulnar collateral ligaments may be seen in cases of lateral epicondylitis.[39]

The sonographic appearance of lateral ligament injuries is identical to that of medial UCL injuries, with partial-thickness tears demonstrating an area of hypoechoic incomplete fiber disruption, and full-thickness tears demonstrating a hypoechoic or anechoic region of fiber discontinuity. The annular ligament is infrequently injured and should have a uniform echogenic appearance. Radial head subluxation in children, more commonly known as nursemaid's elbow, may be visualized sonographically as a widened radiocapitellar joint.[40] Occasionally, the annular ligament can be seen interposed between the hypoechoic epiphyses of the capitellum and radial head. Following a successful reduction maneuver, the radiocapitellar joint space should return to its normal dimensions and the annular ligament will be visualized in its anatomic position surrounding the radial head. Comparison to the contralateral elbow is often helpful in these cases.

c. Peripheral Nerve Pathology

i. Ulnar Nerve – Cubital tunnel syndrome refers to ulnar nerve compression at the elbow and is the second most common upper extremity compressive neuropathy following carpal tunnel syndrome.[41] Patients typically report paresthesias affecting the small finger, ulnar half of the ring finger, and the dorsal ulnar aspect of the hand. In chronic cases, clawing of the ring and small fingers and weakness with gripping and pinching may be noted. Elbow flexion increases the pressure within the cubital tunnel and may exacerbate symptoms. Activities associated with repetitive elbow flexion or direct pressure over the medial elbow may predispose patients to the development of this condition.

Compression of the ulnar nerve at the elbow may occur at one of several sites including the medial intermuscular septum at the mid-arm, posterior to the medial epicondyle at the entrance to the cubital tunnel as the nerve passes beneath Osborne's ligament, within the cubital tunnel itself, and between the two heads of the flexor carpi ulnaris muscle deep to the flexor-pronator aponeurosis.[42]

A potential source of ulnar nerve compression within the cubital tunnel is the anconeus epitrochlearis, an anomalous muscle found in an estimated 34% of the population.[43] It has a hypoechoic appearance on sonography and extends from the triceps brachii towards to the medial epicondyle along the posterior aspect of the cubital tunnel. It is most easily seen with the elbow in extension as no muscle tissue should typically be visualized adjacent to the medial epicondyle. This is in contrast to elbow flexion in which the medial triceps is often within the field of view. The anconeus epitrochlearis may result in compression of the ulnar nerve against the medial epicondyle or olecranon and sometimes manifests with a snapping sensation similar to that seen in snapping triceps syndrome. Other abnormal space-occupying conditions within the cubital tunnel include synovial hypertrophy/joint cyst (Figure 49 and Figure 50), loose bodies, and hemorrhage secondary to trauma.

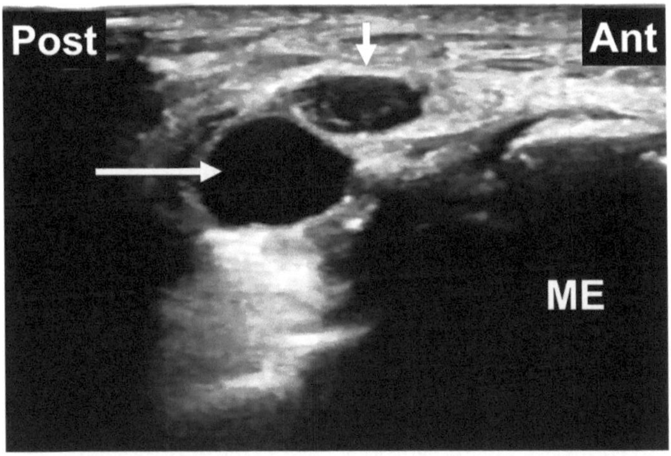

Figure 3-49: Transverse ultrasound image of the medial elbow showing a case of a degenerative elbow cyst (long arrow) causing compression of the ulnar nerve (short arrow) in the cubital tunnel. ME = medial epicondyle.

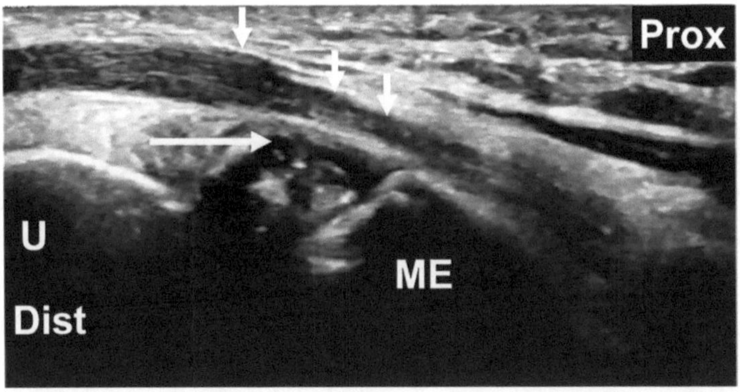

Figure 3-50: Longitudinal ultrasound image of the medial elbow showing a case (same case as Figure 49) of a degenerative elbow cyst (long arrow) causing compression of the ulnar nerve (short arrows) in the cubital tunnel. Narrowing of the ulnar nerve near the cyst can be appreciated. ME = medial epicondyle. U = ulna.

Ulnar neuritis is recognized sonographically by hypoechoic enlargement of the ulnar nerve (Figure 51). The typical appearance will be that of increased nerve caliber just proximal to the site of compression (with a lower cross-sectional area) (Figure 50) with gradual transition to normal size distally. A measurement of the cross-sectional area of the nerve at the site of maximal enlargement should be compared to the diameter of the nerve at a normal proximal location or the diameter of the unaffected contralateral ulnar nerve. While a range of values have been reported in the literature, a meta-analysis of 14 studies demonstrated that a cross-sectional area greater than 10 mm^2 at the site of maximal enlargement should be considered an abnormal finding.[44] Additionally, an increase in the ratio of abnormal to normal cross-sectional area greater than 2.8 has also been suggested as a possible diagnostic cutoff.[45] In one small study of four patients with clinical symptoms of cubital tunnel syndrome without EMG findings showed severe increase in the ulnar nerve cross-sectional area in all patients averaging 20mm^2.[46] If comparing the dimensions of the contralateral nerve, the measurement should be taken with the elbow in the same degree of flexion as increased flexion results in decreased nerve cross-sectional area.

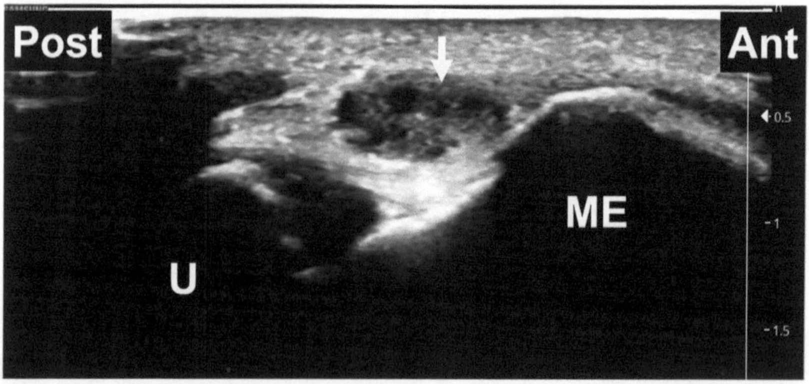

Figure 3-51: Transverse ultrasound image of the medial elbow showing a case of severe ulnar nerve hypertrophy (white arrow) in the cubital tunnel from cubital tunnel syndrome. ME = medial epicondyle. U = ulna.

Recurrent subluxation of the ulnar nerve anterior and medial to the medial epicondyle is another risk factor for ulnar neuritis. It is estimated that this condition occurs in approximately 20% of asymptomatic individuals,[47] therefore it is important to correlate the sonographic findings with the patient's reported symptoms. Abnormal subluxation of the nerve may be perceived by the patient as a snapping sensation which occurs during elbow flexion. The nerve typically returns to its normal position posterior to the medial epicondyle with elbow extension resulting in a frictional neuritis secondary to these repetitive subluxations. The possibility of an associated snapping triceps syndrome (discussed previously) should be considered in any patient who presents with snapping over the medial elbow. A dynamic sonographic evaluation with the transducer placed transversely over the cubital tunnel can confirm ulnar nerve dislocation.[48,49] As the elbow is slowly brought into flexion, the ulnar nerve translates anteriorly over the apex of the medial epicondyle and returns to its normal posterior location with elbow extension. One study showed that dynamic ultrasound predicted the intraoperative amount of subluxation of the ulnar nerve during cubital tunnel release in 88% of patients.[48]

ii. Median Nerve – Compression of the median nerve around the elbow can occur at several sites, although all are less common than compression within the carpal tunnel at the wrist.[50] The first, and most uncommon, potential site of compression is beneath the ligament of Struthers as it runs from the medial epicondyle to an anteromedial bony prominence termed the supracondylar process of the humerus, an anatomic variant present in approximately 1% of individuals. The second potential site of compression is beneath a thickened biceps aponeurosis (lacertus fibrosus). The third potential site of compression is at the level of the elbow joint between the humeral and ulnar heads of the pronator teres; this is the most common site of median nerve compression proximal to the wrist and is termed pronator syndrome. The fourth potential site of compression of the median nerve is at the level of the proximal forearm as it passes under a thickened proximal edge of the flexor digitorum superficialis. The anterior interosseous nerve branches from the median nerve approximately 4 to 6 cm distal to the medial epicondyle and can be compressed by the proximal edge of flexor digitorum superficialis or the ulnar head of the pronator teres.

Similar to carpal tunnel syndrome, patients with pronator syndrome present with paresthesias in the thumb, index, middle finger, and radial half of the index finger. However, unlike carpal tunnel syndrome, these patients report pain and paresthesia involving the proximal volar forearm and altered sensation over the palm of the hand.[51] Symptoms may be reproduced by resisted forearm pronation with the elbow in extension. Symptom reproduction with resisted elbow flexion and forearm supination is more suggestive of the biceps aponeurosis as the site of compression. Sonographic findings of median nerve entrapment at the elbow are typically absent.

The presentation of anterior interosseous nerve syndrome differs from that of pronator syndrome in that the former presents with motor deficits only. The anterior interosseous nerve supplies the flexor digitorum profundus to the index and middle fingers, the flexor pollicis longus, and the pronator quadratus. Loss of innervation to these muscles manifests as weakness in resisted pronation with the elbow flexed and weakness of grip and pinch. As the condition progresses, the affected muscles may atrophy; this typically involves the pronator quadratus initially, followed by the flexor digitorum profundus and the flexor pollicis longus. This is reflected sonographically by increased echogenicity and decreased muscle bulk.[52]

iii. Radial Nerve – Compression of the deep branch of the radial nerve may occur at one of several locations around the elbow. From proximal to distal these include: fibrous bands extending from the brachioradialis muscle to the joint capsule at the level of the radial head; the vascular arcade consisting of branches of the radial recurrent artery referred to as the Leash of

Henry just distal to the radial head; the proximal tendinous edge of the extensor carpi radialis brevis muscle; the fibrous proximal aspect of the supinator muscle known as the arcade of Frohse; and the distal aspect of the supinator.[53] Nerve compression can lead to either radial tunnel syndrome or posterior interosseous nerve syndrome (sometimes referred to as supinator syndrome) which are differentiated by their clinical presentation.

Radial tunnel syndrome presents with proximal lateral forearm pain, preserved motor function, absent findings on electrodiagnostic testing. This condition may mimic lateral epicondylitis, although the point of maximal tenderness in radial tunnel syndrome is typically 3 to 5 cm distal to the lateral epicondyle.[54] The two symptoms may present concurrently, possibly with compression or irritation of the nerve by the degenerated or torn extensor carpi radialis brevis tendon. One should also keep lateral antebrachial cutaneous neuritis in the differential, although this is a rare diagnosis. Sonographic findings are often absent in radial tunnel syndrome, however atrophy of the supinator muscle may be visualized as hyperechogenicity and decreased muscle bulk.

Posterior interosseous nerve syndrome primarily presents with weakness of the thumb and finger extensors. Pain may be present but is typically not the primary complaint. In contrast to radial tunnel syndrome, abnormal electrodiagnostic test findings are generally present in posterior interosseous nerve syndrome. Chronic cases may present with atrophy of the forearm extensor musculature. Sonographic evaluation may demonstrate swelling of the deep branch of the radial nerve proximal to a potential site of compression, with one study demonstrating a mean diameter of 4.2 mm.[55] Color Doppler imaging may also demonstrate hyperemia of the nerve. The adjacent tissue should be inspected for unusual masses, ganglion cysts, or adjacent elbow joint processes which could contribute to nerve compression. The supinator and extensor musculature should be evaluated for atrophy which would manifest as hyperechogenicity and decreased muscle bulk. Imaging findings should be correlated with the patient's reported symptoms as not all findings may be clinically relevant. A hypertrophic Leash of Henry, for example, was noted in 9 out of 60 asymptomatic elbows in one series.[56]

d. Joint Space and Bursal Pathology

i. Elbow Joint Space – Joint effusions around the elbow may be identified in multiple locations including the coronoid fossa, the annular recess of the radiocapitellar joint, and the olecranon fossa. Effusions are typically hypoechoic or anechoic, although heterogeneous joint fluid—such as that caused by hemorrhage or infection—may vary from hypoechoic to hyperechoic and possibly heterogeneous. With the elbow flexed, the olecranon fossa demonstrates the highest sensitivity for detection of a joint effusion.[57] If an effusion is present, imaging of the olecranon fossa in the longitudinal axis will usually demonstrate superior and posterior displacement of the hyperechoic fat pad. Displacement of the anterior fat pad within the anterior joint recess may be noted as well.

Synovial hypertrophy is frequently a response to an active infectious or inflammatory process. It is often diffuse, with extension into the joint recesses and a hypoechoic appearance relative to the subcutaneous fat. Color Doppler may demonstrate hyperemia in acute processes, but this finding may be absent in chronic synovial hypertrophy. Significant joint distension can be appreciated in chronic presentations and may potentially cause compression of the radial or ulnar nerves. Cortical irregularities may indicate bone erosions and are occasionally seen underlying regions of synovitis. In synovial chondromatosis, hyperechoic calcifications can be identified within the synovial tissue. Complex fluid and synovial hypertrophy can have a similar appearance in many clinical presentations. Findings that suggest complex fluid rather than synovial hypertrophy include the ability to redistribute the joint recess contents with transducer pressure, joint recess compressibility, and lack of flow on color Doppler imaging.

Loose bodies may be identified within the joint recesses around the elbow, including the olecranon fossa, the coronoid fossa, and the annular recess. When mineralized, they appear hyperechoic superficial to the cartilage layer with posterior shadowing. The presence of an effusion may improve the visibility of a calcified loose body, although ultrasound identification of purely cartilaginous loose bodies remains challenging. Cartilaginous loose bodies appear hypoechoic and are often obscured by the presence of a surrounding hypoechoic effusion. The articular cartilage should be inspected, as an irregularity may represent the donor site of the associated loose body, or osteochondritis dissecans lesions. Particular attention should be directed to the anterior aspect of the capitellum, as this is a common donor site. In cases of trauma, a fracture of the radial head of neck may be visualized as a cortical step-off. Ultrasound may be most helpful in pediatric radial head fractures where the bone is not ossified yet, as these fractures in adults are easily seen on multiplanar radiographs.

ii. Olecranon Bursa – The main bursa of clinical concern around the elbow is the olecranon bursa. The olecranon bursa lies superficial to the posterior olecranon. It may be distended as a result of mechanical irritation or due to a chronic inflammatory process such as gout. It is difficult to identify in its normal state but becomes conspicuous when distended. The transducer should be placed over the bursa with a thick layer of gel to minimize pressure and displacement of any associated fluid. The bursal distension may be the result of simple fluid, complex fluid, or synovial hypertrophy. Simple fluid appears uniformly hypoechoic or anechoic (Figure 52), while the appearance of complex fluid and synovial hypertrophy can range from hypoechoic to hyperechoic. As with evaluation of joint recess distension, findings that suggest complex fluid rather than synovial hypertrophy include the ability to redistribute the bursal contents with transducer pressure, bursal compressibility (Figure 53 and Figure 52), and lack of flow on color Doppler imaging. Gout is a frequent cause of olecranon bursitis and has a characteristic appearance of hyperechoic synovium with internal hyperechoic foci.[58] In general, the borders of the olecranon bursa are well defined, which differentiates it from an abscess or other nonspecific fluid collection.

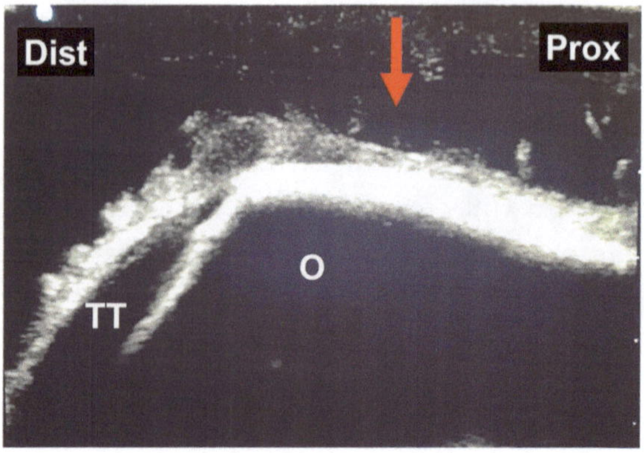

Figure 3-52: Longitudinal ultrasound image of the posterior elbow showing a large hypoechoic homogeneous olecranon bursitis (red arrow). O = olecranon. TT = triceps tendon.

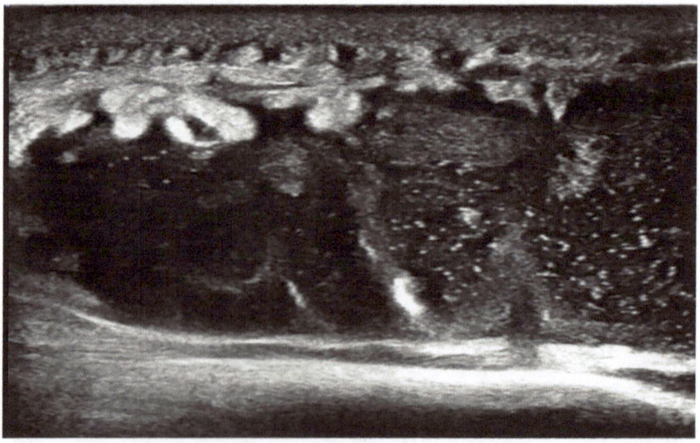

Figure 3-53: Possible substitute for 52. Long axis view of recurrent olecranon bursitis that turned out to be infection with an atypical mycobacterium. The skin is the top of the image with some "cobble-stoning" of the subcutaneous fat. The ulna lies at the bottom with a complex fluid between the bone and skin.

4. Ultrasound-Guided Interventions in the Elbow and Forearm:

a. **Elbow Joint Injection:**

i. While aspiration or injection of the elbow joint is not technically difficult, ultrasound can provide some advantages. Ultrasound allows for needle localization which can lead to more accurate placement.[59] It also can lead to less pain due to visualization of the appropriate trajectory which helps to avoid hitting extra-articular bony structures. One prospective randomized-controlled trial of 80 patients with elbow arthritis showed that ultrasound improved the accuracy of intra-articular steroid injections from 78% to 100% using a posterior approach.[59]

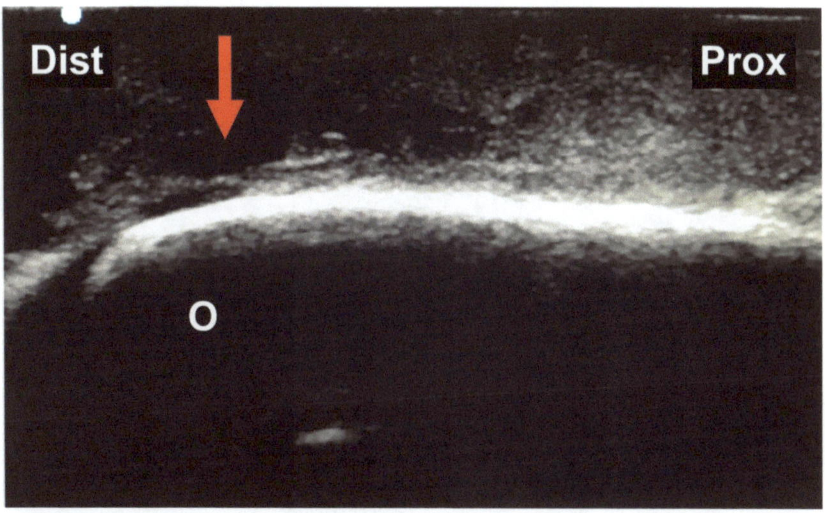

Figure 3-54: Same case as Figure 52, showing a longitudinal ultrasound image of the posterior elbow with compression demonstrating a compressed olecranon bursa (red arrow) indicating it is full of fluid and not synovitis or deposition disease. O = olecranon.

ii. Technique: The radiocapitellar joint can be easily visualized on the lateral side of the elbow with ultrasound. The middle of the probe can be placed directly between the radial head and the capitellum to assist with accurate needle placement and appropriate trajectory (Figure 54) and can be done in any degree of flexion. This is easily done with the patient's elbow and forearm placed on the table with the patient seated (Figure 17). The needle is then placed collinear with the probe starting in the middle. Another option for injection or aspiration is the posterior elbow joint. The posterior approach for aspiration or injection can be used when imaging is planned to evaluate the lateral ligaments so passing a needle through the lateral joint can be avoided. The olecranon tip is hard to palpate through the triceps tendon, so avoiding the olecranon with posterior elbow needle placement can be difficult with palpation alone. The olecranon tip and the olecranon fossa are visualized on this approach allowing for appropriate needle placement towards the olecranon fossa but avoiding the olecranon tip (Figure 55).

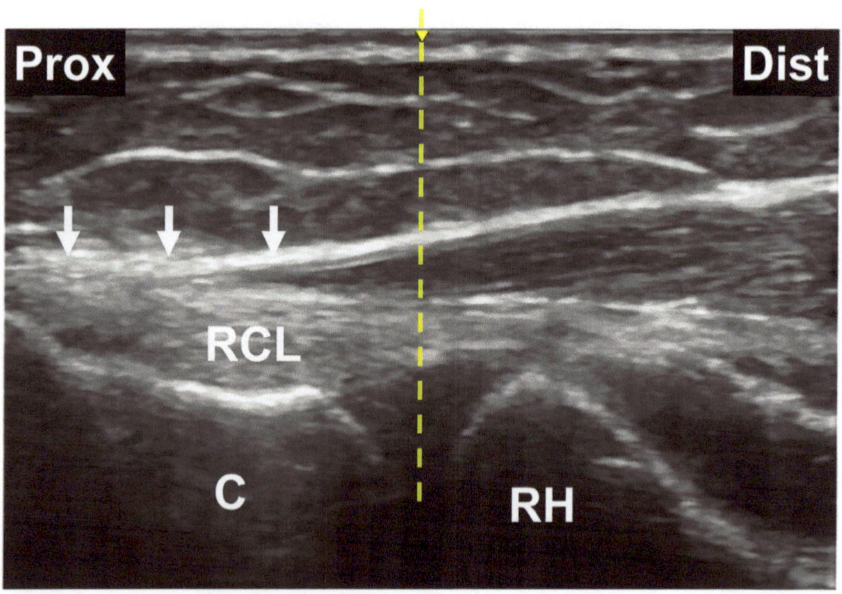

Figure 3-55: Longitudinal ultrasound image of the lateral elbow showing the joint space from the lateral view between the capitellum (C) and the radial head (RH). The yellow dotted line is the needle trajectory in the middle of the probe using this ultrasound view. RCL = radial collateral ligament. White arrows represent the common extensor tendon.

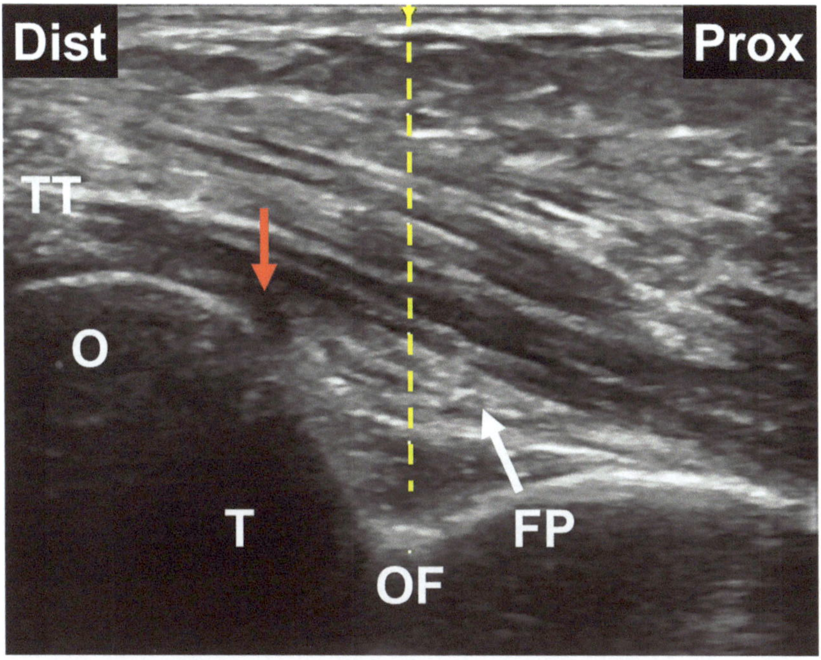

Figure 3-56: Longitudinal ultrasound image of the posterior elbow showing the joint space fat the olecranon fossa (OF). The yellow dotted line is the needle trajectory in the middle of the probe using this ultrasound view. Ultrasound is useful for avoiding the olecranon tip (red arrow) and to make sure the injection is to the correct depth deep to the posterior fat pad (FP). T = trochlea. TT = triceps tendon.

b. **Lateral Epicondylitis Intervention:**

i. Percutaneous treatments are the mainstays of nonoperative management of recalcitrant lateral epicondylitis including needle tenotomy, steroid injections, platelet-rich plasma (PRP) injections, autologous whole blood injection, and percutaneous bone drilling.[30,60] In addition, newer techniques are available such as ultrasonic percutaneous tenotomy.[61] The benefits of ultrasound include appropriate localization of the ECRB tendon/common extensor tendon to assist in an adequate needle tenotomy and placement of injectable treatments, such as steroid or PRP on the middle and anterior aspects of the lateral epicondyle corresponding with the most common areas of disease. In addition, true partial-thickness, common, extensor tendon tears can be localized for injection and/or needle tenotomy. One cadaver study showed adequate injection localization under ultrasound (98% of the common extensor tendon insertion) even using 1mL of injection material using a single pass injection.[62] Another study looked at ultrasound guided PRP injections (LE and ME) and found that all injections were given within the tendon with injectate spread a mean of 12.6mm from the injection site.[63] Another study of ultrasound-guided dry needling and autologous blood injections showed decreased hypoechoic changes and neovascularity with this treatment as well as improved outcomes.[64] With regard to needle tenotomy and/or injections to induce healing, multiple areas of the common extensor tendon can be visualized and treated using ultrasound instead of the shotgun approach which is used based on anatomic landmarks only. One study of ultrasound guided needle tenotomy and steroid injection showed an 87% good to excellent result, as well as a decrease in calcification in the majority of patients.[65]

ii. Technique: The middle of the probe can be placed following visualization of the partial tear or anterior aspect of the lateral epicondyle (Figure 56) and can be done in any degree of flexion. The needle is then placed collinear with the probe starting in the middle, moving the probe as needed to identify other aspects of the tear or just passing it on the anterior aspect of the lateral epicondyle in the area of the ECRB tendon. Hyperechoic regions can be seen after the injection and needle tenotomy in this case assuring the appropriate area was treated (Figure 57).

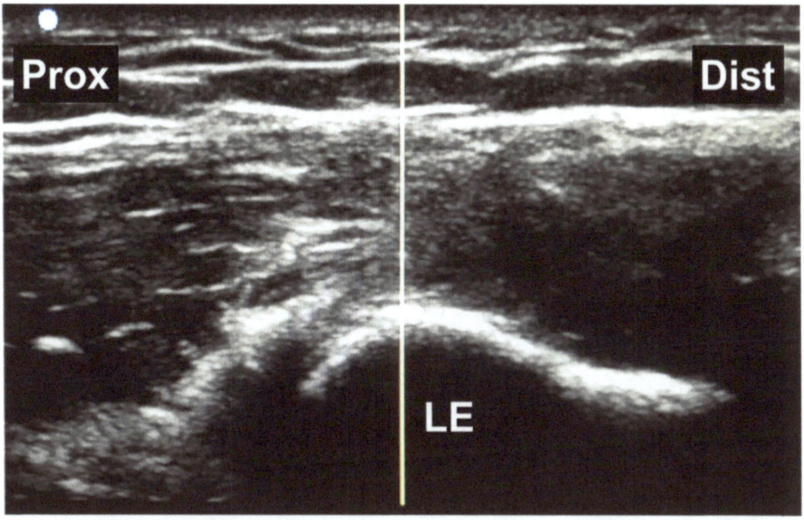

Figure 3-57: Longitudinal ultrasound image of the lateral elbow showing the lateral epicondyle (LE) with the yellow line being the needle trajectory (probe centered over the LE as in this image).

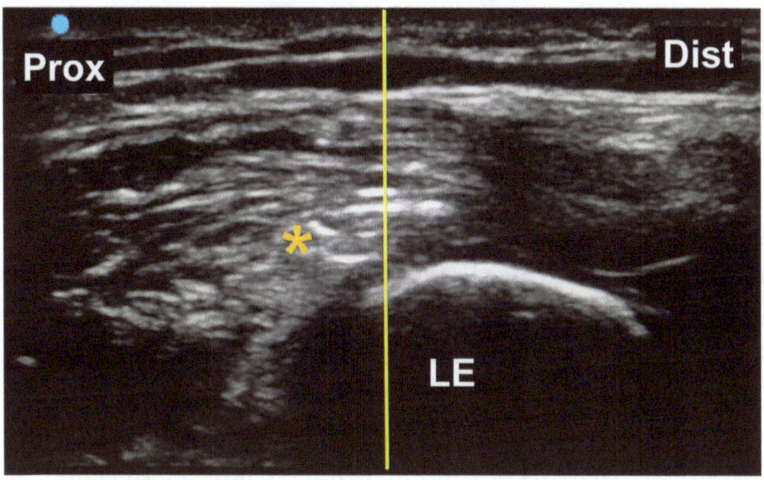

Figure 3-58: Longitudinal ultrasound image of the lateral elbow showing the anterior aspect of the lateral epicondyle (LE). This image shows the hyperechoic area seen after a needle tenotomy and steroid injection in the region of the lateral epicondyle and proximal to it (star).

c. **Medial Epicondylitis Injection:**

i. Ultrasound can be used for injections and/or needle tenotomy for medial epicondylitis as well. Benefits of ultrasound here include better visualization of the entire medial epicondyle and the ability to assess the location of the ulnar nerve in reference to the medial epicondyle in order to avoid placing the needle or injectate near the ulnar nerve (Figure 58). We recommend that the elbow in question is placed in maximum extension for this injection to avoid injury or fluid extravasation around the ulnar nerve.

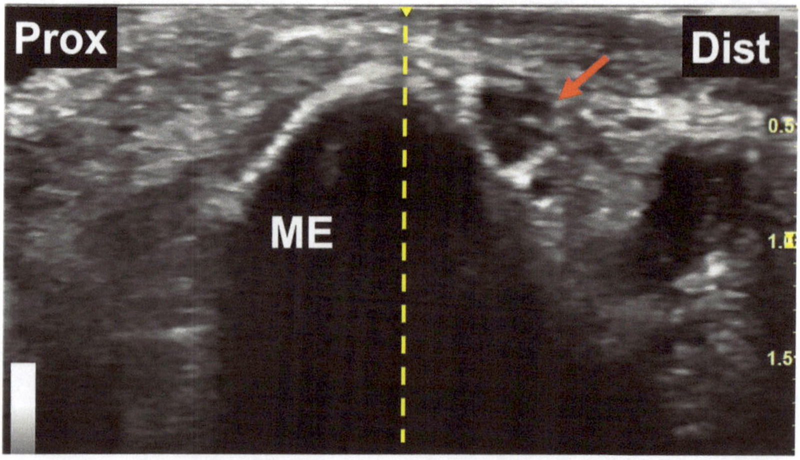

Figure 3-59: Oblique ultrasound image of the medial elbow in full extension showing the medial epicondyle (ME) with the yellow dotted line being the needle trajectory (probe centered over the ME as in this image). Ultrasound allows for visualization of and avoidance of injection around the ulnar nerve (red arrow).

d. **Ulnar Neuritis or Cubital Tunnel Syndrome Injection:**

i. Steroid injection for ulnar neuritis or cubital tunnel syndrome is an option for patients with significant symptoms who are looking to avoid surgical intervention. Efficacy of cubital tunnel injection in cubital tunnel syndrome (diagnosed by EMG) has reported short-term clinical success of 57-63%[66,67] and has been documented as safe [66-69] in small-case series. In order to avoid direct injury to the ulnar nerve, we recommend that ulnar nerve injections within the cubital tunnel be done always with ultrasound.[66] Ultrasound can avoid intraneural injection of lidocaine and steroid which may further damage the ulnar nerve, and can allow for accurate injection next to the ulnar nerve, as opposed to injecting into the UCL or the elbow joint (Figure 59).

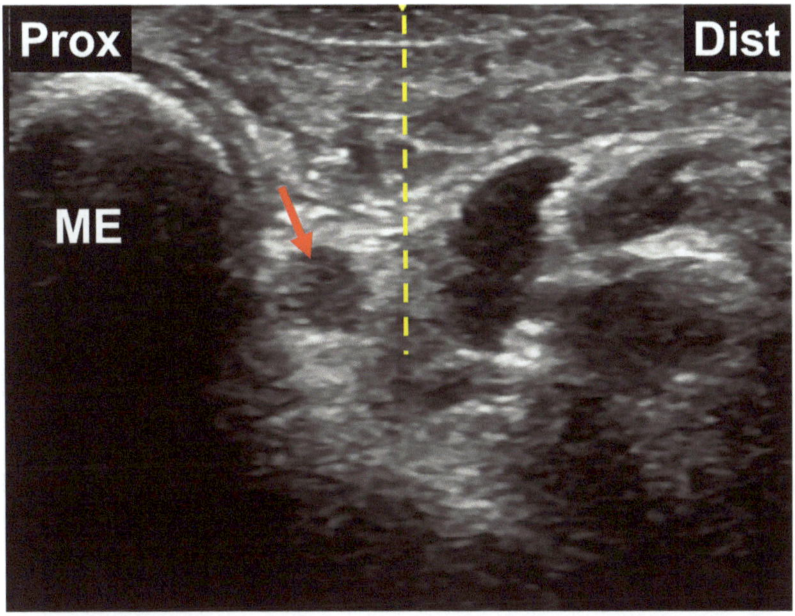

Figure 3-60: Oblique ultrasound image of the medial elbow in full extension showing the cubital tunnel, with the yellow dotted line being the needle trajectory (probe centered over the cubital tunnel as in this image). Ultrasound allows for visualization of and avoidance of injection directly into the ulnar nerve (red arrow).

ii. Technique: Adequate access to the medial elbow is necessary with the shoulder in abduction with the patient sitting or supine. Positioning can be difficult, but we recommend choosing a position where the patient is comfortable, with the elbow supported to avoid patient movement during the injection. We recommend low volume injection of 1-2mL of lidocaine and 1ml of steroid which is supported in the literature. Transducer is placed transversely with adequate visualization of the ulnar nerve and the needle is placed in the middle of the probe adjacent to the ulnar nerve (Figure 60)

e. **Ulnar Collateral Ligament Sprain or Partial Tear**

i. More common in overhead athletes, persistent symptoms of ulnar collateral ligament sprains or tears can continue to be painful. PRP has been recommended as a treatment for these less severe injuries compared to full-thickness tears. Ultrasound allows localization of the partial tears or thickened ligament areas[70] which can allow for more accurate placement of the PRP injection. Also, assessing the depth of the injection with ultrasound can avoid a large amount of PRP injected into the joint instead of around the ligament (Figure 61). In addition, visualization of the ulnar nerve is possible to avoid iatrogenic injury.

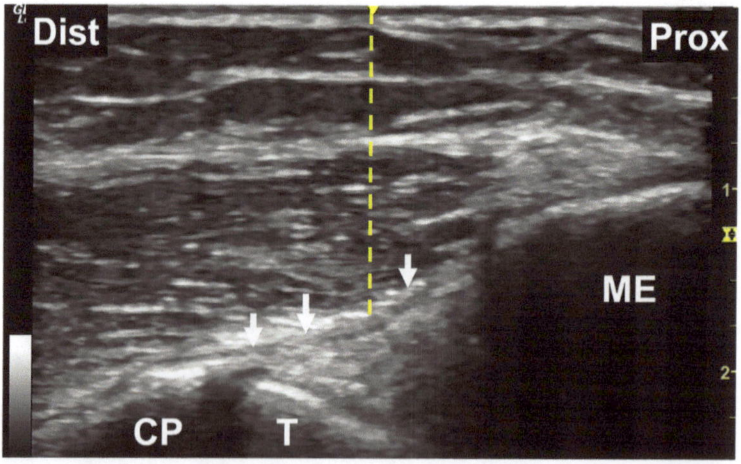

Figure 3-61: Longitudinal ultrasound image of the medial elbow in full extension showing the ulnar collateral ligament (white arrows), with the yellow dotted line being the needle trajectory for UCL injection. Once the area of the UCL is found, the probe can be turned obliquely to make sure that the site of injection is not overlying the ulnar nerve. CP = coronoid process. T = trochlea. ME = medial epicondyle.

ii. Technique: Adequate access to the medial elbow is necessary with the shoulder in abduction with the patient sitting or supine. Positioning can be difficult, but wc recommend choosing a position where the patient is comfortable with the elbow supported to avoid patient movement during the injection. Transducer is placed transversely with adequate visualization of the ulnar nerve and the needle is placed in the middle of the probe overlying the UCL.

f. Radial Tunnel Injection:

i. The radial tunnel and its contents are more easily localized on ultrasound compared to just surface anatomy. Visualization of the radial nerve proximally and of the supinator and PIN distally along are possible with ultrasound (Figure 20). The ability to avoid the superficial radial nerve during needle placement is possible as well with ultrasound. Ultrasound-guided injections of the radial tunnel allow more accurate needle placement in all planes (especially to the appropriate depth) and allows for the provider to visualize the injection fluid surrounding the neurovascular structures dynamically during the injection to assure accurate placement. Aspiration of ganglion cysts causing radial nerve entrapment has also been reported using ultrasound [71,72] with one case also reporting a steroid injection.[73] Successful treatment of chronic radial tunnel syndrome using ultrasound-guided perineural hydro-dissection[74] as well as hydro-dissection with steroid injection[75] have been reported.

ii. Technique: Patient should be supine or sitting with the elbow on the table or bed and the forearm pronated. The needle can be placed obliquely, with the transducer placed transversely following the needle during placement to assure an accurate path (Figure 62).

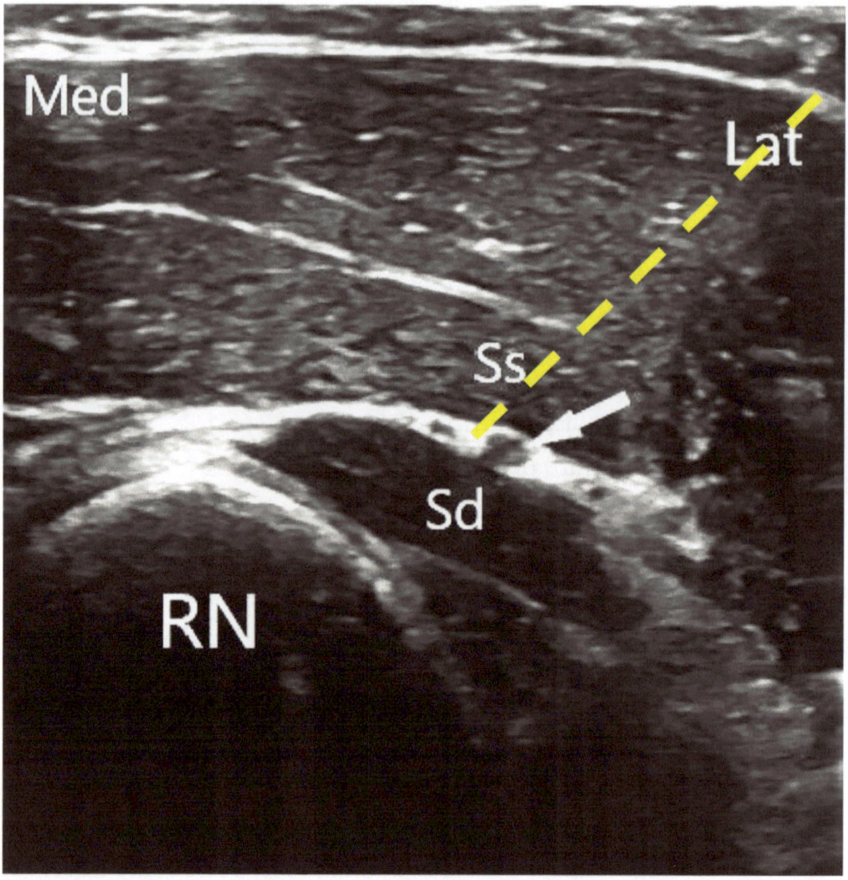

Figure 3-62: Transverse ultrasound image of the anterolateral elbow showing the radial tunnel (white arrow) between the deep (Sd) and superficial (Ss) heads of the supinator muscle. RN = radial neck. The yellow dotted line shows the trajectory of the needle in the same plane as the ultrasound probe so that the entire needle can be visualized prior to injection.

g. **Distal Biceps Tendon Injection:**

   i. The distal biceps tendon can be difficult to evaluate using ultrasound given its oblique course and deep location in the antecubital fossa and attachment to the radial tuberosity on the ulnar and posterior side of the proximal radius. In addition, the surrounding neurovascular structures, including the radial recurrent artery and multiple deep veins (relatively small structures), make anterior access difficult. While injection of the distal biceps tendon is not a common treatment, it is an option in partial-thickness tears (preferably low-grade) or tendonitis. Ultrasound-guided PRP[76,77] as well as corticosteroid injections[78] have been reported in recalcitrant cases of distal biceps tendinopathy with good results.

ii. Technique: If PRP or steroid injection of the distal biceps tendon is indicated, then we recommend the posterior approach for the injection. This technique avoids the possibility of injury to the anterior neurovascular structures. The patient's elbow is flexed and pronated and the transducer is placed transversely on the posterior aspect of the proximal forearm. The middle of the transducer can be placed over the distal biceps tendon and the needle can then be passed (Figure 63).

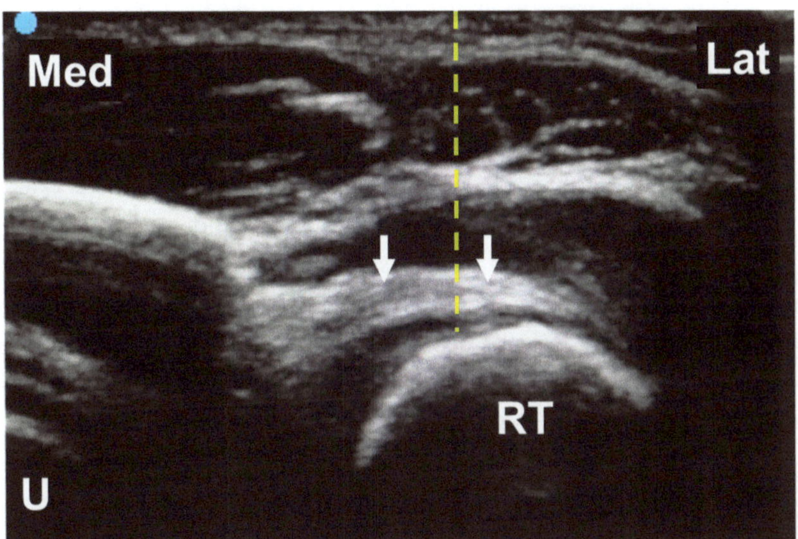

Figure 3-63: Transverse ultrasound image of the posterior elbow showing the trajectory (yellow dotted line) for injection of the distal biceps tendon (white arrows) near the radial tuberosity (RT). U = ulna.

h. Olecranon Bursitis Aspiration:

i. While aspiration of an inflamed olecranon bursa is not technically difficult, in patients with overlying indurated tissue due to cellulitis, inflammatory arthropathy, or crystalline deposition involvement, fluid pockets can exist in these scenarios that are easily missed by blind aspiration. Ultrasound may help identify fluid pocket locations in certain cases of olecranon bursitis that may then facilitate fluid aspiration, helping to make a more accurate diagnosis and decreasing the patient's pain. Doppler can also show hyperemic flow signals around fluid pockets.

ii. Technique: Adequate access to the posterior elbow is needed which can be accomplished by hanging it over the end of a table or bed or adding padding under the medial arm/forearm (Figure 33). Once the fluid collection is identified, it can then be aspirated by placing the middle of the transducer over the fluid collection and aspirating it

i. Biopsy of Deep Soft Tissue Mass of the Elbow or Forearm:

i. Smaller masses may be imaged with ultrasound which can help determine the layer affected or even the structure in some cases (Figure 64). MRI generally should be used to evaluate deep soft tissue masses in the elbow and forearm routinely. However, when an MRI is not available or when the diagnosis appears benign, based on the patient history of benign lesions or on MRI, then a needle biopsy may be appropriate to confirm the diagnosis. Ultrasound can help localize these deeper masses to obtain a more accurate needle biopsy. In low risk or likely benign cases, this may help avoid an open procedure when complete excision of mass is not planned to obtain a diagnosis. Ultrasound can also be used to localize and aspirate deep abscesses around the elbow and in the forearm in cases where surgical debridement and irrigation is delayed or cannot be performed.

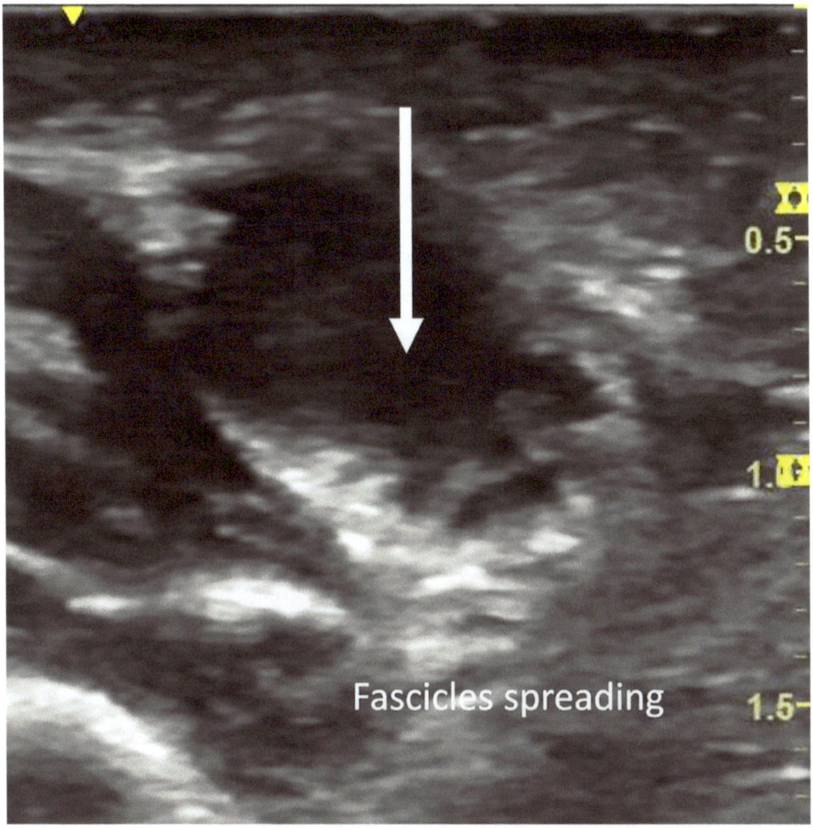

Figure 3-64: Transverse ultrasound image of the medial elbow showing the ulnar nerve (white arrow) with a lesion involving the ulnar nerve. The nerve fascicles are being spread by the tumor. As the fascicles are so close to the tumor this one was biopsied open.

Figure 63: Transverse ultrasound image of the medial elbow showing the ulnar nerve (white arrow) with a lesion involving the ulnar nerve. The nerve fascicles are being spread by the tumor.

a. **Removal of Foreign Body**

i. Ultrasound can be used to identify foreign bodies (especially helpful in radiolucent foreign bodies). Ultrasound can help identify the number and location of foreign bodies including their depth and relationship to the neurovascular structures. A common clinical scenario seen is broken needles in the antecubital fossa which ultrasound can help identify for removal.

b. **Nerve Blocks**

i. Ultrasound can assist in identifying and facilitating perineural injection of anesthetic around peripheral nerves in order to perform hand procedures. The ulnar nerve can be blocked at or proximal to the cubital tunnel to perform small ulnar-sided forearm and hand procedures. The median nerve just proximal to the elbow crease can be blocked to perform radial-sided hand procedures. The radial sensory nerve distal to the elbow crease can be blocked to perform dorsal-radial forearm and hand procedures.

5. **Postoperative Evaluation:**

a. **UCL Reconstruction Integrity:**

i. Ultrasound can be used to evaluate the UCL graft in cases of postoperative concern for pain or instability after UCL reconstruction.[79]

b. **Ulnar Nerve Subluxation:**

i. Ultrasound can be used to assess the ulnar nerve in cases of prior cubital tunnel release with recurrent symptoms. This includes at the presence of subluxation which can be assessed dynamically. Please see Cubital Tunnel Syndrome diagnosis section for complete information.

c. **Nerve Evaluation:**

i. Ultrasound can be used to evaluate the integrity of the radial, ulnar, or median nerves as needed if there is concern for nerve injury or laceration postoperatively.

6. Acknowledgements

The authors would like to acknowledge the following for their assistance in this chapter: Marissa Pazik, MS, ATC; Randy Zinnerman; Aimee Struk, MBA, MEd, ATC; Nicole Riley, aRNP; Silvia Hunkins, aRNP; Steve Hare, PA-C; and the Gainesville VA Musculoskeletal Radiology department. We would also like to thank Christopher Jobe, MD for providing some of the ultrasound cases.

References:

1. Tagliafico AS, Bignotti B, Martinoli C. Elbow US: anatomy, variants, and scanning technique. *Radiology.* 2015;275(3):636-650.

2. Chiavaras MM, Jacobson JA, Billone L, Lawton JM, Lawton J. Sonography of the lateral antebrachial cutaneous nerve with magnetic resonance imaging and anatomic correlation. *J Ultrasound Med.* 2014;33(8):1475-1483.

3. Blasi M, de la Fuente J, Martinoli C, et al. Multidisciplinary approach to the persistent double distal tendon of the biceps brachii. *Surg Radiol Anat.* 2014;36(1):17-24.

4. Smith CD, Guyver P, Bunker TD. Indications for reverse shoulder replacement: a systematic review. *J Bone Joint Surg Br.* 2012;94(5):577-583.

5. Giuffre B, Lisle D. Tear of the distal biceps branchii tendon: a new method of ultrasound evaluation. *Australas Radiol.* 2005;49(5):404-406.

6. Brigido MK, De Maeseneer M, Jacobson JA, Jamadar DA, Morag Y, Marcelis S. Improved visualization of the radial insertion of the biceps tendon at ultrasound with a lateral approach. *Eur Radiol.* 2009;19(7):1817-1821.

7. Teixeira PAG, Omoumi P, Trudell DJ et al. Ultrasound assessment of the lateral collateral ligamentous complex of the elbow: imaging aspects in cadavers and normal volunteers. *Eur Radiol.* 2011;21(7):1492-1498.

8. Jacobson JA, Chiavaras MM, Lawton JM, Downie B, Yablon CM, Lawton J. Radial collateral ligament of the elbow: sonographic characterization with cadaveric

dissection correlation and magnetic resonance arthrography. *J Ultrasound Med.* 2014;33(6):1041-1048.

9. Cerezal L, Rodriguez-Sammartino M, Canga A et al. Elbow synovial fold syndrome. *Am J Roentgenol.* 2013;201(1):W88-W96.

10. Rosenberg ZS, Beltran J, Cheung YY. Pseudodefect of the capitellum: potential MR imaging pitfall. *Radiology.* 1994;191(3):821-823.

11. Stewart B, Harish S, Oomen G, Wainman B, Popowich T, Moro JK. Sonography of the lateral ulnar collateral ligament of the elbow: study of cadavers and healthy volunteers. *Am J Roentgenol.* 2009;193(6):1615-1619.

12. Konjengbam M, Elangbam J. Radial nerve in the radial tunnel: anatomic sites of entrapment neuropathy. *Clinical Anatomy: The Official Journal of the American Association of Clinical Anatomists and the British Association of Clinical Anatomists.* 2004;17(1):21-25.

13. Ward SI, Teefey SA, Paletta Jr GA et al. Sonography of the medial collateral ligament of the elbow: a study of cadavers and healthy adult male volunteers. *Am J Roentgenol.* 2003;180(2):389-394.

14. Jacobson JA, Propeck T, Jamadar DA, Jebson PJ, Hayes CW. US of the anterior bundle of the ulnar collateral ligament: findings in five cadaver elbows with MR arthrographic and anatomic comparison—initial observations. *Radiology.* 2003;227(2):561-566.

15. De Smet AA, Winter TC, Best TM, Bernhardt DT. Dynamic sonography with valgus stress to assess elbow ulnar collateral ligament injury in baseball pitchers. *Skeletal Radiol.* 2002;31(11):671-676.

16. Safran MR, Graham SM. Distal biceps tendon ruptures: incidence, demographics, and the effect of smoking. *Clinical Orthopaedics and Related Research (1976-2007).* 2002;404:275-283.

17. Nesterenko S, Domire ZJ, Morrey BF, Sanchez-Sotelo J. Elbow strength and endurance in patients with a ruptured distal biceps tendon. *J Shoulder Elbow Surg.* 2010;19(2):184-189.

18. Miller TT, Adler RS. Sonography of tears of the distal biceps tendon. *Am J Roentgenol.* 2000;175(4):1081-1086.

19. Lobo LDG, Fessell DP, Miller BS, et al. The role of sonography in differentiating full versus partial distal biceps tendon tears: correlation with surgical findings. *Am J Roentgenol.* 2013;200(1):158-162.

20. Festa A, Mulieri PJ, Newman JS, Spitz DJ, Leslie BM. Effectiveness of magnetic resonance imaging in detecting partial and complete distal biceps tendon rupture. *The Journal of hand surgery.* 2010;35(1):77-83.

21. Yeh PC, Dodds SD, Smart RL, Mazzocca AD, Sethi PM. Distal triceps rupture. *JAAOS-Journal of the American Academy of Orthopaedic Surgeons.* 2010;18(1):31-40.

22. Roles N, Maudsley R. Radial tunnel syndrome: resistant tennis elbow as a nerve entrapment. *The Journal of bone and joint surgery British volume.* 1972;54(3):499-508.

23. Shiri R, Viikari-Juntura E, Varonen H, Heliövaara M. Prevalence and determinants of lateral and medial epicondylitis: a population study. *Am J Epidemiol.* 2006;164(11):1065-1074.

24. Regan W, Wold LE, Coonrad R, Morrey BF. Microscopic histopathology of chronic refractory lateral epicondylitis. *The American journal of sports medicine.* 1992;20(6):746-749.

25. Miller TT, Shapiro MA, Schultz E, Kalish PE. Comparison of sonography and MRI for diagnosing epicondylitis. *J Clin Ultrasound.* 2002;30(4):193-202.

26. Connell D, Burke F, Coombes P et al. Sonographic examination of lateral epicondylitis. *Am J Roentgenol.* 2001;176(3):777-782.

27. Levin D, Nazarian LN, Miller TT et al. Lateral epicondylitis of the elbow: US findings. *Radiology.* 2005;237(1):230-234.

28. G-Y, Lee S-M, Lee MY. Diagnostic value of ultrasonography for clinical medial epicondylitis. *Arch Phys Med Rehabil.* 2008;89(4):738-742.

29. Dones VC, Grimmer K, Thoirs K, Suarez CG, Luker J. The diagnostic validity of musculoskeletal ultrasound in lateral epicondylalgia: a systematic review. *BMC Med Imaging.* 2014;14(1):10.

30. Shergill R, Choudur HN. Ultrasound-Guided Interventions in Lateral Epicondylitis. *J Clin Rheumatol.* 2019;25(3):e27-e34.

31. Ferreira FB, Fernandes ED, Silva FD, Vieira MC, Puchnick A, Fernandes AR. A sonographic technique to evaluate the anterior bundle of the ulnar collateral ligament of the elbow: imaging features and anatomic correlation. *J Ultrasound Med.* 2015;34(3):377-384.

32. Miller TT, Adler RS, Friedman L. Sonography of injury of the ulnar collateral ligament of the elbow—initial experience. *Skeletal Radiol.* 2004;33(7):386-391.

33. Bica D, Armen J, Kulas AS, Youngs K, Womack Z. Reliability and precision of stress sonography of the ulnar collateral ligament. *J Ultrasound Med.* 2015;34(3):371-376.

34. Nazarian LN, McShane JM, Ciccotti MG, O'Kane PL, Harwood MI. Dynamic US of the anterior band of the ulnar collateral ligament of the elbow in asymptomatic major league baseball pitchers. *Radiology.* 2003;227(1):149-154.

35. Sasaki J, Takahara M, Ogino T, Kashiwa H, Ishigaki D, Kanauchi Y. Ultrasonographic assessment of the ulnar collateral ligament and medial elbow laxity in college baseball players. *JBJS.* 2002;84(4):525-531.

36. Ciccotti MG, Atanda Jr A, Nazarian LN, Dodson CC, Holmes L, Cohen SB. Stress sonography of the ulnar collateral ligament of the elbow in professional baseball pitchers: a 10-year study. *The American journal of sports medicine.* 2014;42(3):544-551.

37. Roedl JB, Gonzalez FM, Zoga AC et al. Potential utility of a combined approach with US and MR arthrography to image medial elbow pain in baseball players. *Radiology.* 2016;279(3):827-837.

38. McKee MD, Schemitsch EH, Sala MJ, O'Driscoll SW. The pathoanatomy of lateral ligamentous disruption in complex elbow instability. *J Shoulder Elbow Surg.* 2003;12(4):391-396.

39. Bredella M, Tirman P, Fritz R, Feller J, Wischer T, Genant H. MR imaging findings of lateral ulnar collateral ligament abnormalities in patients with lateral epicondylitis. *AJR American journal of roentgenology.* 1999;173(5):1379-1382.

40. Kosuwon W, Mahaisavariya B, Saengnipanthkul S, Laupattarakasem W, Jirawipoolwon P. Ultrasonography of

pulled elbow. *The Journal of Bone and Joint Surgery British volume.* 1993;75(3):421-422.

41. Bartels R, Verbeek A. Risk factors for ulnar nerve compression at the elbow: a case control study. *Acta Neurochir (Wien).* 2007;149(7):669.

42. Elhassan B, Steinmann SP. Entrapment neuropathy of the ulnar nerve. *J Am Acad Orthop Surg.* 2007;15(11):672-681.

43. Byun SD, Kim CH, Jeon IH. Ulnar neuropathy caused by an anconeus epitrochlearis: clinical and electrophysiological findings. *J Hand Surg Eur Vol.* 2011;36(7):607-608.

44. Chang K-V, Wu W-T, Han D-S, Özçakar L. Ulnar nerve cross-sectional area for the diagnosis of cubital tunnel syndrome: a meta-analysis of ultrasonographic measurements. *Arch Phys Med Rehabil.* 2018;99(4):743-757.

45. Yoon JS, Walker FO, Cartwright MS. Ultrasonographic swelling ratio in the diagnosis of ulnar neuropathy at the elbow. *Muscle & Nerve: Official Journal of the American Association of Electrodiagnostic Medicine.* 2008;38(4):1231-1235.

46. Yoon JS, Walker FO, Cartwright MS. Ulnar neuropathy with normal electrodiagnosis and abnormal nerve ultrasound. *Arch Phys Med Rehabil.* 2010;91(2):318-320.

47. Okamoto M, Abe M, Shirai H, Ueda N. Morphology and dynamics of the ulnar nerve in the cubital tunnel: observation by ultrasonography. *The Journal of Hand Surgery: British & European Volume.* 2000;25(1):85-89.

48. Rutter M, Grandizio LC, Malone WJ, Klena JC. The use of preoperative dynamic ultrasound to predict ulnar nerve stability

following in situ decompression for cubital tunnel syndrome. *The Journal of hand surgery.* 2019;44(1):35-38.

49. Babusiaux D, Laulan J, Bouilleau L et al. Contribution of static and dynamic ultrasound in cubital tunnel syndrome. *Orthopaedics & Traumatology: Surgery & Research.* 2014;100(4):S209-S212.

50. 50. Dellon A, Mackinnon SE. Musculoaponeurotic variations along the course of the median nerve in the proximal forearm. *J Hand Surg Am.* 1987;12(3):359-363.

51. Rodner CM, Tinsley BA, O'Malley MP. Pronator syndrome and anterior interosseous nerve syndrome. *JAAOS-Journal of the American Academy of Orthopaedic Surgeons.* 2013;21(5):268-275.

52. Hide IG, Grainger AJ, Naisby GP, Campbell RS. Sonographic findings in the anterior interosseous nerve syndrome. *J Clin Ultrasound.* 1999;27(8):459-464.

53. Tsai P, Steinberg DR. Median and radial nerve compression about the elbow. *JBJS.* 2008;90(2):420-428.

54. Moradi A, Ebrahimzadeh MH, Jupiter JB. Radial tunnel syndrome, diagnostic and treatment dilemma. *Archives of Bone and Joint Surgery.* 2015;3(3):156.

55. Bodner G, Harpf C, Meirer R, Gardetto A, Kovacs P, Gruber H. Ultrasonographic appearance of supinator syndrome. *J Ultrasound Med.* 2002;21(11):1289-1293.

56. Husarik DB, Saupe N, Pfirrmann CW, Jost B, Hodler J, Zanetti M. Elbow nerves: MR findings in 60 asymptomatic subjects—normal anatomy, variants, and pitfalls. *Radiology.* 2009;252(1):148-156.

57. De MAESENEER M, Jacobson JA, Jaovisidha S et al. Elbow effusions: distribution of joint fluid with flexion and extension and imaging implications. *Invest Radiol.* 1998;33(2):117-125.

58. Fernandes EA, Lopes MG, Mitraud SA, Ferrari AJ, Fernandes AR. Ultrasound characteristics of gouty tophi in the olecranon bursa and evaluation of their reproducibility. *Eur J Radiol.* 2012;81(2):317-323.

59. Kim TK, Lee JH, Park KD, Lee SC, Ahn J, Park Y. Ultrasound versus palpation guidance for intra-articular injections in patients with degenerative osteoarthritis of the elbow. *J Clin Ultrasound.* 2013;41(8):479-485.

60. Yoo SH, Cha JG, Lee BR. Ultrasound-guided percutaneous bone drilling for the treatment of lateral epicondylitis. *Eur Radiol.* 2018;28(1):390-397.

61. Boden AL, Scott MT, Dalwadi PP, Mautner K, Mason RA, Gottschalk MB. Platelet-rich plasma versus Tenex in the treatment of medial and lateral epicondylitis. *J Shoulder Elbow Surg.* 2019;28(1):112-119.

62. Evans JP, Metz J, Anaspure R et al. The spread of Injectate after ultrasound-guided lateral elbow injection–a cadaveric study. *Journal of experimental orthopaedics.* 2018;5(1):27.

63. Park G-Y, Kwon DR, Cho HK, Park J, Park JH. Distribution of platelet-rich plasma after ultrasound-guided injection for chronic elbow tendinopathies. *J Sports Sci Med.* 2017;16(1):1.

64. Connell DA, Ali KE, Ahmad M, Lambert S, Corbett S, Curtis M. Ultrasound-guided autologous blood injection for tennis elbow. *Skeletal Radiol.* 2006;35(6):371-377.

65. Zhu J, Hu B, Xing C, Li J. Ultrasound-guided, minimally invasive, percutaneous needle puncture treatment for tennis elbow. *Adv Ther.* 2008;25(10):1031-1036.

66. Alblas C, van Kasteel V, Jellema K. Injection with corticosteroids (ultrasound guided) in patients with an ulnar neuropathy at the elbow, feasibility study. *Eur J Neurol.* 2012;19(12):1582-1584.

67. Rampen AJ, Wirtz PW, Tavy DL. Ultrasound-guided steroid injection to treat mild ulnar neuropathy at the elbow. *Muscle Nerve.* 2011;44(1):128-130.

68. Hamscha UM, Tinhofer I, Heber S, Grisold W, Weninger WJ, Meng S. A reliable technique for ultrasound-guided perineural injection in ulnar neuropathy at the elbow. *Muscle Nerve.* 2017;56(2):237-241.

69. Choi CK, Lee HS, Kwon JY, Lee W-J. Clinical implications of real-time visualized ultrasound-guided injection for the treatment of ulnar neuropathy at the elbow: a pilot study. *Annals of rehabilitation medicine.* 2015;39(2):176.

70. Van Duijn AJ, Felton SD. Ultrasound imaging of ulnar collateral ligament injury. *J Orthop Sports Phys Ther.* 2016;46(12):1086-1086.

71. Erol B, Cakir T, Kose O, Ozyurek S. Radial nerve entrapment caused by a ganglion cyst at the elbow: treatment with ultrasound-guided aspiration. *Am J Phys Med Rehabil.* 2014;93(11):e6-e7.

72. Seki Y. Posterior interosseous nerve palsy caused by a ganglion: conservative treatment with ultrasound-guided needle aspiration. *Journal of Ultrasonography.* 2017;17(68):73.

73. Kara M, Tiftik T, Yetişgin A, Ural G, Özçakar L. Ultrasound in the diagnosis and treatment of posterior interosseous nerve entrapment: a case report. *Muscle Nerve.* 2012;45(2):299-300.

74. Su DCJ, Yeh M-c, Chou W. Poster 142 radial tunnel syndrome treated by ultrasound guided perineural hydrodissection: a case report. *PM&R.* 2016;9(8):S207-S208.

75. García N, Rosales J, Greene C, Droppelmann G, Verdugo MA. Ultrasound-Guided Hydraulic Release Associated With Corticosteroids in Radial Tunnel Syndrome: Description of Technique and Preliminary Clinical Results. *J Ultrasound Med.* 2020;39(1):165-168.

76. Sanli I, Morgan B, van Tilborg F, Funk L, Gosens T. Single injection of platelet-rich plasma (PRP) for the treatment of refractory distal biceps tendonitis: long-term results of a prospective multicenter cohort study. *Knee Surg Sports Traumatol Arthrosc.* 2016;24(7):2308-2312.

77. Barker SL, Bell SN, Connell D, Coghlan JA. Ultrasound-guided platelet-rich plasma injection for distal biceps tendinopathy. *Shoulder & elbow.* 2015;7(2):110-114.

78. Mautner K, Stafford II CD, Nguyen P. Ultrasound-guided distal bicep tendon injection using a posterior approach. *PM&R.* 2015;7(9):1007-1010.

79. Daniels SP, Mintz DN, Endo Y, Dines JS, Sneag DB. Imaging of the post-operative medial elbow in the overhead thrower: common and abnormal findings after ulnar collateral ligament reconstruction and ulnar nerve transposition. *Skeletal Radiol.* 2019:1-18.

Chapter 4 Hand and Wrist

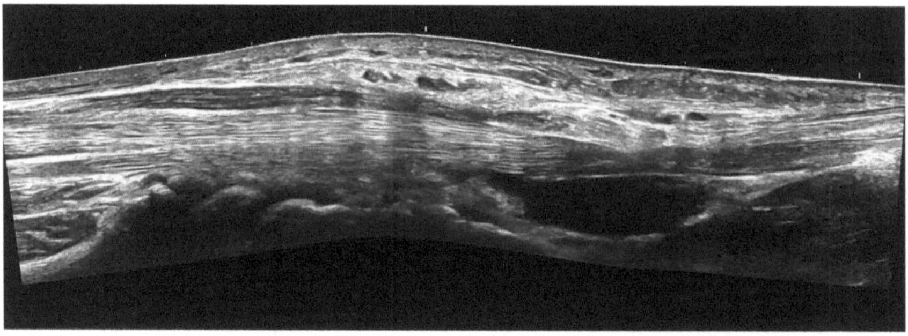

- John Fowler,MD
- Christopher M Jobe, MD, RMSK
- Robert Vercio, MD

Introduction:

The hand and wrist are usually the subject of a limited exam. While many shoulder conditions produce a rotator type of shoulder pain benefiting from a systematic exam, carpal tunnel syndrome, for example, does not require a full evaluation of their six extensor compartments for diagnosis and evaluation.

An astute examiner can confirm carpal tunnel syndrome, evaluate tendon ruptures, including location of proximal tendon stump, and provide accurate injections for treatments of De Quervain's, trigger fingers, and joints. Bilateral examinations and dynamic testing are helpful adjuncts for the beginning ultrasonographer.

Diagnostic Evaluation:

We recommend breaking down the hand/wrist and finger exam into volar and dorsal components. Some areas and features, such as the thumb collateral ligament, can be evaluated on an as-needed basis and do not require a complete exam. This section will briefly describe the main areas of focus, how to image them and what you can evaluate within each region.

Hand/Wrist

Volar Exam:

The examiner is seated across from the patient. The patient places the forearm in full supination with the elbow in approximately 60-70 degrees of flexion and rests the dorsum of the forearm on the examination table. The wrist is in neutral flexion-extension and the fingers are placed in a normal resting posture/cascade. The ultrasound probe is placed perpendicular to the long axis of the forearm (short-axis view) at the level of the wrist crease (Fig. 1A fowler).

The wrist can be divided into three sections: radial, middle, and ulnar. In the middle section of the wrist (Fig. 1B), which contains the carpal tunnel, the bony floor will be the lunate and the capitate. The median nerve and flexor tendons will be located superficial to the bony structures and deep to the transverse carpal ligament. In the forearm, the nerve is sandwiched between the FDS and FDP tendons, which provide sources of stark contrast and facilitate identification of the nerve. The median nerve can be distinguished by its hypoechogenciity (relative to the tendons) and being stable during dynamic examination. Proximally, the nerve is radial and oval shaped in cross-section and flattens as it approaches the level of the hook of the hamate.

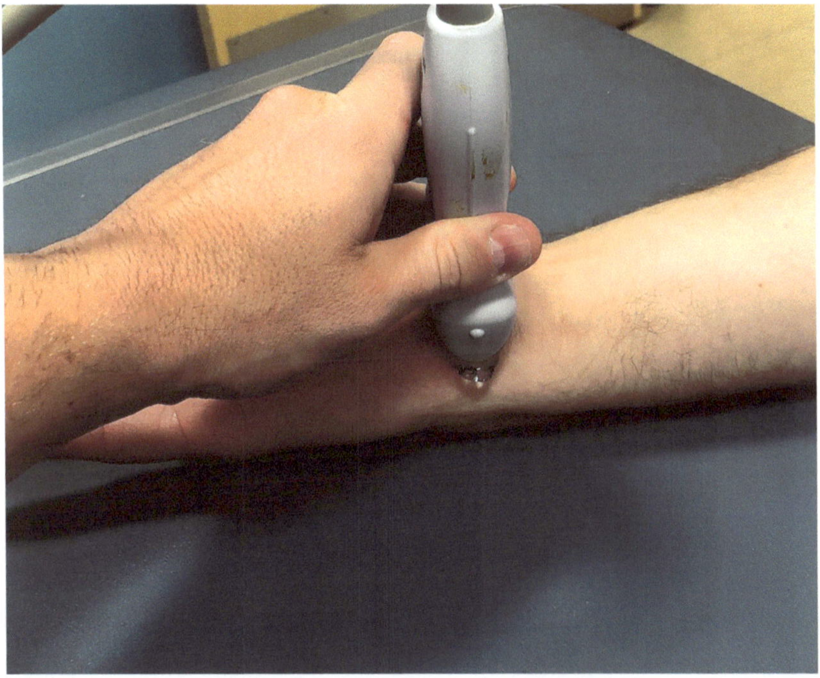

Figure 4-1a: The probe position for examining the wrist in short axis

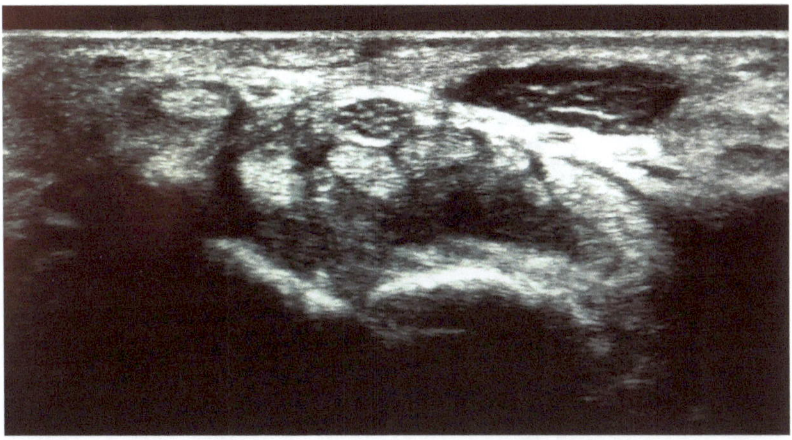

Figure 1b: A short-axis view of the wrist at the level of the lunate. The median nerve is seen superficially in the center with flexor tendons immediately below. The hypoechoic thenar muscles are to the upper right.

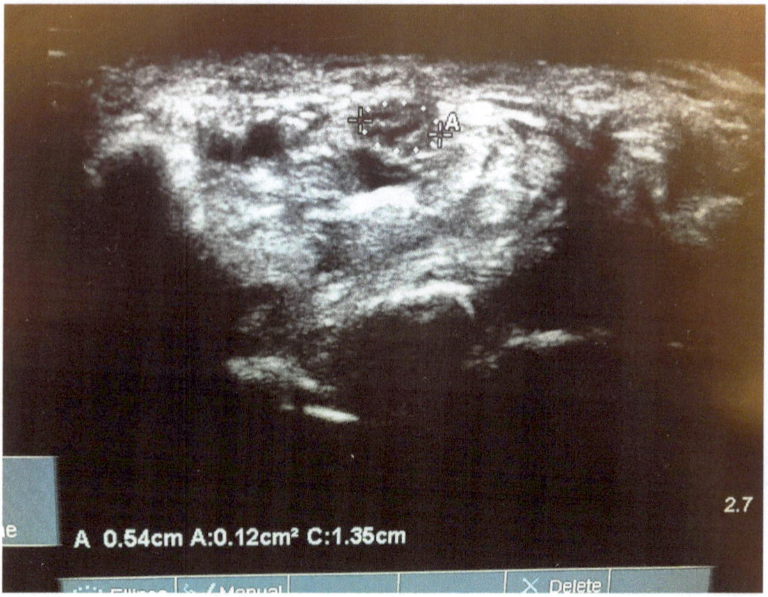

Figure 4-1c: The ellipse, or trace tool, is used to measure the cross-sectional area of the median nerve in the forearm and again at the level of the lunate (as shown here). Enlargement of the nerve just proximal to the entrance of the carpal tunnel points to nerve compression in the tunnel.

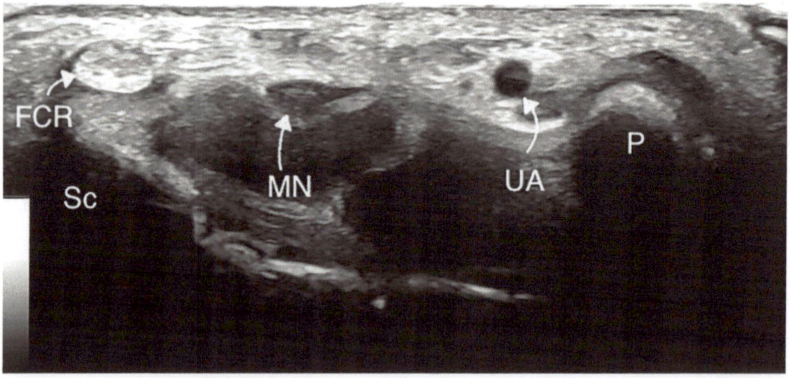

Figure 4-1d: A short-axis view of the proximal row. On the left the FCR is seen in cross section on top of the volar pole of the scaphoid. On the right the ulnar artery and the pisiform are seen.

The median nerve lies under the transverse carpal ligament just to the left of the middle.

The radial side of the volar wrist allows for visualization of the scaphoid, FCR, radial artery, and thenar musculature. This is also a common area to visualize a volar ganglion cyst.

The ulnar side of the volar wrist allows for visualization of the ulnar nerve and artery and the hypothenar musculature.

In the long axis (2a and 2b), we can see the nerve and flexor tendons, and determine the path of an injection relative to the fascia and the TCL.

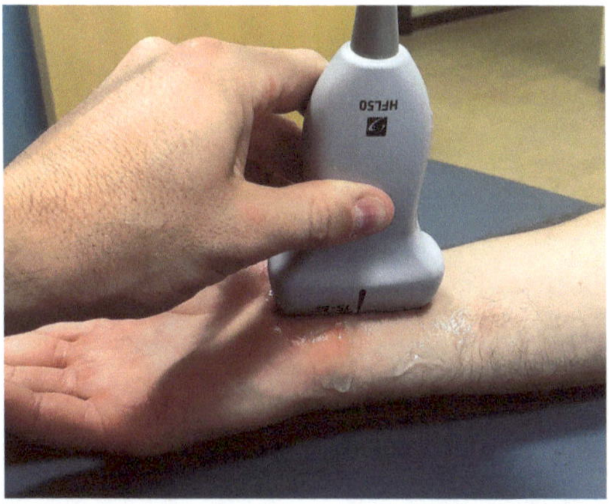

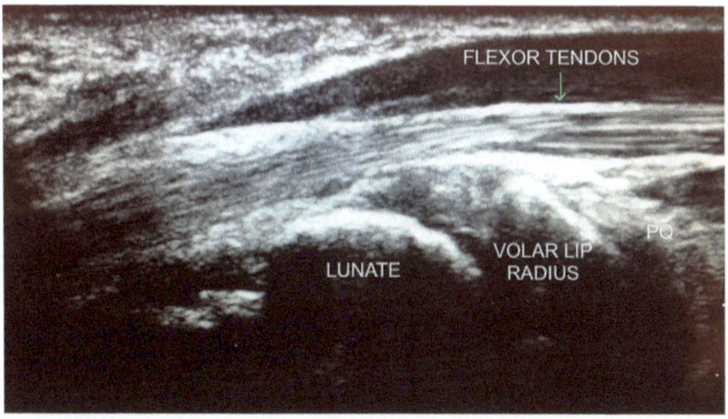

Figure 4-2a: The position for examining the wrist in long axis. B. A long axis view showing the bony landmarks with the tendons and the nerve.

Dorsal Exam:

The examiner is seated across from the patient. The shoulder needs to be partially abducted and forearm in pronation to help position the dorsal surface for good visibility. There are three dorsal sections of the hand/wrist to evaluate. The proximal radial dorsal section allows you to see the extensor tendons and leading distally to the dorsal joint recesses. The distal radial dorsal section allows you to see the carpal bones, scapholunate ligament and to check for a dorsal ganglion cyst. The ulnar dorsal section allows for better visualization of the ECU tendon and the TFCC (though the TFCC is not easily visualized)

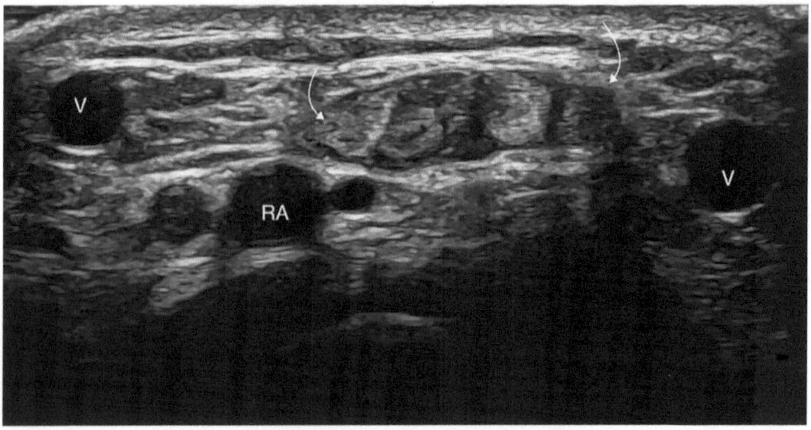

Figure 4-3a: The first dorsal compartment is seen here, between the arrows, where it is about to cross over the radial artery (RA). It is common to have more than two tendons, but this subject has four, as we look distal to the fibro-osseus canal. The abductor pollicis longus tendons are those closer to the RA, while the extensor pollicis brevis tendons are to the right (or more dorsal aspect) closer to the cephalic vein, V.

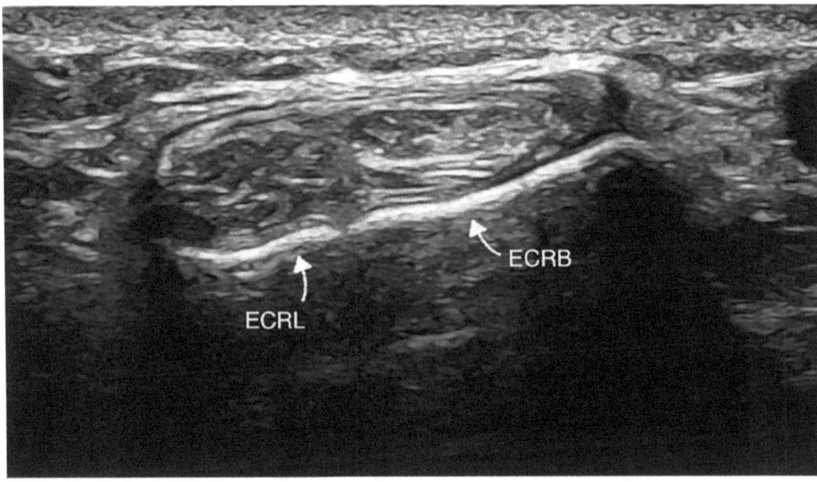

Figure 4-3b: The second compartment contains the two radial wrist extensors. The longus is more radial (left) while the brevis is more central (right).

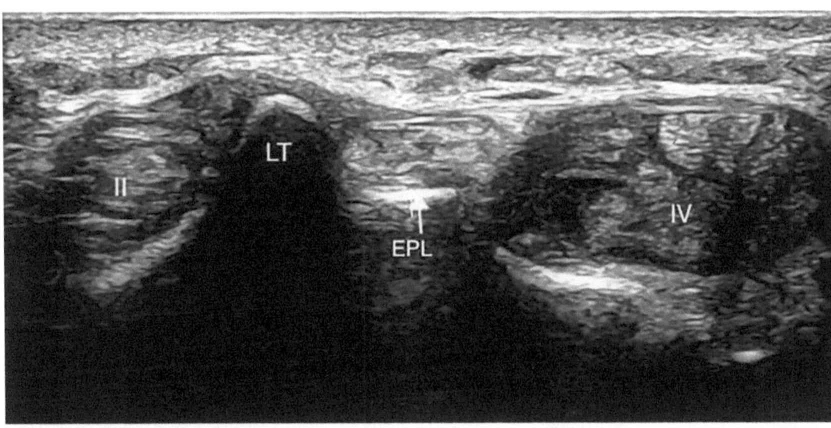

Figure 4-3c: The third compartment contains the extensor pollicis longus, EPL, and lies just ulnar to Lister's tubercle, LT.

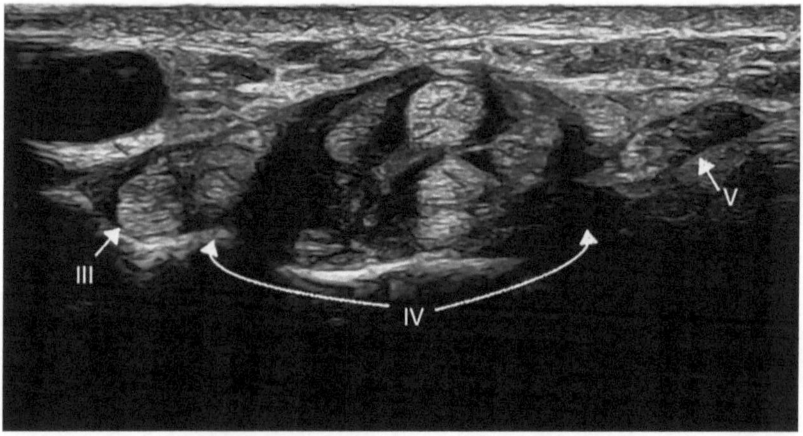

Figure 4-3d: The fourth compartment with EDC and EIP lies directly superficial to the central wrist. The fifth, containing the extensor digiti minimi, V, is also seen on the right over the DRUJ.

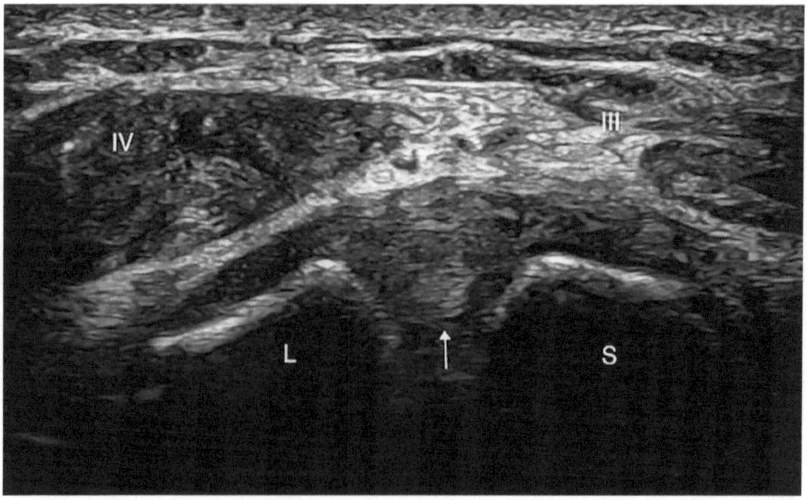

Figure 4-3e: The scapholunate joint is seen distal to the radius between the third and fourth compartment.

Fingers

Volar Exam:

The examiner is seated across from the patient. The patient places the forearm in full supination with the elbow in approximately 60-70 degrees of flexion, and rests the dorsum of the forearm on the examination table. The wrist is in neutral flexion-extension and the fingers are placed in full extension. This position will enable you to visualize the flexor tendons, tendon pulleys, the volar plate, and the joint recesses.

Dorsal Finger Exam:

The examiner is seated across from the patient. The shoulder needs to be partially abducted with the forearm in pronation to help position the dorsal surface for good visibility. This will enable you to visualize the extensor tendon, hood mechanism, and joint recesses. While the shape of the fingers can preclude the imager's ability to position the probe in such a way to obtain a wide image, the dorsal fingers are notoriously difficult, and we would recommend stand-off pads or thick gel to aid in imaging. We recommend using high frequency probes to aid in structure visualization in this region, as most of the dorsal structures are superficial and without significantly contrasting layers.

Surgical Planning:

An additional benefit to ultrasound is the opportunity to prepare for surgical approaches in areas where there may be concern of differing anatomy or unfamiliar approaches. Ultrasound allows you to visualize the recurrent motor branch of the median nerve prior to injection or carpal tunnel release to confirm safety of approach. As the examiner becomes more proficient with ultrasound, the opportunities become limitless.

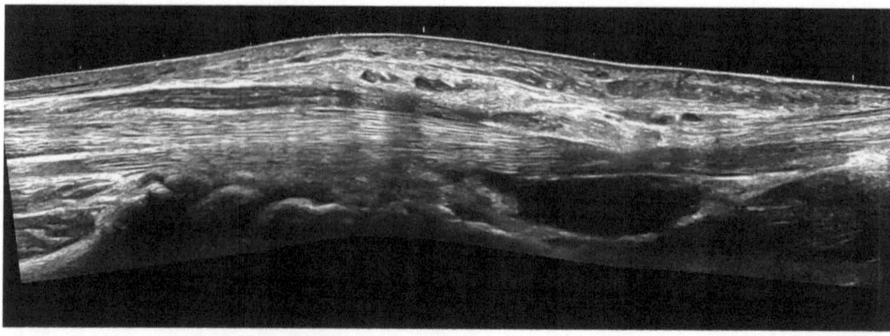

Figure 4-4a: The title figure for the hand chapter, if broken into segments, can serve as a summary of many of the ideas covered in the diagnostic section. Left is proximal and right is distal. This view is broken into segments and enlarged in the next three figures.

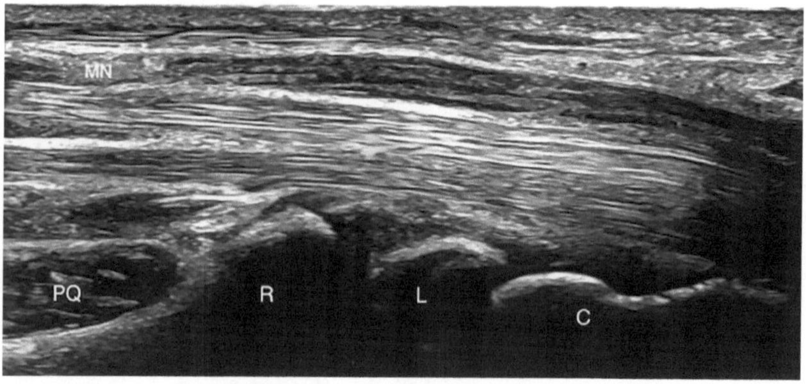

Figure 4-4b: The proximal third of the volar wrist and hand shows how the tendons, T, with their multiple internal layers are echogenic, yet transmit sound through to the deeper structures. Deeper structures includes 1. the carpal bones: radius (R), lunate (L), and capitate (C), as well as 2. the pronator quadratus (PQ) muscle. The bones are more echogenic and therefore do not transmit through. The median nerve (MN) is less bright as it has fewer layers, and moves far less than the tendons on the dynamic view. Also note that the skin is not entirely parallel to the deeper structures, so some toggling will be needed to

get the best view. The need for toggling will be the greatest for the tendons, which are the most anisotropic because of their internal organization. Note also the narrowing of the nerve at about the lunate-capitate joint where it enters the canal in this patient with CTS.

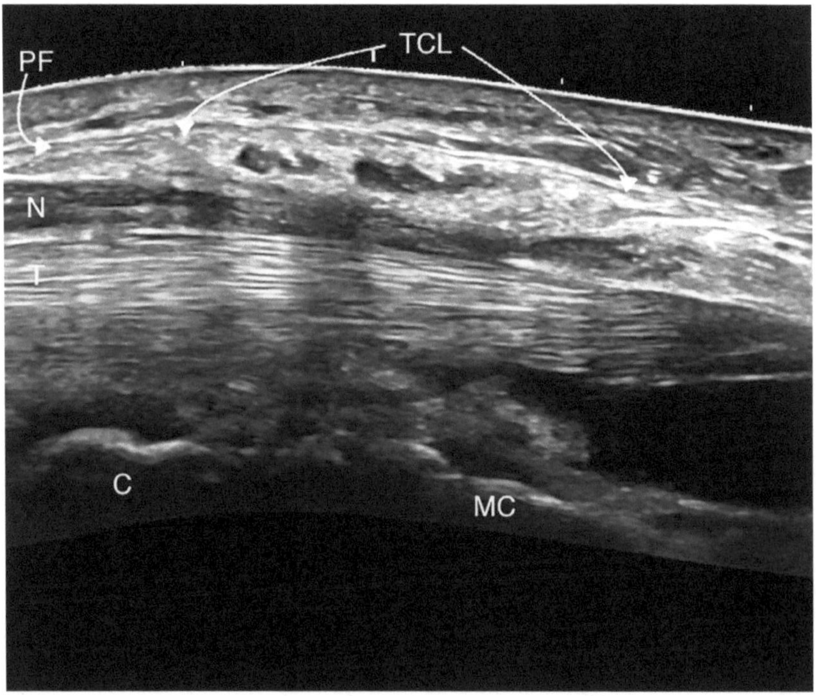

Figure 4-4c: The transverse carpal ligament (TCL), seen here in its short axis of the ligament which is the long axis of the wrist, marks the location of the narrowing of the nerve in CTS. The whole region is covered by the relatively thinner palmar fascia (PF) which resembles ligament and tendon in its appearance. As the nerve lies in radial aspect of the TCL, some of the less echogenic thenar muscles fibers are also seen. As muscle transmits more sound, the underlying nerve and tendons appear brighter under the muscle than under the more collagenous regions of the ligament. C: capitate; MC base of the metacarpal.

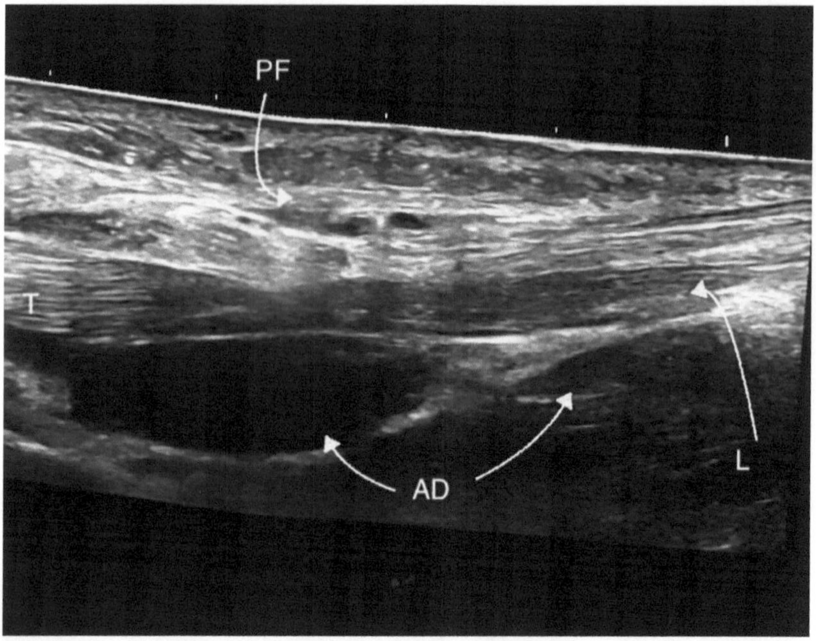

Figure 4-4d: In the distal third of the palm, the palmar fascia (PF) continues over fat that contains vessels and nerves. Deviating the probe a little off the deep flexor (T) on the right, we see the long finger lumbrical (L). In the deeper area are the two heads of the adductor pollicis (AD) oblique on the left and direct on the right. In this deeper area the muscles are quite dark, indicating that the sonographer should transition to the time gain compensation (TGC) on the ultrasound machine to enhance and more easily visualize the deeper images.

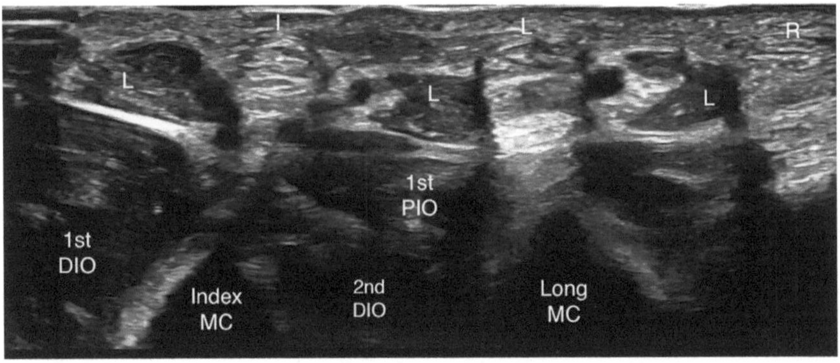

Figure 4-4e: In this short-axis view of the hand, one can see almost all of the way dorsally to the skin. The index, long, and ring finger flexor tendons (I, L, and R, respectively) are two flexor tendons, superficial and deep, to each digit. The lumbricals (L) are just radial to their respective tendons. Two metacarpals and three interosseus muscles, dorsal and palmar, are also labeled.

Pathology:

Carpal Tunnel Syndrome

Compression of the median nerve within the carpal tunnel results in swelling of the nerve proximal and distal to the site of compression, but especially proximally. The nerve swelling can be measured with axial imaging (short axis), and if the cross-sectional area (CSA) of the nerve exceeds a specific threshold, the diagnosis of carpal tunnel syndrome is confirmed. The most sensitive and specific geographical level to measurement is at the wrist crease/level of the pisiform (1). Some have suggested that a wrist-forearm ratio (the ratio of the CSA of the median nerve at the wrist crease to the CSA of the median nerve 12 cm proximal to the wrist crease) of ≥ 1.4 is a more sensitive and specific diagnostic test compared to the CSA area of the median nerve at the wrist alone (2). Additionally, it appears quantification of the flexor retinaculum bowing, the nerve flattening ratio, and color Doppler to evaluate for hypervascularity of the nerve also provide independent diagnostic utility (3).

The examiner is seated across from the patient. The patient places the forearm in full supination with the elbow in approximately 60-70 degrees of flexion, and rests the dorsum of the forearm on the examination table with neutral wrist rotation and resting finger cascade. The ultrasound probe is placed perpendicular to the long axis of the forearm (short-axis view) at the level of the wrist crease (Figure 1a). The pisiform and distal pole scaphoid are identified. The median nerve is identified, and the CSA of the median nerve is measured using the trace function on the ultrasound machine (Figure 1b). The CSA is measured just inside the hyperechoic epineurium. In general, a CSA of ≥ 10 mm^2 is diagnostic for carpal tunnel syndrome (4). The long axis view is not typically utilized for diagnosis of carpal tunnel syndrome, although it can be useful to help identify space-occupying lesions within the carpal tunnel (Figure 2a, b). The long axis may also help in finding the motor branch, which traditionally can be localized at the distal end of the tunnel, but may occur after the nerve has branched or in the canal.

Ultrasound guidance for carpal tunnel injections improves accuracy and mitigates risk of injury to the median nerve during injection. A large series performed by Green and colleagues, demonstrated that typical landmark-guided (without US) needle placement for carpal tunnel injections resulted in direct injury/penetration of the median nerve in ~8% and completely missing the carpal tunnel in ~25%.(5) The technique for ultrasound guided carpal tunnel injection involves placing the probe in the short axis at the level of the wrist crease and identifying the median nerve. Nearly all ultrasound machines have a function that places a vertical line down the center of the screen, and this line corresponds with a mark at the center of the ultrasound probe (Figure 5a). This line is typically placed just ulnar to the median nerve, however, in some patients the median nerve sits very close ulnar in the carpal tunnel. In these cases, the injection is performed radial to the median nerve. The ulnar neurovascular bundle is identified, and the vertical line is confirmed to be radial to these structures. After sterile skin prep, a 25-gauge needle is inserted in line with the targeting mark at a 45 degree angle from proximal to distal. The position of the needle within the carpal tunnel can be confirmed on a long axis view (Figure 5b). Despite ultrasound guidance, the author still asks patients to vocalize if there are having any shooting/tingling pains with needle insertion. The location of the needle within the carpal tunnel (and not in a tendon) is confirmed and the steroid/anesthetic mixture injected.

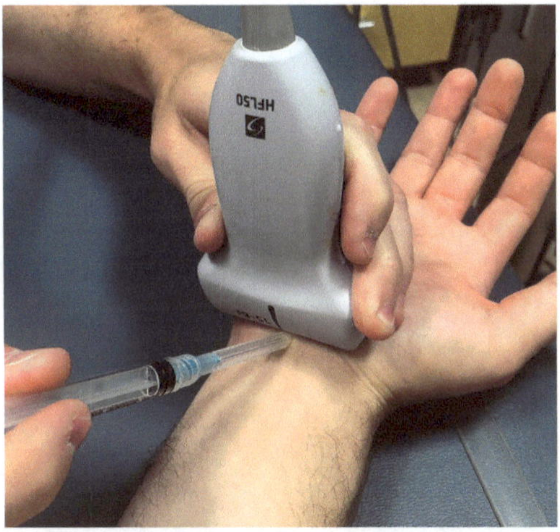

Figure 4-5a: The starting position of the probe and needle for carpal tunnel injection. The marker on the probe corresponds to a marker, or centerline, on the ultrasound monitor. The needle enters midway between median nerve and ulnar artery.

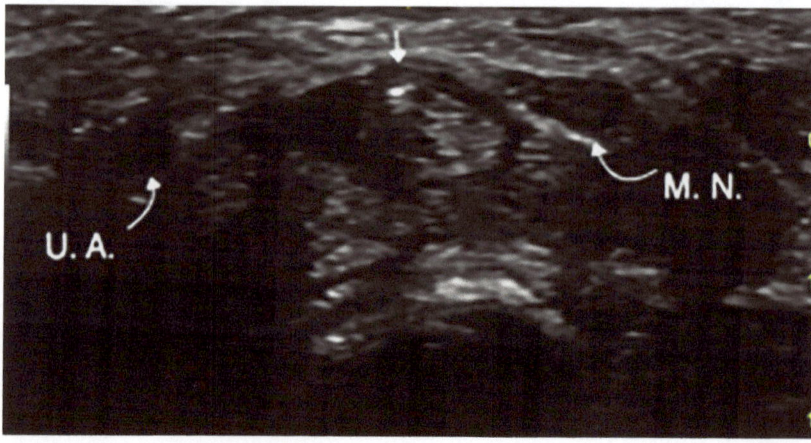

Figure 4-5b: The needle position (arrow) in short axis between median nerve (M.N.) and ulnar artery (U.A.)

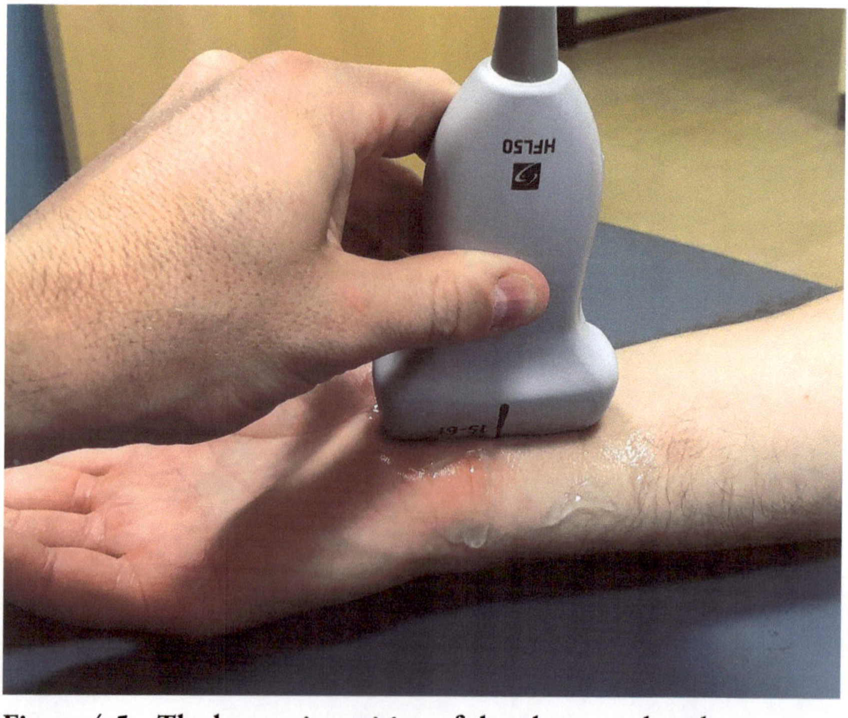

Figure 4-5c: The long axis position of the ultrasound probe.

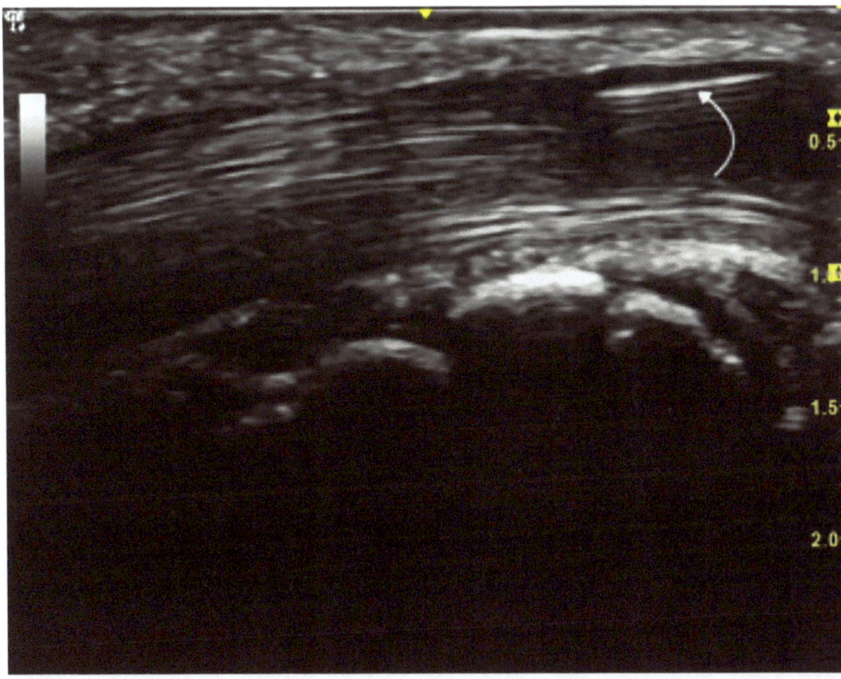

Figure 4-5d: In the long axis, the needle is followed on the deep surface of the forearm fascia and the proximal TCL. The injection is visualized on the monitor as the medication is administered.

Ultrasound guided release

US guided carpal tunnel release, USCTR, allows confirmation of the diagnosis, evaluation of safety, location of structures at risk, and surgical release in a single visit.

Diagnosis confirmation

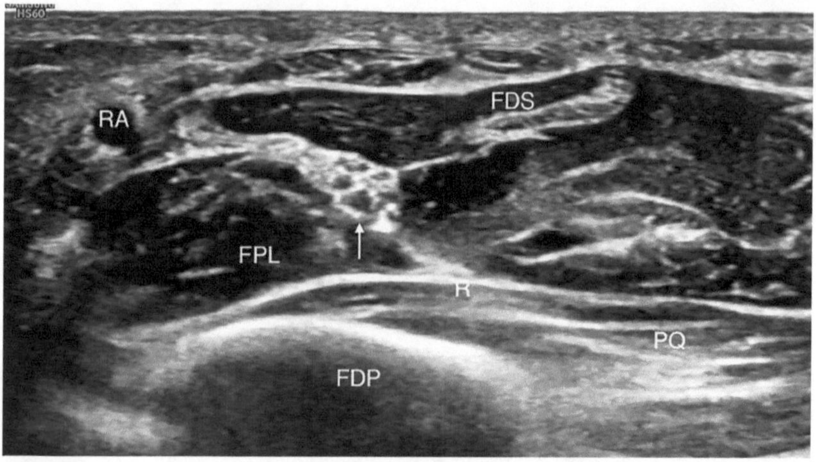

Figure 4-6a: A left wrist cross-sectional area of the median nerve is measured where it overlies the pronator quadratus, or even more proximal. The cross-sectional area can be measured at this level to determine the normal size for this patient.

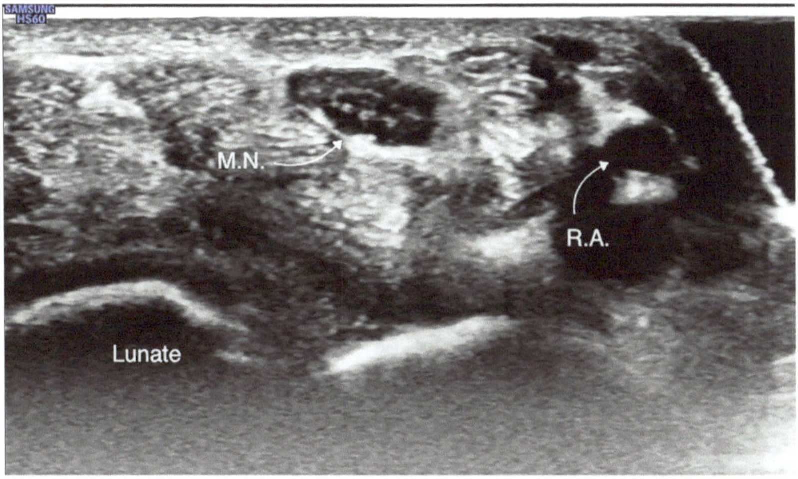

Figure 4-6b: This right wrist cross-sectional area demonstrates the location where the nerve is again measured near the canal entrance to look for enlargement. This is roughly at the level of the lunate. Median nerve (M.N.); Radial artery (R.A). If this is >40% or 2 mm2 enlarged compared to the nerve in the forearm, or grossly larger than 10 mm2 the diagnosis is confirmed. Generally the difference is larger than 2 mm2 and is easily seen.

Assessing the safe zone.

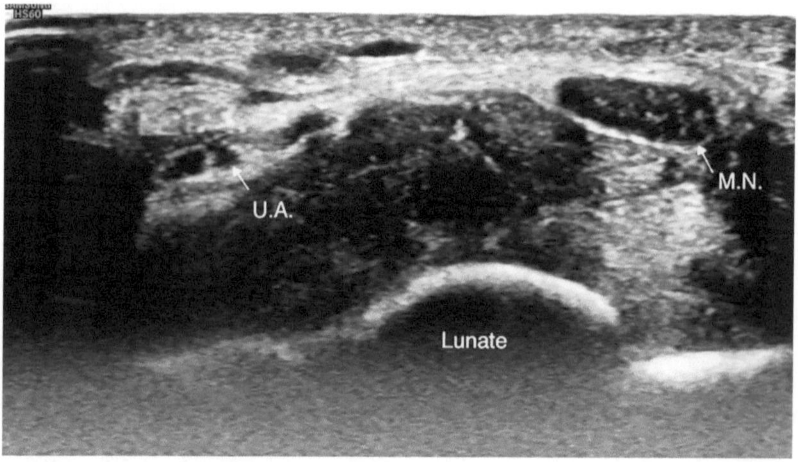

Figure 4-7a: The 'safe zone' is the space between the enlarged median nerve and the ulnar artery. At the entrance over the lunate, as seen here, the zone can be quite wide. We look at the entire course of the median nerve and ulnar artery to ensure that there is some space between them.

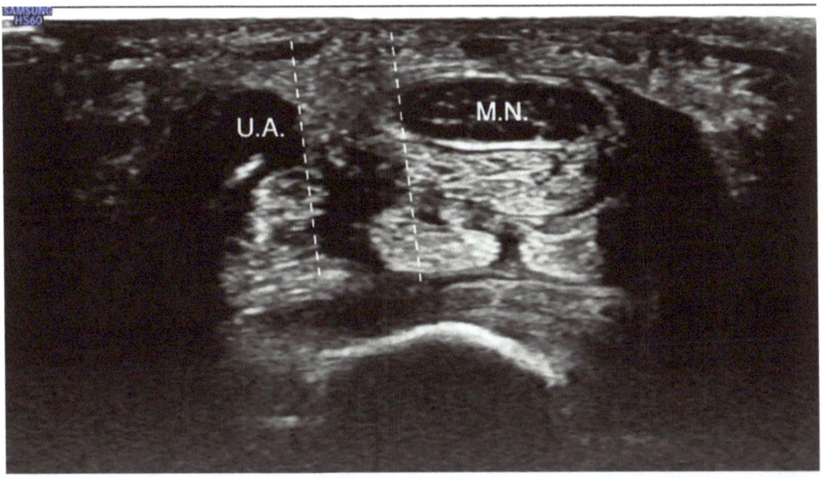

Figure 4-7b: In other individuals, the safe zone can be narrow. A transverse skin incision may be utilized if there is a wide safe zone. However when it is narrow, a longitudinal incision must be used. If a transverse incision is used, only the dermis is cut transversely. The fascia is exposed by blunt dissection because of the number of small veins in the subcutaneous fat.

In addition, the safe zone can be encroached by other structures at risk: the third common digital nerve, the motor branch to the thenar muscles, and the superficial palmar arch. The third common digital nerve crosses the long finger flexors to reach the ring-long finger interspace. Ideally, that crossing will be distal to the canal so that the flexors are not pushed into the path of the cutting instrument. In 1% of cases, the motor branch may come off the ulnar side of the median nerve.

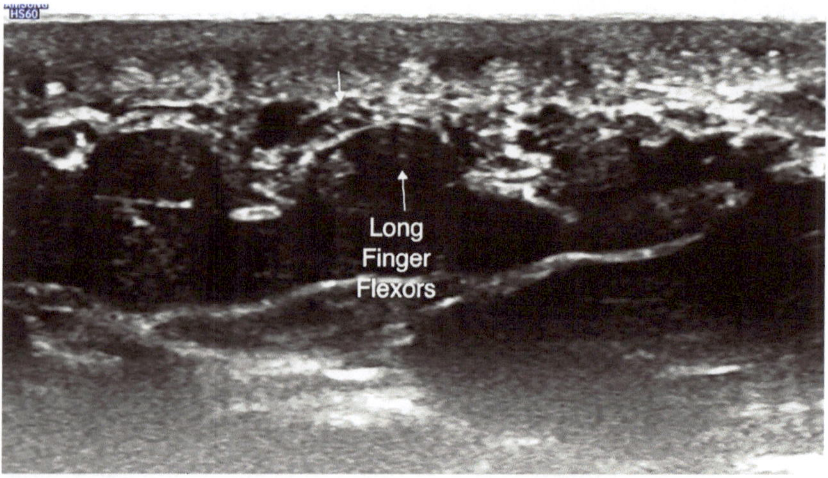

Figure 4-8a: Third common digital nerve (down arrow) of the right hand (the ulnar side is to the left). This nerve can be picked up distally in the palm where it lies ulnar to the long finger flexors. The site where it crosses the long finger flexors is noted. As in this case, utilizing anisotrophy to darken the flexor tendons dark may help with visualization.

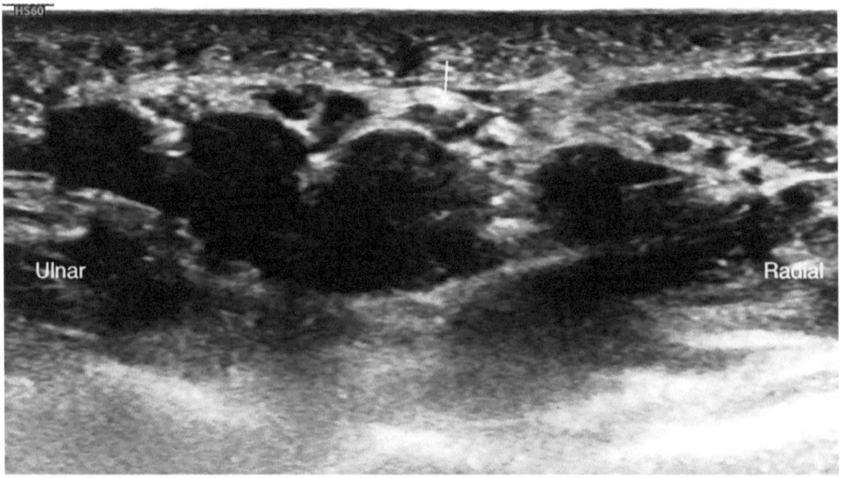

Figure 4-8b: Third common digital nerve (down arrow) crossing the long finger flexors to the radial side on the right. We see this crossing as we move the transducer proximally toward the canal. We want to make sure that this crossing is distal to the canal. Again, note the negative anisotropy of the flexor tendons.

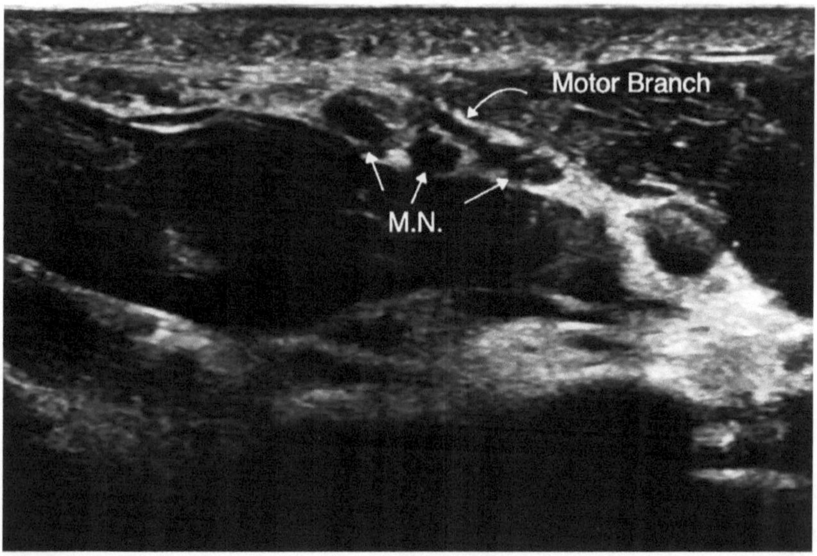

Figure 4-9: Fortunately, in some patients, the motor branch can be followed for some distance in the canal distally. This image is distal to the transverse carpal ligament where the main median nerve divides into the common digital nerves. We want the motor branch to be toward the radial side (as it is in this patient), and not on the ulnar side.

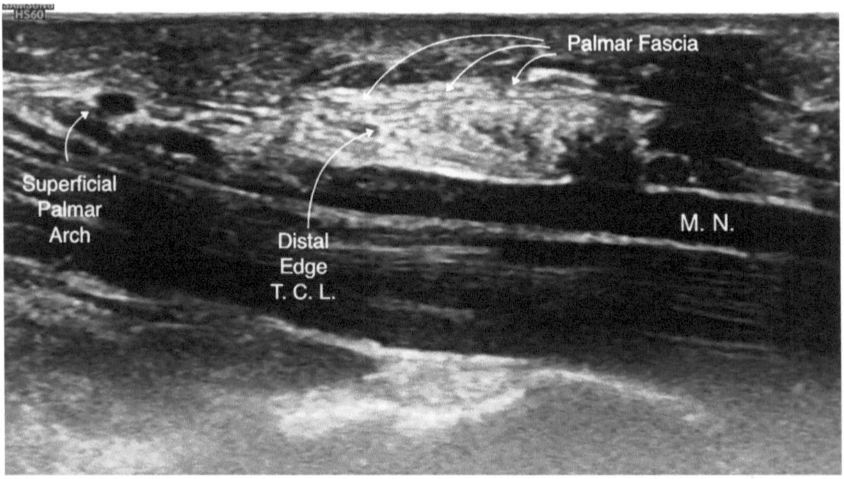

Figure 4-10: The superficial palmar arch is another structure at risk. In this patient, the arch is safely distal to the distal edge of the transverse carpal ligament (T.C.L.), which is the distal limit of our release. This is the desired position for the artery. An artery in the area of release would be a contraindication.

Injection and hydro-dissection

Most of these procedures are done under local anesthesia. In addition to the anesthesia, the local anesthetic solution provides a negative contrast medium to aid in visualization.

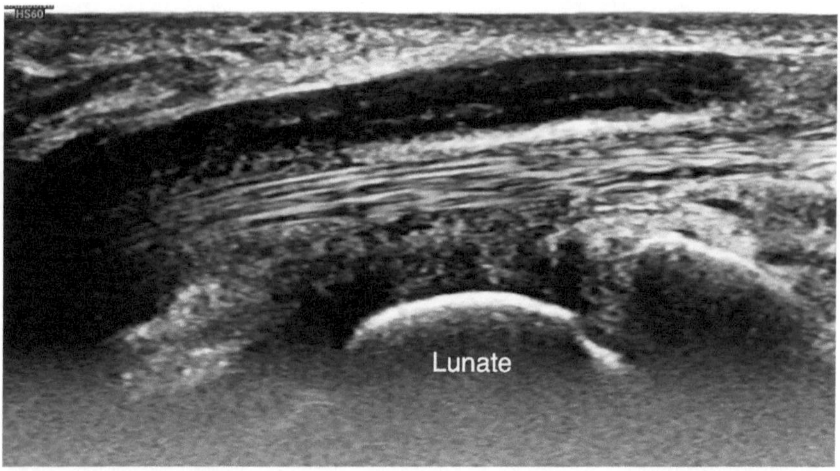

Figure 4-11a: In the long axis, the starting point for injection and incision is roughly over the volar apex of the lunate. A transverse line is drawn on the skin at this level. Almost always, this is the proximal flexion crease of the wrist.

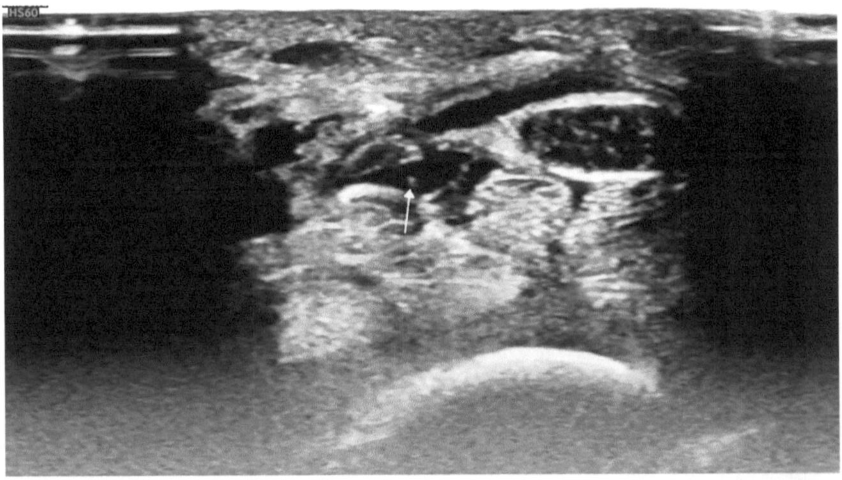

Figure 4-11b: The starting point in the short axis is between median nerve and ulnar artery, somewhat closer to the nerve than the artery. The initial injection is into the subcutaneous fat and a little deep to the forearm fascia with a 27G needle. Note the swelling in the subcutaneous fat compared with Fig. 11a. Lidocaine with epinephrine is injected to provide hemostasis in addition to anesthesia. The arrow points to some injectate deep to the forearm fascia. Always check to make sure there are no air bubbles in your needle as air blocks the sound.

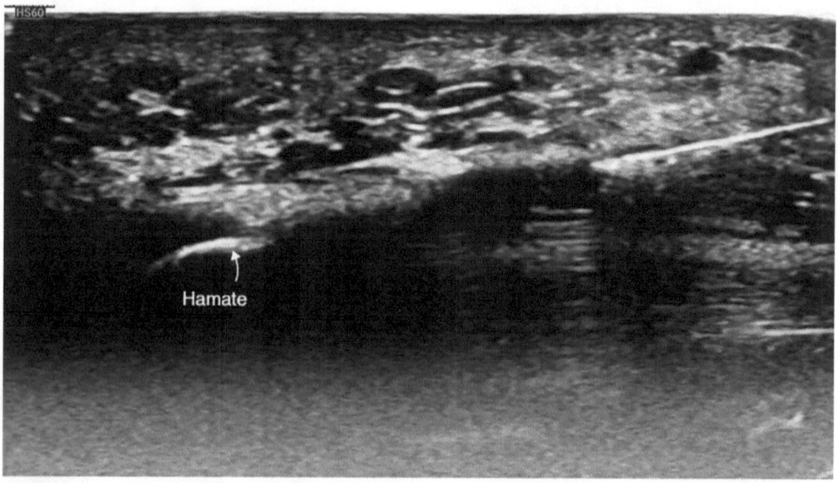

Figure 4-12a:22G needle is then introduced and its alignment confirmed before proceeding. We want the needle in the long axis to be flat, and close to both the fascia and transverse carpal ligament. In this long view, we see the tip of the needle appropriately beneath and against the fascia. But even before we move to the short-axis view, we can tell the needle is directed too far to the ulnar as it is pointing towards the hook of the hamate.

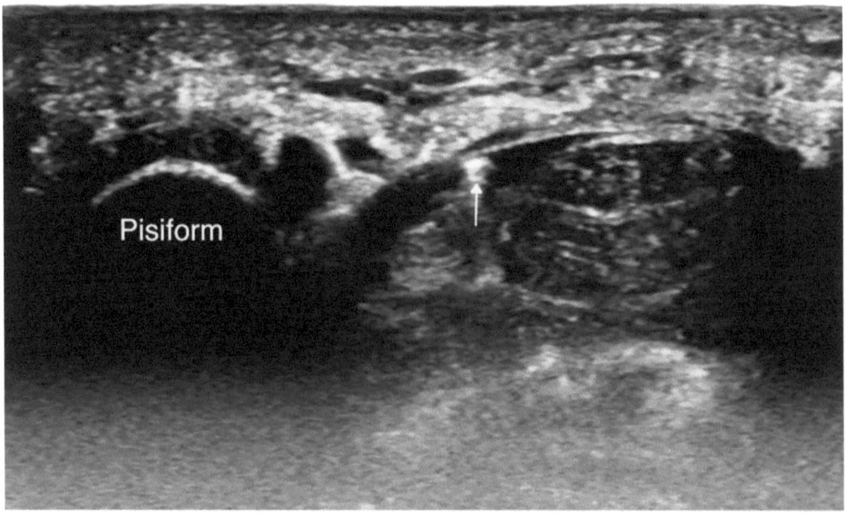

Figure 4-12b:A short-axis view of the needle in the canal. It is far enough away from the nerve to be safe. In addition, it is still under the more horizontal portion of the TCL, where both the needle and ligament are more easily visualized together. Because of spatial compounding (US beams at different angles), we more easily identify the needle and overlying ligament together in the short axis of the needle than in the long axis where the ultrasound beams are all parallel.

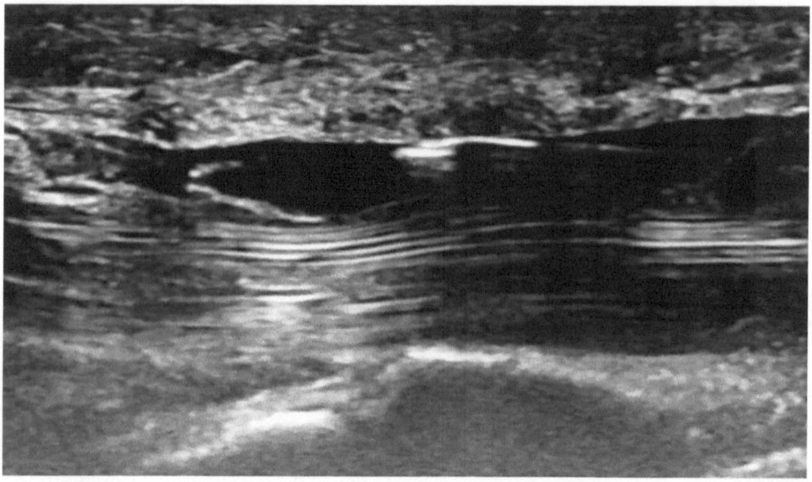

Figure 4-12c: A clean hydro-dissection with lidocaine. Only about 2mL is required for anesthesia, but 6-8 mL may be used as the lidocaine serves as a negative contrast medium. This hydro-dissection is done with lidocaine without epinephrine. If epinephrine is used, the anesthetic may last ten hours or longer

A good technique to create a clean hydro-dissection includes first starting by injecting the ligament, and then applying pressure as the needle is withdrawn. A bit more wrist dorsiflexion may be required to direct the needle into the ligament.

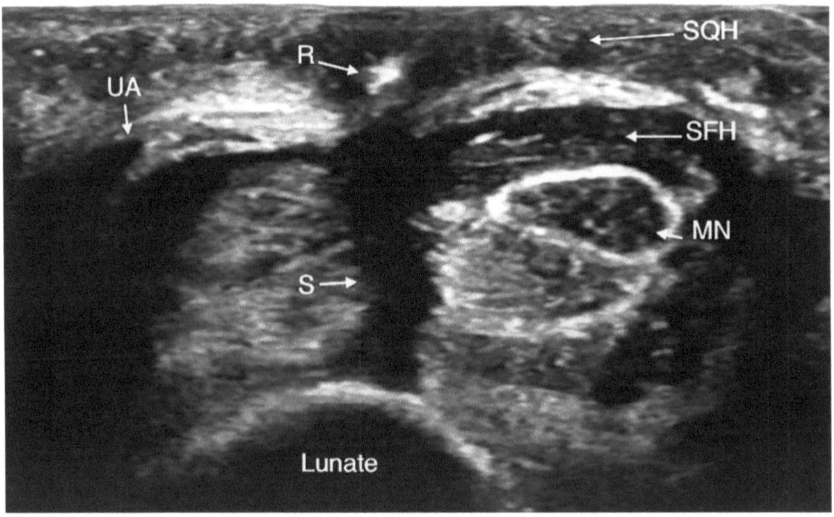

Procedure

Figure 4-13a: A longitudinal incision, 4-5mm in length, is made under ultrasound control at the starting point. A little extra distal fascia is released under the skin in line with the incision. The reflection (R) and the shadow (S) of the blade can be seen passing through the subcutaneous hydro-dissection (SQH) to the subfascial (SFH) hydro-dissection. Note the incision is intentionally made closer to the nerve than the artery. Of note, a transverse incision can also be used, and as previously mentioned, this is done in patients with a wide safe zone. Only the dermis is cut, then the subcutaneous fat is spread. The forearm fascia is released with tenotomy scissors in a longitudinal direction under ultrasound guidance.

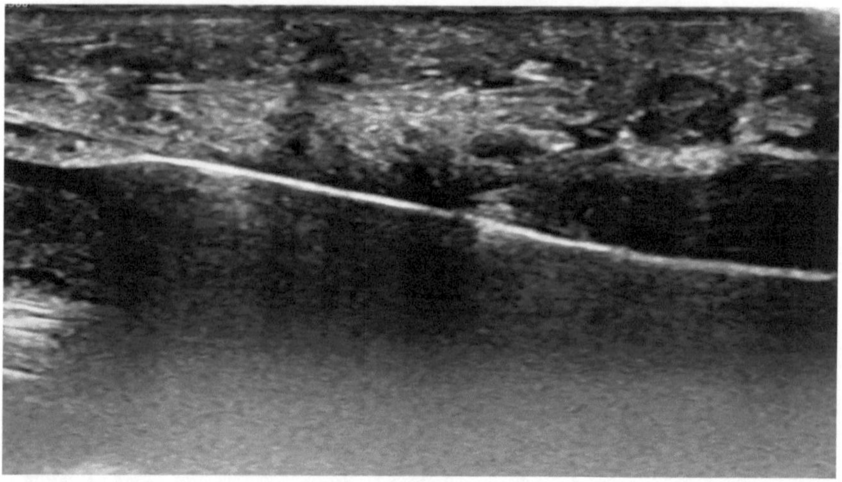

Figure 4-13b: A long axis view of a 3-4 mm. uterine dilator against the TCL passing from the right to the left.

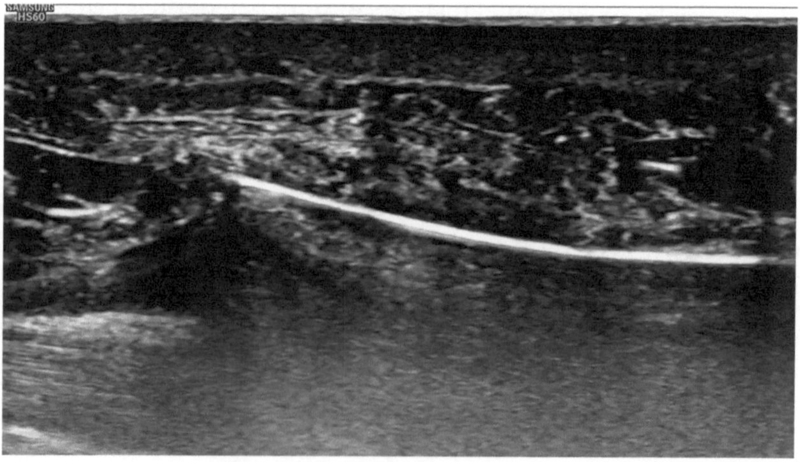

Figure 4-13c: Long axis view of a freer elevator cleaning the back of the TCL. The tip of the freer is located precisely at the distal edge of the ligament. This requires only a few seconds. Note how well the freer conforms to the back of the ligament.

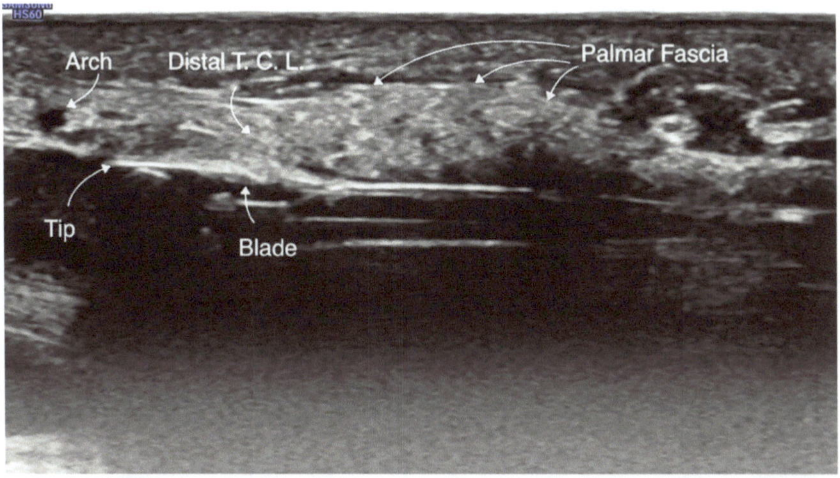

Figure 4-13d: The micro-knife is advanced to where the blade is at the level of the distal edge of the TCL. The tip of the knife retracts other tissues. While we may increase dorsiflexion during the injection phase, in this phase, we may consider decreasing dorsiflexion so that the more proximal portion of the knife lies flat against the ligament and fascia so that no other tissue can pass between the ligament and our cutting device.

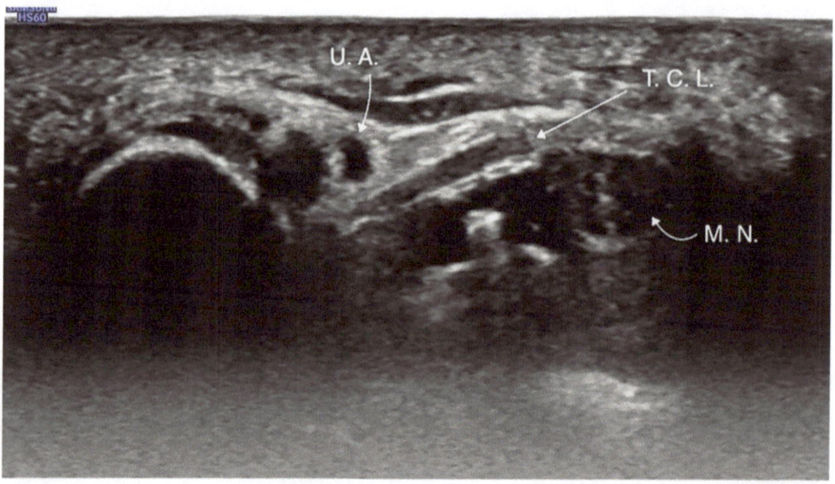

Figure 4-13e: After inflating the balloons with saline, the knife can be rotated ulnar to place it flat against the transverse carpal ligament (T.C.L.). The more radial balloon is used to exclude the nerve from the cutting surface. This rotation is seen best at the level of the pisiform, and then followed distally. The position of the ulnar artery (U.A) can also be noted.

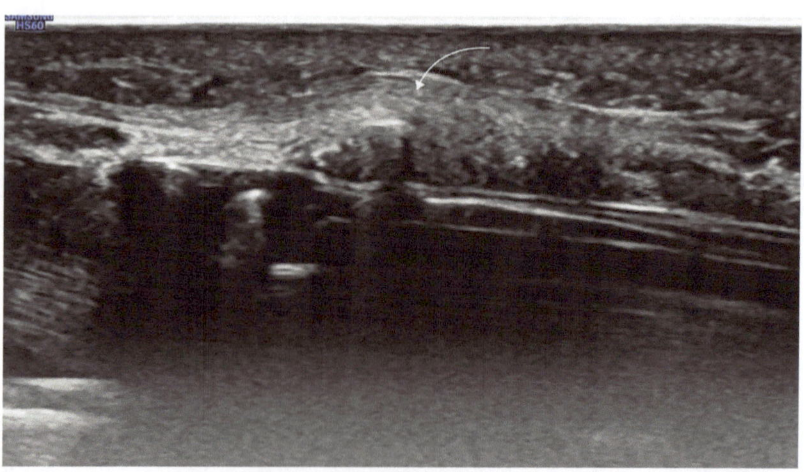

Figure 4-13f: After confirming the safety of the at-risk structures, the blade is activated (arrow). In the long axis, the blade can be followed proximally without moving the probe.

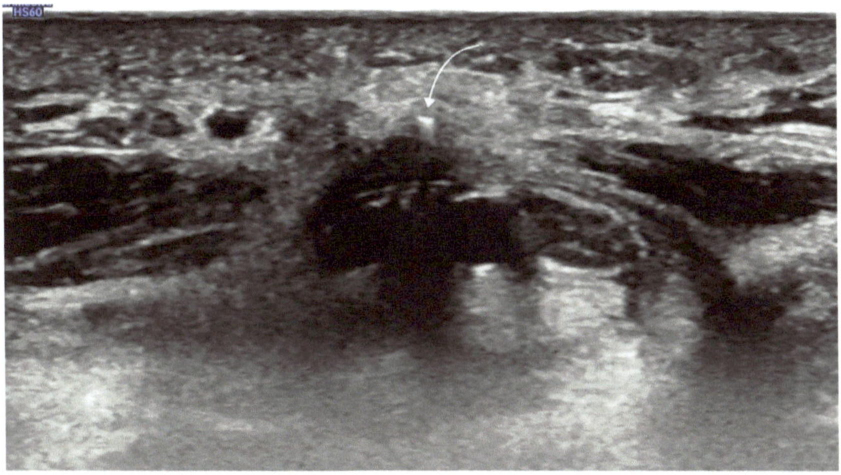

Figure 4-13g: The tip of the blade can also be followed proximally in the short axis in a technique called the 'inch-worm' technique. The blade and the ultrasound probe are moved in increments proximally. The advantage of the inch worm technique is that it puts the broadest exposure over the track of the blade, another advantage of spatial compounding. Note on the left the shadowing of the ulnar balloon by the hamate, which itself is not seen.

Aftercare

The excess lidocaine is milked from the wound, so that the wound is dry, or as dry as possible. An acrylic skin glue or a single stitch can be used to close the skin. After the glue hardens, a clear plastic dressing is applied. Often, in a case done under local, the case is over before the block fully sets up, and the motor branch can be tested before the patient leaves the OR. The patient should be advised that the numbness may last 6 hours or longer. Frequent finger motion is encouraged. In the immediate post-operative weeks, the wrist can be loaded if it is held in a straight line, or dorsiflexed. So, to get up from a chair the patient should use a clenched fist as pulling with the wrist in volar flexion may be uncomfortable for several weeks.

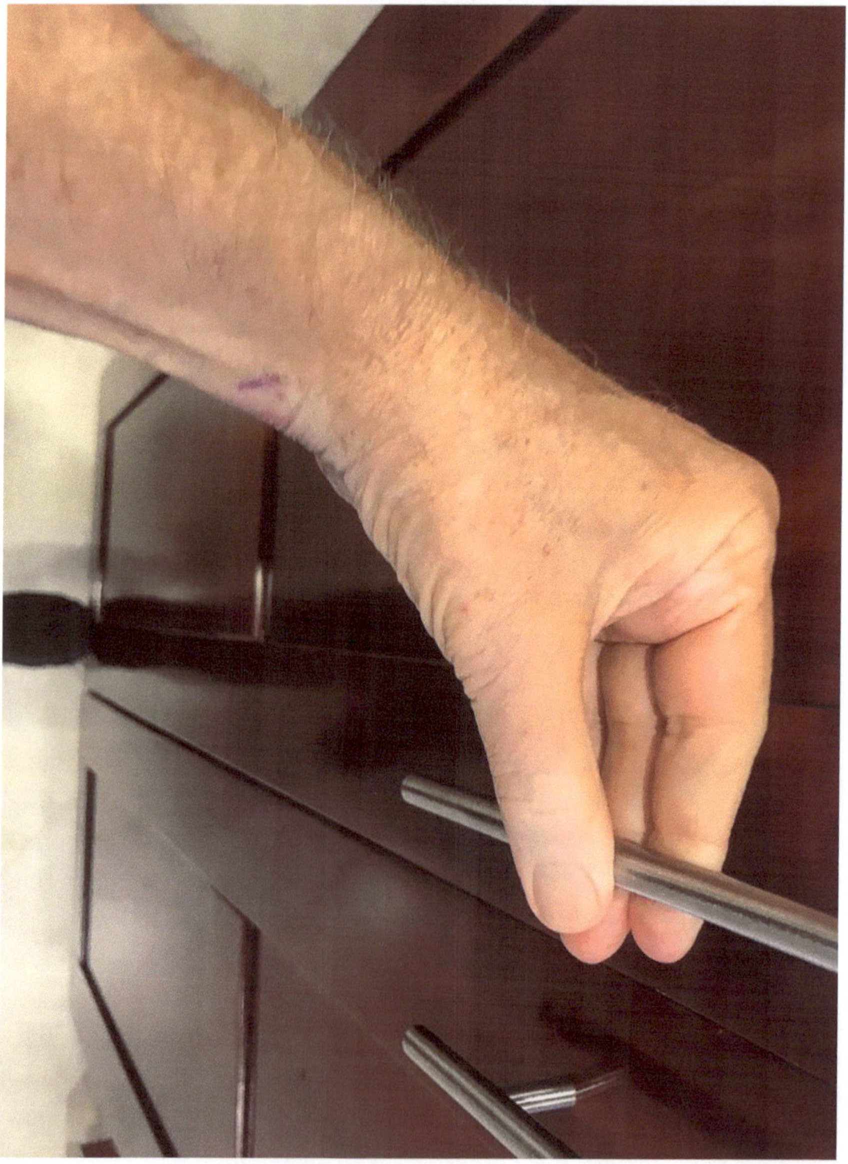

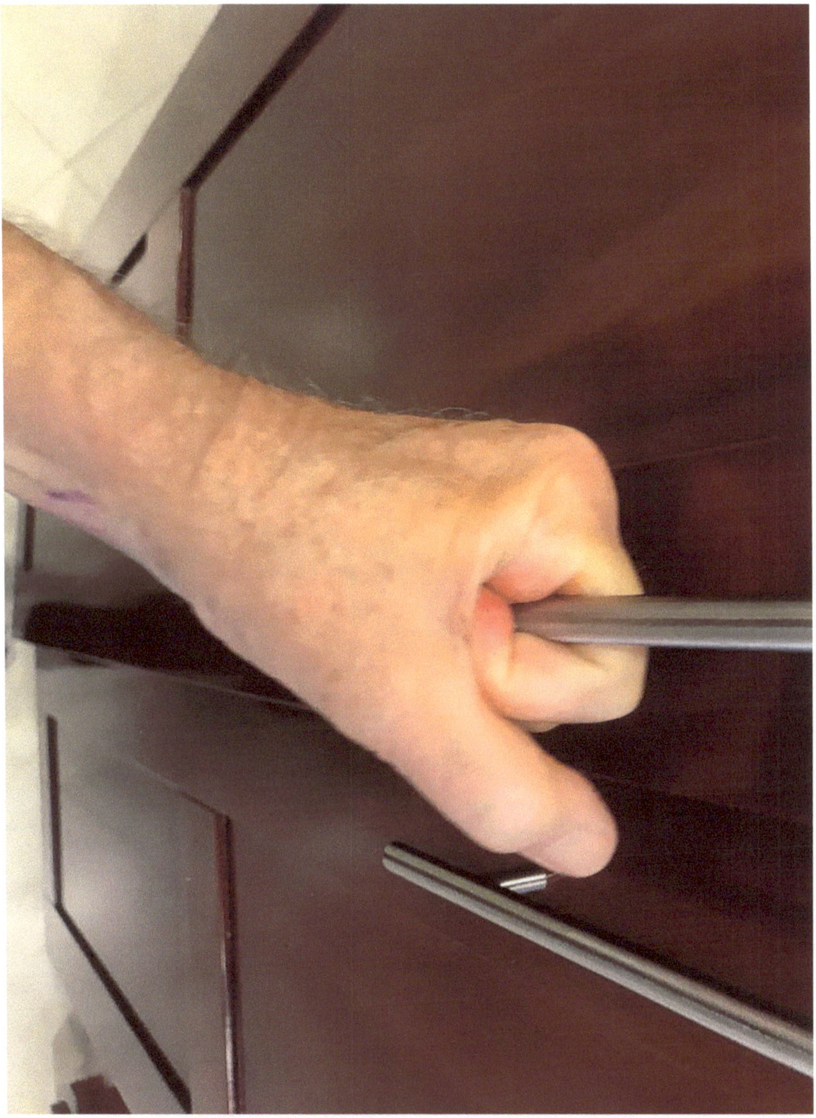

Figure 4-14a and b: Painful position for activity (top) and the painless position for activity (bottom) on day one as experienced by the author (CMJ) on POD #1.

Acute CTS on previously asymptomatic CTS in mildly angulated distal radius fracture

Carpal tunnel release is recommended for acute carpal tunnel syndrome in distal radius fractures. In some complex fractures, the release is sometimes done open at the two trapezial attachments of the transverse carpal ligament, as part of the approach to the very distal radius.

This case is unusual in that the carpal tunnel symptoms arose in a patient with a relatively minor (in terms of displacement or angulation) distal radius fracture. She had no previous carpal tunnel symptoms. Two hours after arrival in the ER, she developed numbness in the median nerve distribution.

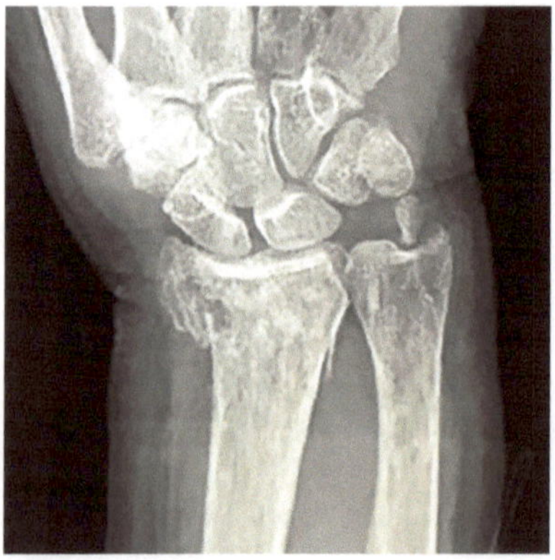

Figure 4-15a

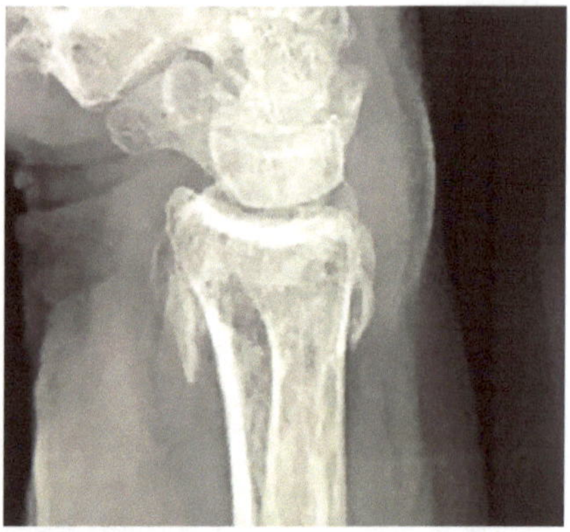

Figure 15b

Figs. 15a and b: AP and Lateral x-rays of the right wrist of a 72 year-old female with no neurologic symptoms pre- or immediately post-injury.

After induction of anesthesia, while preparing for an external fixator, a diagnostic ultrasound was carried out to look for a cause of the acute CTS, such as a hematoma or bone fragment.

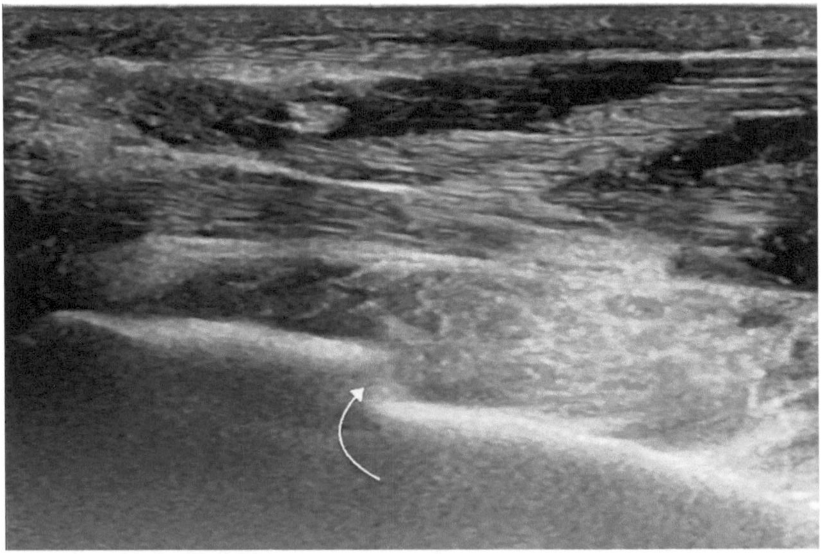

Figure 4-16a: On US, we see the small displacement of the fracture (arrow), minor angulation, and some swelling of the overlying pronator quadratus. Note the increased echogenicity of the pronator compared to the overlying flexors. We do not see any hematoma or bone fragments. There was no traumatic source for her nerve symptoms and so a routine carpal tunnel ultrasound evaluation was performed.

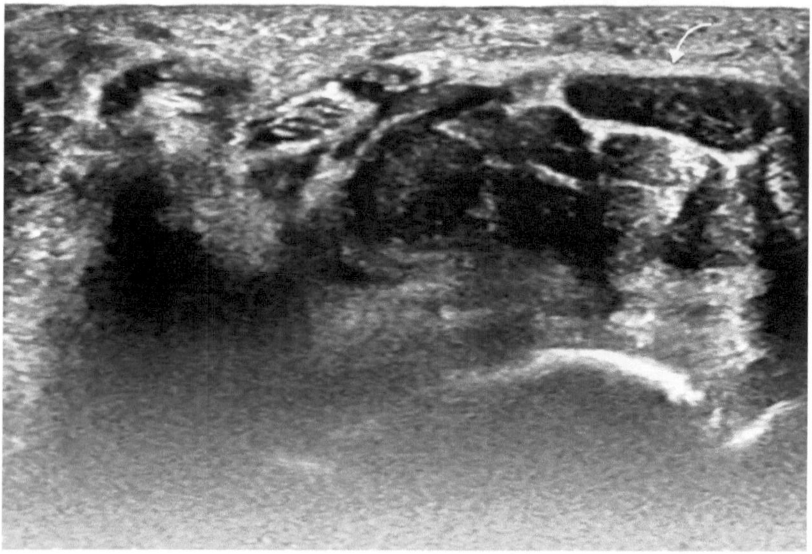

Figure 4-16b: A short-axis view of the nerve (arrow) taken at the entrance to the canal over the lunate, at the bottom. The cross-sectional area is at least twice what was seen over the pronator, and the "honey comb" architecture is gone, indicating a pre-existing chronic CTS.

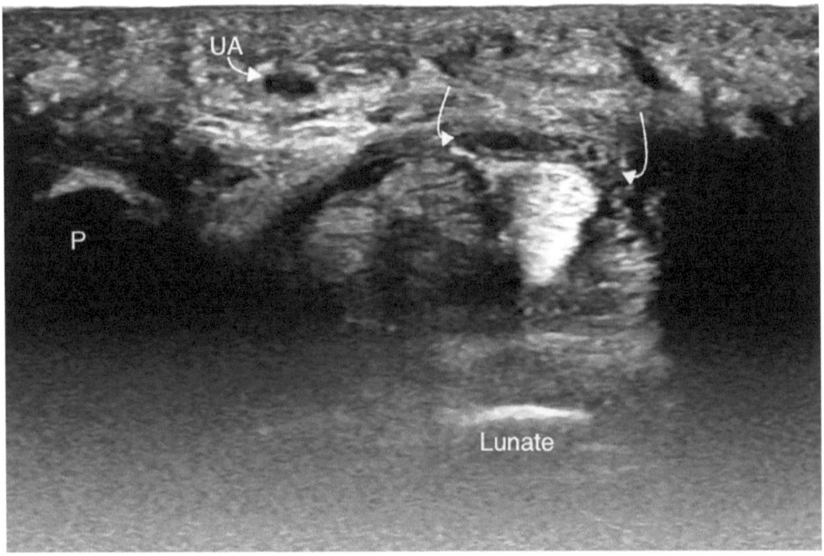

Figure 4-16c: A short-axis view of the narrowed and especially flattened median nerve in the canal, at the level of the pisiform (P) where the ulnar artery (UA) is visualized in the top left. Compare the degree of narrowing with large cross section seen proximal to the canal in Figure16b.

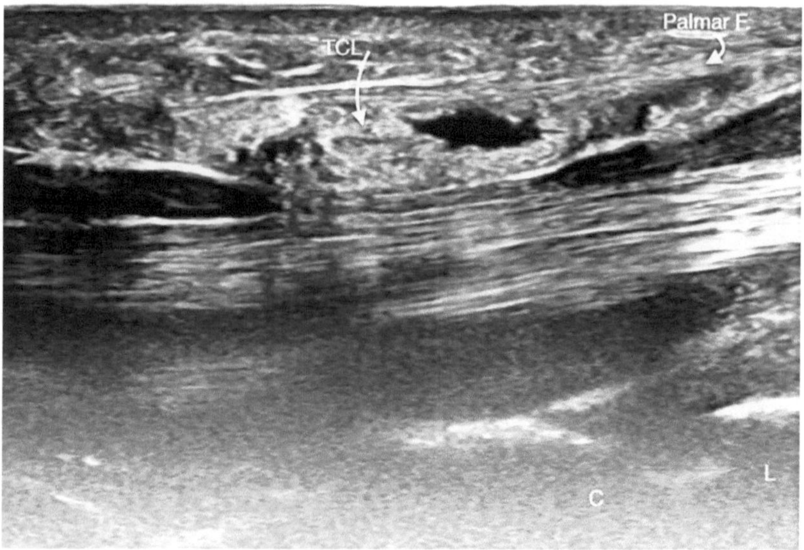

Figure 4-16d: Traditionally, compression in the long axis is not the proper way to diagnose CTS, but this is a dramatic demonstration of the compression under the transverse carpal ligament (TCL) and the lack of any other abnormality impinging on the nerve. L: lunate; C: capitate.

Though her chronic CTS was found in an unusual way as the fracture appeared to only cause slight worsening of local swelling, concomitant release was done under ultrasound guidance during the same operation the radial fixator was applied, and she had no numbness on post op day one.

Canal abnormalities
Possible contraindications
Rheumatoid Tenosynovitis
"Horseshoe Synovitis"
An absolute contraindication for USCTR

Open teno-synovectomy for rheumatoid arthritis is now rarely performed, but it may be required when the site-specific inflammation is resistant to treatment that is otherwise efficacious to other joints. This patient was referred with carpal tunnel symptoms. On physical exam she had only mild swelling, whereas, on ultrasound, there was significant synovitis (Figs. 17a and b) causing compression. Additionally, the synovitis appeared to be a source of scarring around the nerve. This would be a contraindication to the minimally invasive approach.

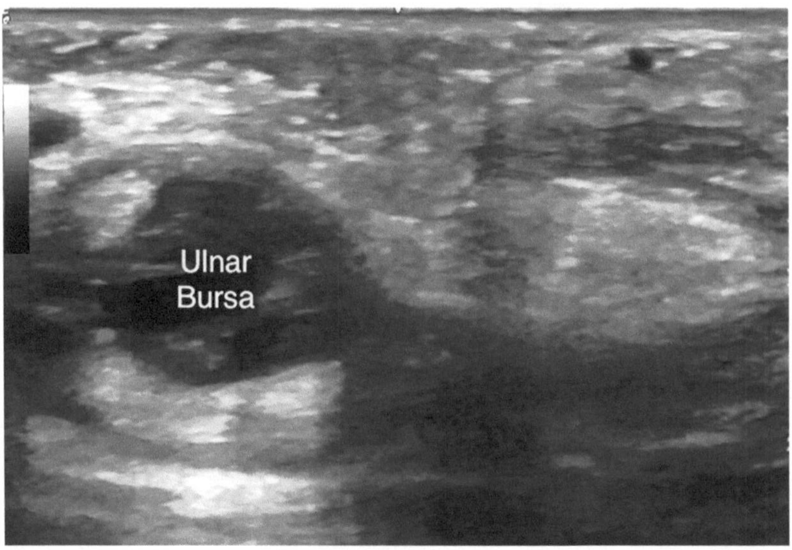

Figure 4-17a: Ulnar bursa. The hypoechoic ulnar bursa is seen on the left with the hyperechoic tendons, one to the volar-ulnar corner (upper left) and three on the dorsum (lower).

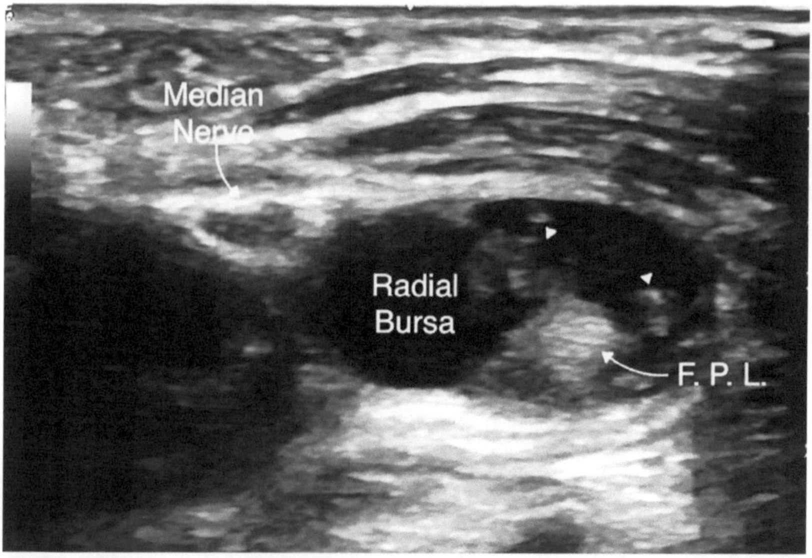

Figure 4-17b: Radial bursa. The radial bursa is on the right with the flexor pollicis longus (F.P.L.) underneath the thenar muscles. The arrowheads point to small 'rice bodies' in the bursa. The junction of the two bursae is deep to the median nerve, and proximal to the canal. The sheaths of the index, long, and ring fingers were free of disease in this hand. An open release and synovectomy were performed.

Carpal Tunnel Release
Reverse Palmaris Longus
Probably not a contraindication

A reverse palmaris might appear to be a significant obstacle to the release of the carpal tunnel when scanning proximal to the TCL. However, at this proximal end of the tunnel, there are more pliable surrounding soft tissues that allow maneuverability on hydro-dissection. In addition, the muscle seems to end on the proximal TCL.

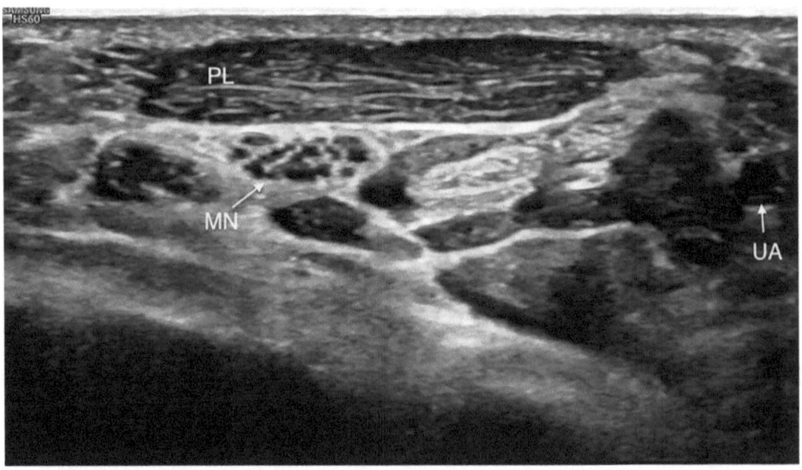

Figure 4-18a: Just proximal to the wrist, the muscle belly of the reverse palmaris would seem to obliterate the safe zone between median nerve (MN) and ulnar artery (UA).

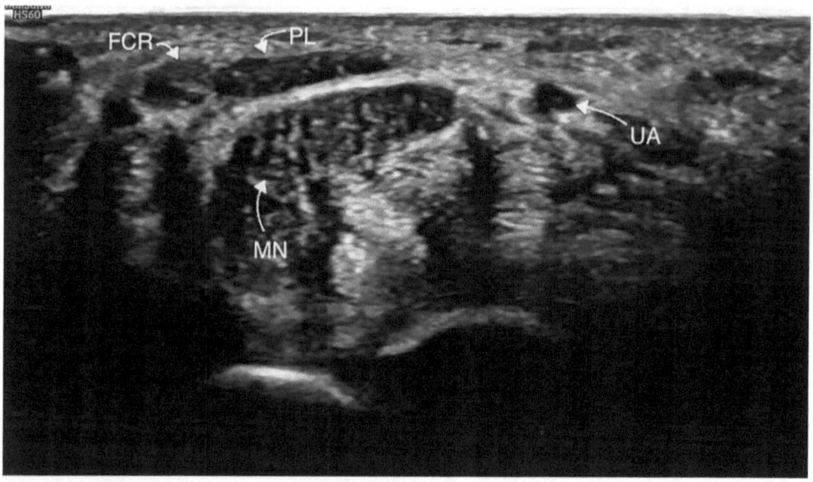

Figure 4-18b: At the level of the lunate, the palmaris (PL) is much narrower, but the large swollen median nerve (MN) is now narrowing the safe zone between nerve and ulnar artery.

Note that the normal "honeycomb" appearance of the MN is altered, especially when compared to the cross section area of that in Figure 18A.

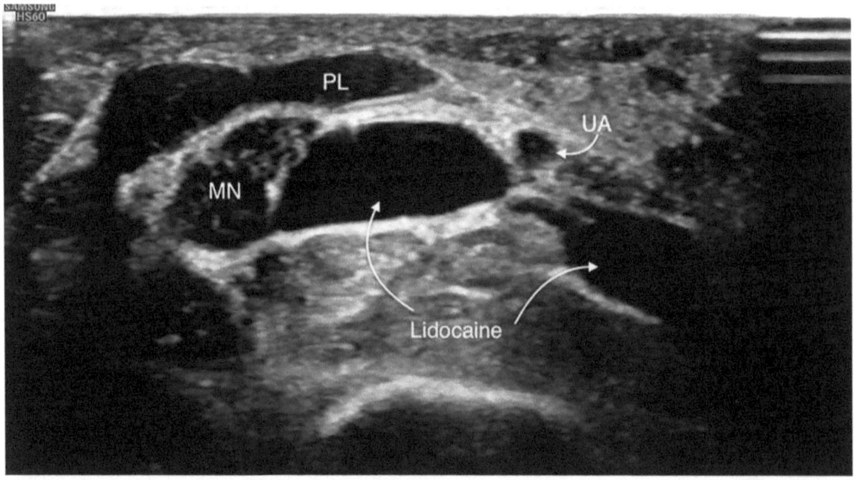

Figure 4-18c: In the proximal hydro-dissection, the anesthetic separates the nerve and artery creating a wider space. As the carpal tunnel arrangement was more typical from this point distally, the release was performed under ultrasound guidance in the usual fashion.

With the anesthetic pushing the palmaris radially, there is enough room for the usual ultrasound guided release technique. A contraindication to this technique would be inability to create adequate space at this level due to palmaris immobility.

Large Median Artery
Contraindication

Blood vessels, especially veins, can be at risk in the carpal canal. This danger can be obviated if hydro-dissection pushes the vessel away from the area of release. The median artery, and more importantly, its venae commitantes are unfortunately anchored at both ends of the canal and cannot be moved. In these cases, the decision is based on the size of the vessel. This example illustrates that cross section area of the very large median artery, a vessel larger than the radial artery. This case was done open, which demonstrated veins unseen in the pre-op US.

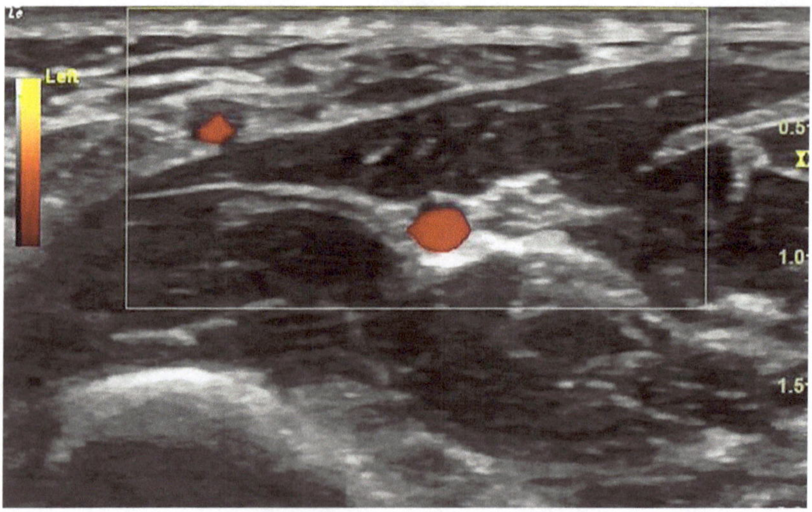

Figure 4-19: The larger of the two arteries is the median artery traveling just to the left of the median nerve. The smaller artery is the radial artery.

A median artery is generally seen only with a bifid medial nerve. In this case we could not see the split in the nerve until a more distal location.

The fact that the veins were compressed would seem to make it difficult to slide instruments past them without tearing them.

Other Encroachments on the Safe Zone

Encroachment on the safe zone may be a relative or absolute contraindication for ultrasound-guided carpal tunnel release (USCTR). This encroachment may be in the form of an unusually placed artery or nerve. With experience these encroachments may become more relative.

Ulnar sided nerve

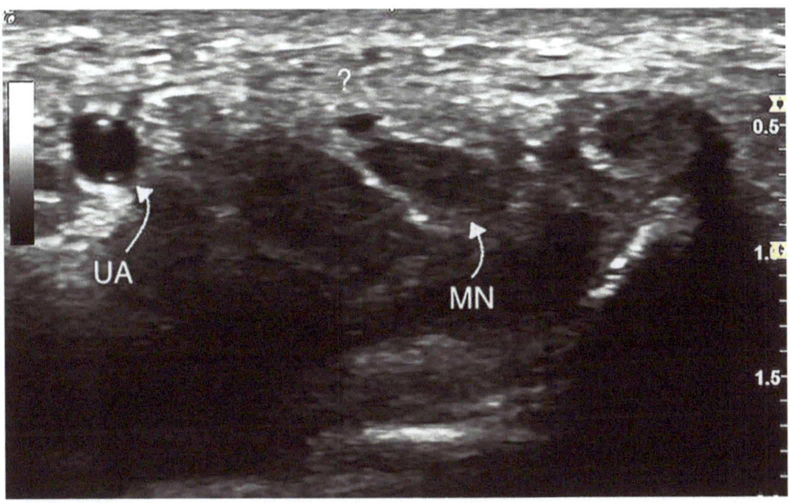

Figure 4-20: A short-axis view of the canal at the proximal end, roughly at the level of the scaphoid. There is an extra nerve to the ulnar side of the median nerve. Tracing the nerve both proximally and distally demonstrates this more likely a long palmar cutaneous branch rather than a motor nerve. In either event, we don't want to cut it, so we want to maintain its visibility.

The decision should be made earlier, during the diagnostic exam, as to the width of the safe zone in order to maintain flexibility to convert to an open procedure at the time of scheduling if necessary.

The artery and nerve are too close: distal

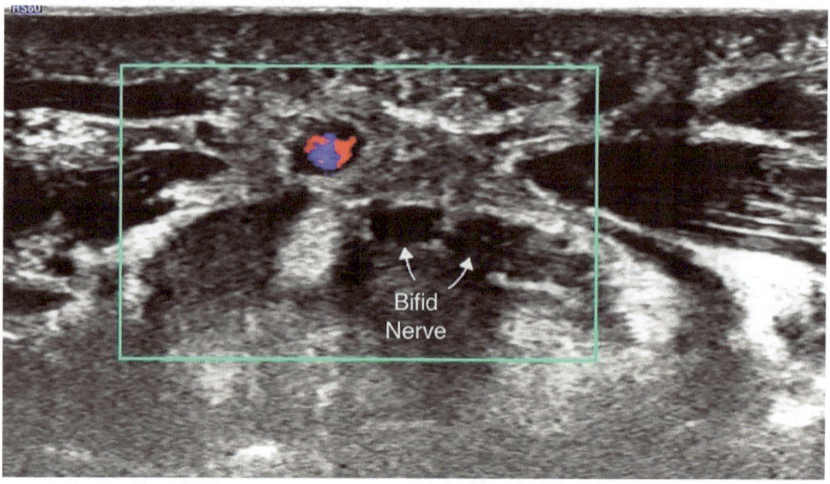

Figure 4-21: The ulnar artery comes out onto the transverse carpal ligament so that at the distal end of the canal there is no space between the artery and the ulnar edge of the bifid nerve.

This hand was released in an open fashion.

De Quervain's Tenosynovitis

De Quervain's tenosynovitis is a painful tendonitis of the first dorsal compartment of the wrist. Traditionally, it was thought to primarily affect females between the ages of 20 and 40, although recent data suggests it may actually be more common after age 40. (6) It typically presents as pain and swelling over the radial side of the wrist, exacerbated by lifting and pinching activities. Patients typically have tenderness to palpation over first dorsal compartment and a positive Finkelstein/Eichoff test.

Examination of the first dorsal compartment is performed by resting the ulnar border of the forearm and wrist against the examination table and allowing the fingers to fall into a normal resting posture. .A) The radial styloid is palpated and the probe is placed in the short axis at this location. Scanning is performed from distal to proximal. The author prefers to utilize a small footprint probe. The abductor pollicis longus (volar) and extensor pollicis brevis (dorsal) are identified (Figure 22b). The first dorsal compartment is evaluated for the presence or absence of an intra-compartmental septum, for multiple splits of the APL, and for inflammatory fluid/tenosynovitis around the tendons (Figure 22c). It is important to evaluate for the septum proximal to the tip of the radial styloid. Of note, a false positive exam for a septum can be mistakenly made distal to the styloid, where the first compartment ends, and the tendons naturally separate, mimicking a septal appearance. Cadaver studies have demonstrated the presence of an intra-compartmental septum in 40-75% of subjects. (7) Presence of an intra-compartmental septum has been associated with failure of non-operative treatment. (8) In addition, identification of an intra-compartmental septum may allow the examiner to simultaneously inject both compartments.

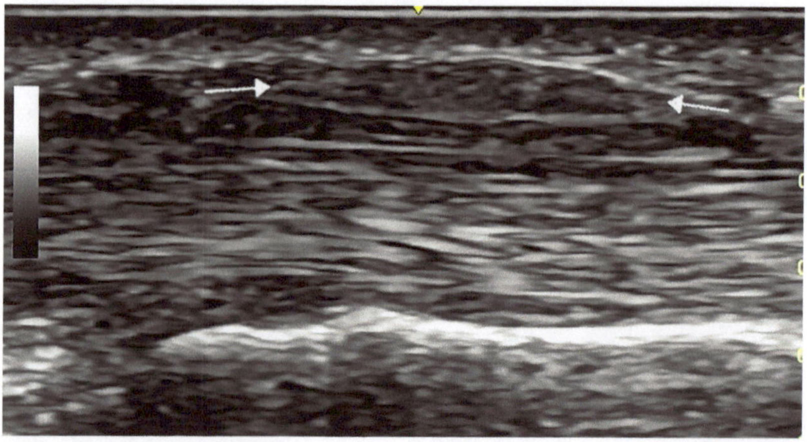

Figure 4-22a: A long axis view of the first extensor compartment. Distal lies to the left. Between the two arrows, we see the thickened pulley of that compartment.

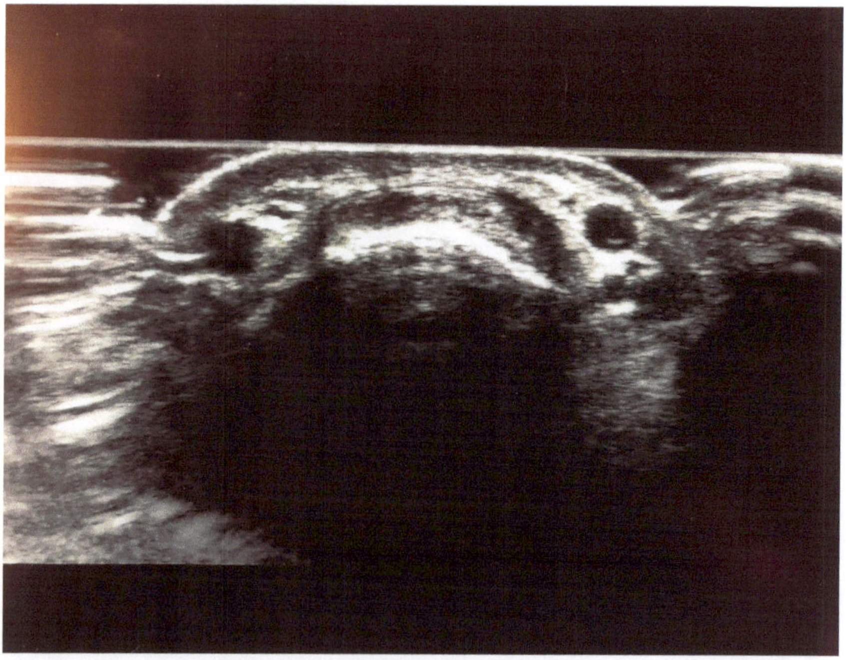

Figure 4-22b: Normal anatomy of the 1st dorsal compartment showing the abductor pollicis longus and extensor pollicis brevis.

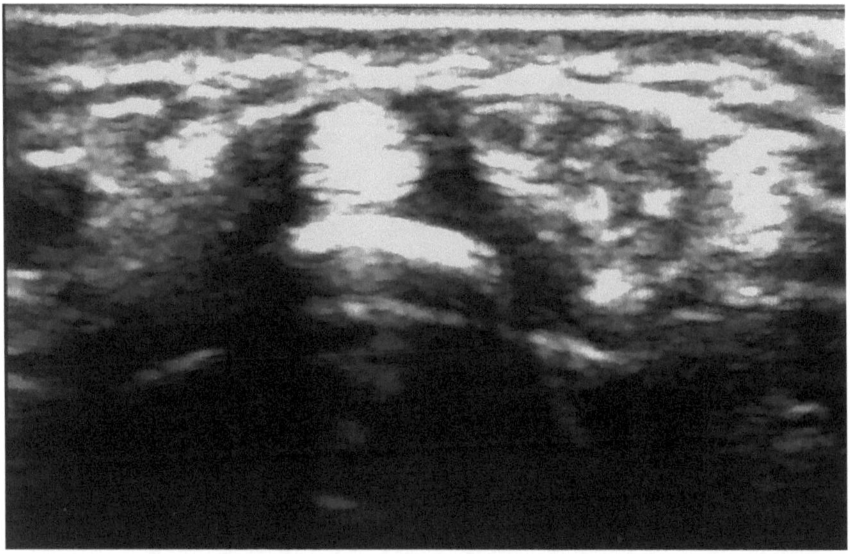

Figure 4-22c: Ultrasound examination showing a separate subcompartment for the extensor pollicis brevis

Ultrasound guidance for injection improves the accuracy of intra-compartment injection, particularly in patients with an intra-compartmental septum. Kutsikovich and Merrell found that ultrasound guidance resulted in injection of dye into both compartments in 75% of patients compared to only 33% using a landmark based technique.(9) A small footprint probe is placed in the short axis just proximal to the radial styloid. After sterile prep, a 25-gauge needle is introduced in line with the probe from the dorsal side. The dorsal approach is preferred to avoid the radial artery, however, there is often a large dorsal vein in this area that also must be avoided. Briefly decreasing the pressure on the ultrasound probe will make the vein more apparent. The needle is advanced under ultrasound guidance into the first dorsal compartment and the injection is performed (Fig. 22d). If an intra-compartmental septum is present, half of the injection is placed in each compartment.

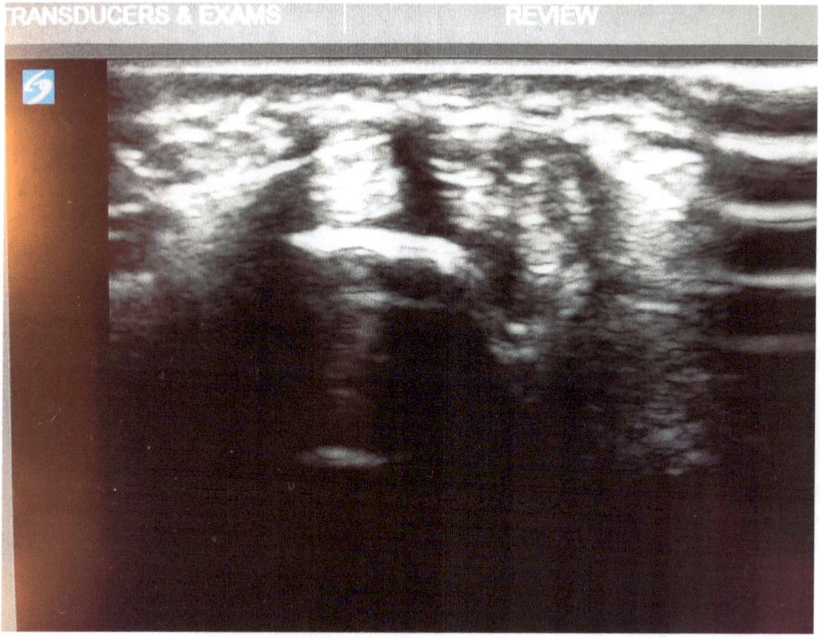

Figure 4-22d: Ultrasound-guided injection of the first dorsal compartment. The needle is typically advanced from dorsal to volar to avoid injury to the radial artery. Note that the long abductor is larger than the round short extensor; additionally, the abductor often has more than one tendon slip.

Wrist Masses

The differential diagnosis for a wrist mass is vast, but most commonly includes ganglion cyst, lipoma, tenosynovitis, giant cell tumor of tendon sheath, hemangioma, and arteriovenous malformation, amongst other. Ganglion cysts are fluid filled masses that emanate from joints or tendon sheaths (Fig. 23A).

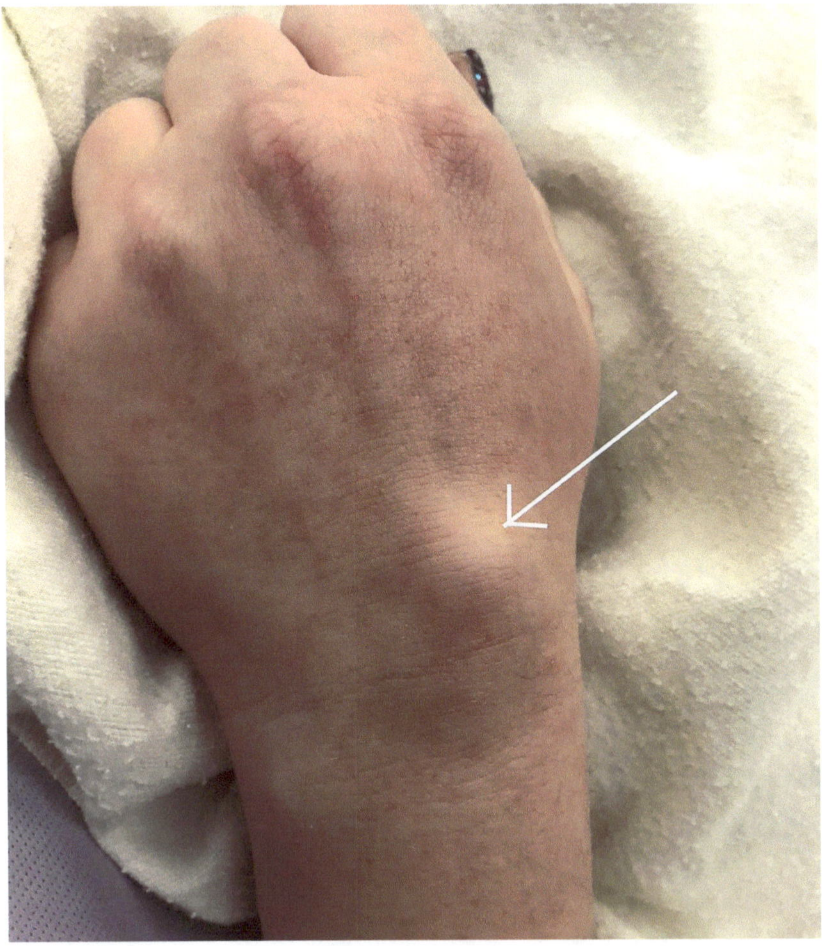

Figure 4-23a: Clinical picture of a typical dorsal ganglion cyst.

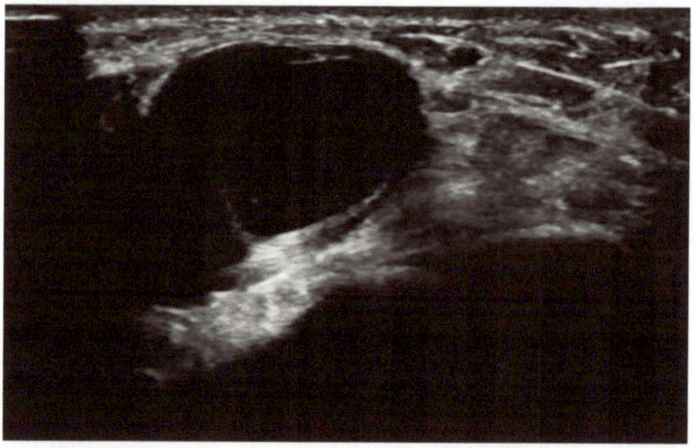

Figure 4-23b: Short axis ultrasound demonstrating a homogenous anechoic mass consistent with a ganglion cyst.

While the diagnosis is often easily made with clinical examination and transillumination, ultrasound can provide confirmation and rule out other diagnoses. In addition, ultrasound can assist in the diagnosis of dorsal occult ganglion cysts in patients who present with dorsal wrist pain without obvious mass (Fig. 23C).

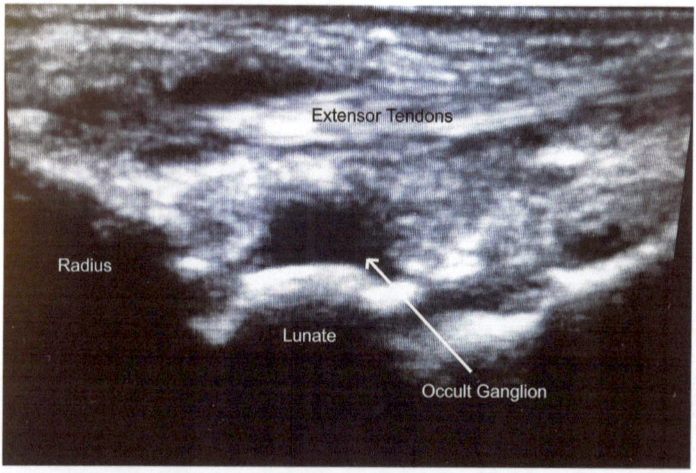

Figure 4-23c: Long axis ultrasound examination of the wrist demonstrating an "occult" ganglion cyst coming off the scapholunate interval, but remaining deep to the extensor tendons.

Extensor tenosynovitis, most commonly of the fourth compartment, is most commonly seen in rheumatoid arthritis (Fig. 24).

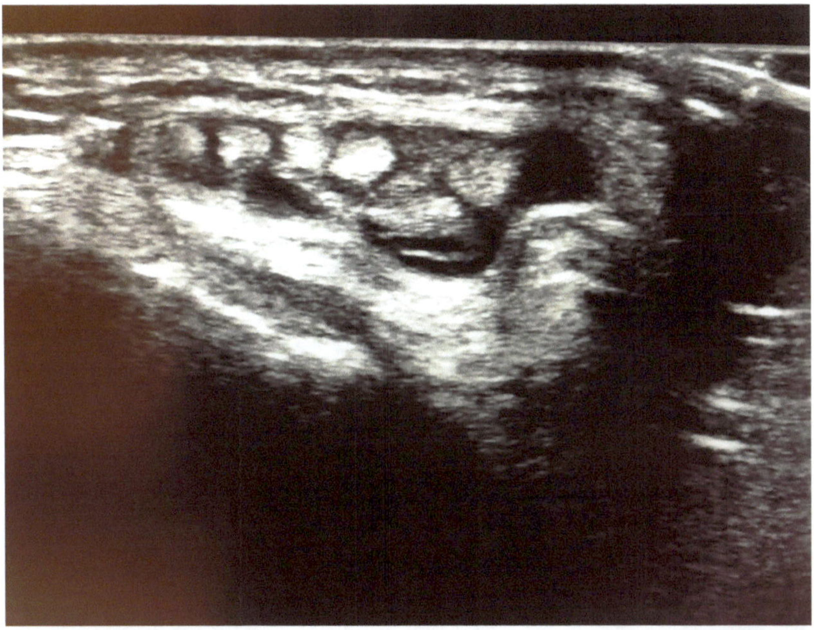

Figure 4-24: Short axis ultrasound examination of the dorsum of the wrist showing extensor tenosynovitis. Note how the hypoechoic fluid is around the extensor tendons rather than directly from the joint, which distinguishes this from a dorsal ganglion cyst.

However, proliferative extensor tenosynovitis an also be found in non-rheumatoid patients.(10) VanHeest described fourth compartment extensor tenosynovitis in athletes who performed repetitive hyperextension activities.(11) Tenosynovitis, particularly extensor tenosynovitis, can be differentiated from a ganglion cyst by lack of transillumination and observable movement with dynamic flexion and extension of the fingers. Ultrasound examination will demonstrate homogenous hypoechogenic fluid around the tendons. An ultrasound-guided injection can be performed into the tenosynovium. Hemangiomas and arteriovenous malformations/aneurysms will demonstrate vascular flow using the color Doppler feature. Hemangiomas may have calcifications within the mass. Giant cell tumor of tendon sheath typically presents as a "spongy" mass in the hand or fingers, distinguishing itself from ganglion cysts by its feel, lack of transillumination, and less distinct borders. Ultrasound examination reveals a hypoechoic nodule with heterogeneous contents, which provides stark contrast from a simple fluid-filled ganglion. These lesions often have vascular flow using color Doppler.(12) A potential benefit of ultrasound examination is determining the extent of the mass (within the tendon sheath, coming from the joint, etc.) to ensure complete excision at the time of surgery. ultrasound can also be used for follow-up for recurrence.

For examination of the dorsum of the wrist, the volar forearm is placed flat on the exam table with the wrist in neutral alignment and fingers fully extended. The probe is first placed in the short axis at the level of Lister's tubercle and the wrist is scanned from proximal to distal (Fig. 25).

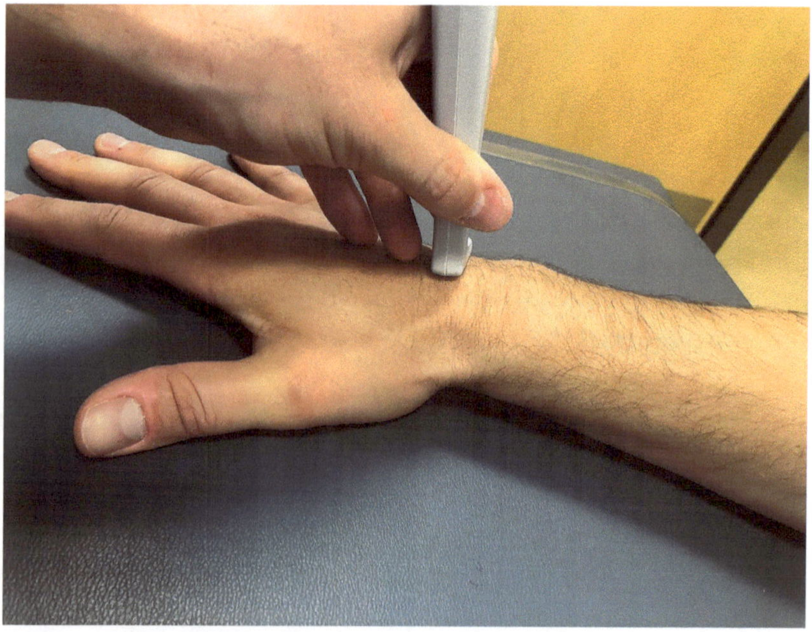

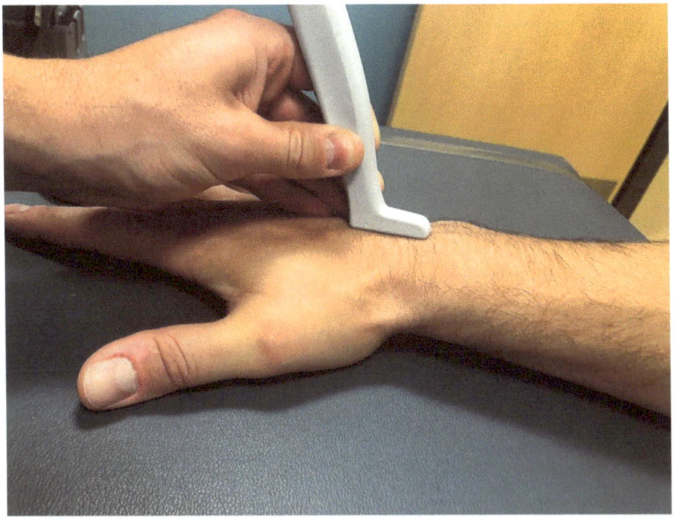

Figure 4-25a and b: Clinical photograph demonstrating positioning for a) short axis and b) long axis examination for dorsal wrist masses.

Ganglion cysts will appear hypoechogenic and homogenous. For typical wrist dorsal ganglion cysts, the connection to the scapholunate ligament (the "stalk") can often be identified. The mass is then scanned in the long axis (Fig. 26).

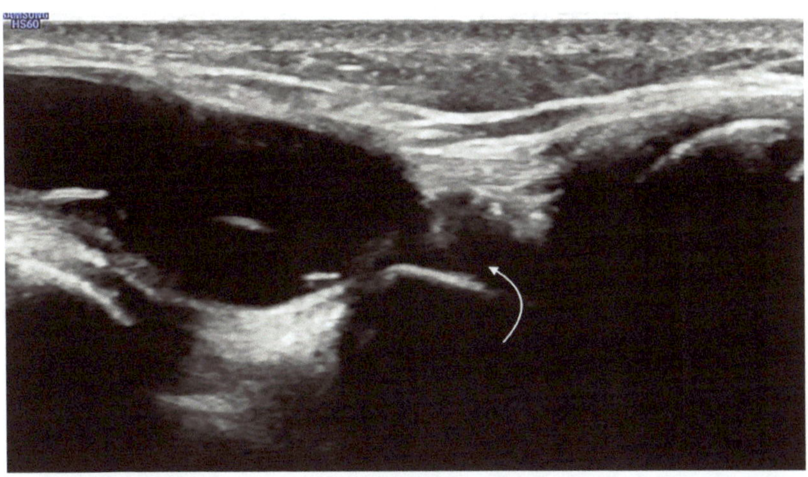

Figure 4-26: Long axis ultrasound demonstrating the "stalk" of a dorsal wrist ganglion coming from the scapholunate interval.

The color Doppler mode is used to ensure that there is no vascular flow through the soft tissue mass, thereby eliminating an arteriovenous malformation and/or hemangioma as the etiologic source. For occult dorsal ganglion cysts, long axis scanning will identify a homogenous hypoechoic mass deep to the extensor tendons, emanating from the scapholunate interval. If desired, ultrasound guidance can be utilized for ganglion aspiration and/or injection.

For volar wrist masses, the dorsal forearm is placed flat on the table with the wrist in neutral alignment and the fingers in the normal resting cascade. As these masses typically originate on the radial side, the examination is focused on this area. The probe is placed in the short axis a few centimeters proximal to the mass and scanning is performed from proximal to distal. Again, ganglion cysts will appear hypoechogenic and homogenous. The color Doppler is used to identify the radial artery and to ensure absence of communication with the mass (Fig. 27). (Fowler 12 is of a short axis ultrasound of a volar ganglion cyst just superficial to the radial artery.)

The mass is also scanned in the long axis. If desired, ultrasound guidance can be utilized for ganglion aspiration and/or injection, taking care to avoid the radial artery.

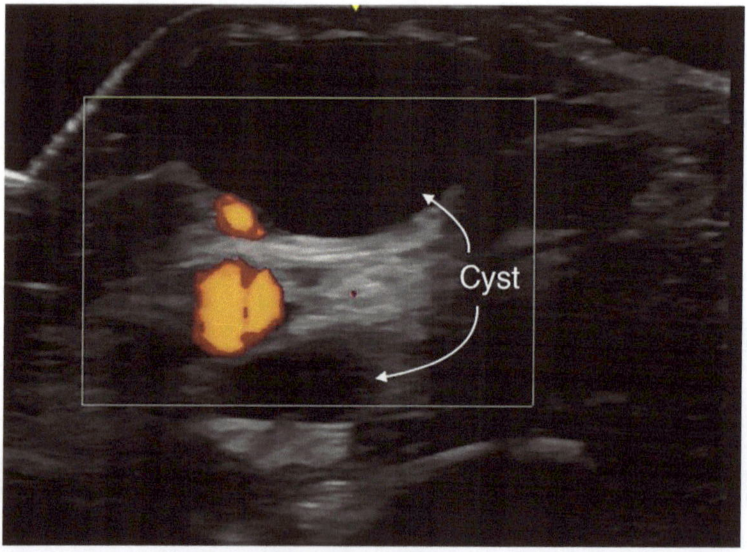

Figure 4-27: For a volar ganglion, the surgeon can appreciate the relationship of the cyst to the radial artery.

Extensor Carpi Ulnaris

The extensor carpi ulnaris (ECU) passes through a fibro-osseus sheath in the sixth dorsal wrist compartment (Figs. 28a and b).

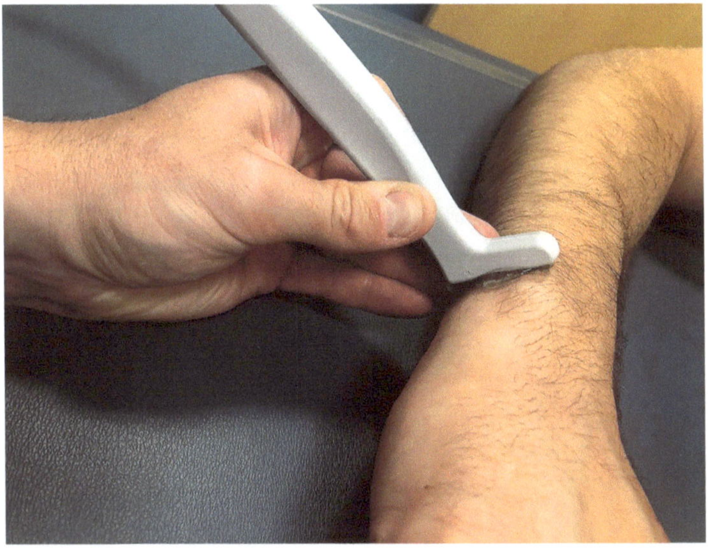

Figure 28a Positioning for short axis evaluation of the extensor carpi ulnaris;

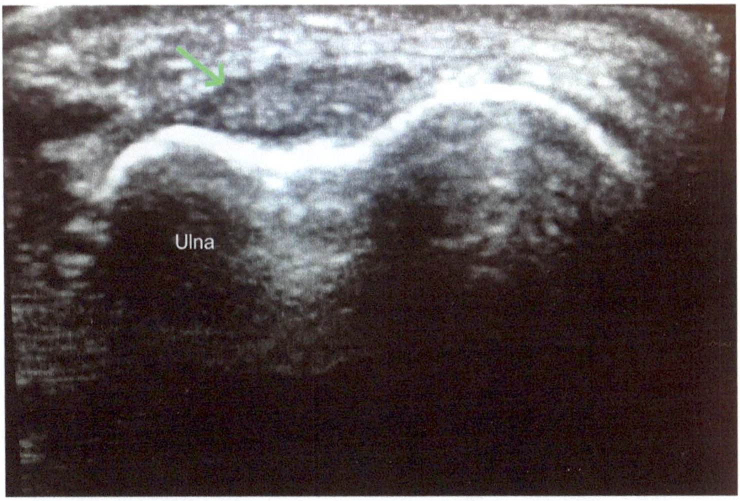

Figure 4-28b Normal appearance of the extensor carpi ulnaris.

The ECU is subject to extensor tenosynovitis, longitudinal split tears, and instability in the form of subluxation and/or frank dislocation. The presence of abnormalities on ultrasound examination should be carefully correlated with the history and physical examination, as there is a high incidence of structural abnormalities in asymptomatic individuals. For example, Sole and colleagues found that 75% of wrists in asymptomatic tennis players had a static abnormality (most commonly a partial-thickness tear), and 42% had dynamic instability (13). In addition, Erickson et al. found that 64% of ECU tendons in a cadaver model had a distal longitudinal split tear(14).

Patients may present with ulnar-sided clicking/clunking with forearm supination and pronation. In particular, ulnar deviation and supination (the "ice-cream scoop" maneuver) may exacerbate the click. Inoue and Tamura described three types of fibro-osseous sheath disruption (Fig. 29. Redraw Inoue and Tamura classification)(15).

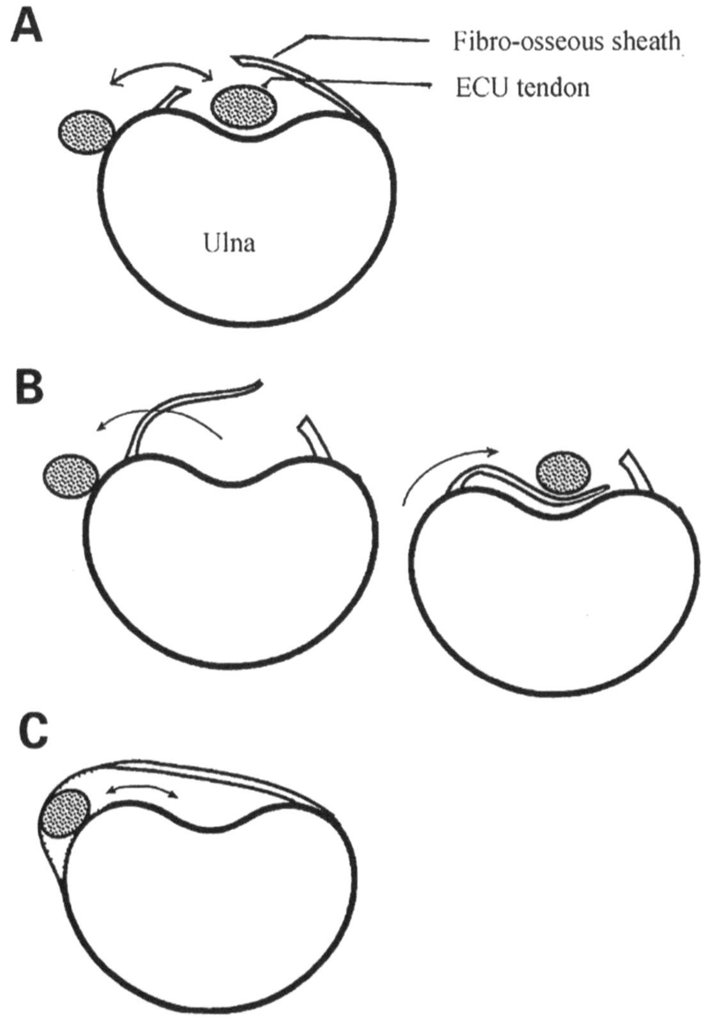

Figure 4-29: Inoue and Tamura classification for extensor carpi ulnaris tendon sheath tears. Type A: the sheath is disrupted from the ulnar side, and the tendon may remain deep to the sheath; Type B" the sheath is disrupted from the radial side and the tendon is superficial to the sheath, preventing healing; Type C: the tendon subluxates or dislocates into a false pouch formed from stripping of the subsheath from the ulna. (Inoue G, Tamura Y. Surgical treatment for recurrent dislocation of the extensor carpi ulnaris tendon. J Hand Surg Br. 2001; 26(6): 556-559.)

Type A disruptions involve rupture of the sheath ulnarly with the sheath still superficial to the ECU tendon. Type B disruptions involve rupture of the sheath radially with the sheath deep to the ECU. Type C involve periosteal detachment of the sheath from the ulnar side resulting in a false pouch into which the ECU dislocates. These abnormalities are able to be visualized using ultrasound, which is demonstrated in Fig. 30.

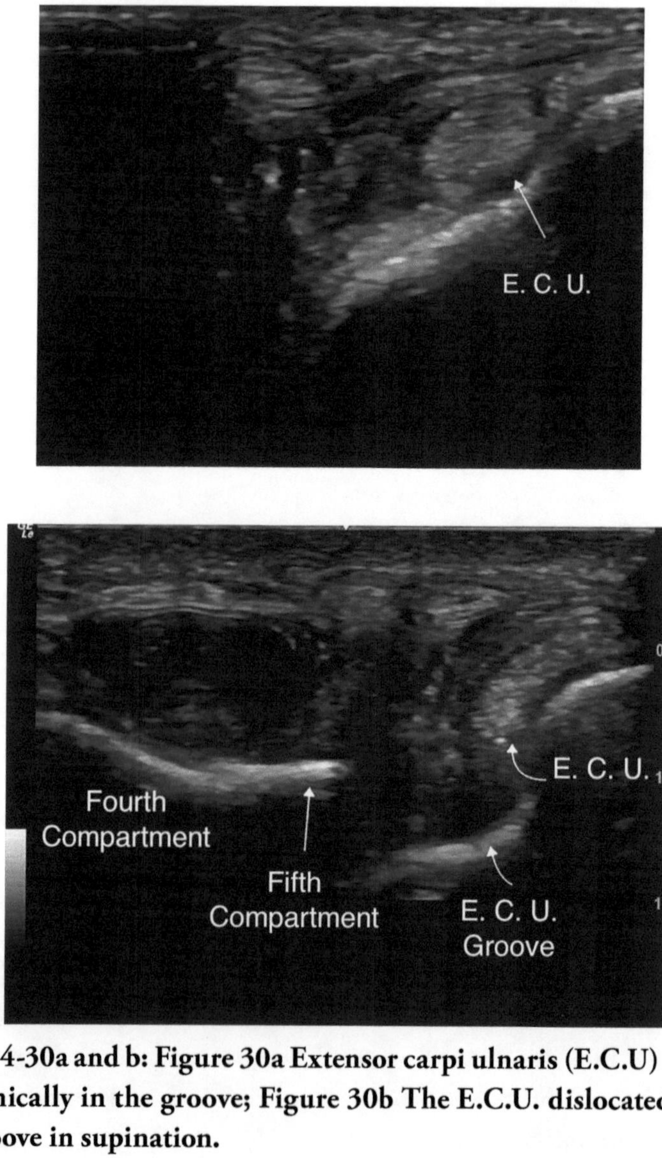

Figure 4-30a and b: Figure 30a Extensor carpi ulnaris (E.C.U) located anatomically in the groove; Figure 30b The E.C.U. dislocated out of the groove in supination.

The patient is seated across from the examiner and has the tip of the olecranon resting on a towel in approximately 90 degrees of flexion. The forearm is in neutral rotation and wrist in neutral flexion/extension. A small footprint probe is placed perpendicular to the long axis of the forearm over the ulnar head. Scanning is then performed in the radial/ulnar plane to identify the groove in the ulnar head, the ECU tendon, and the extensor retinaculum. While holding the probe in place, the forearm can be slowly supinated and pronated, and evaluation for subluxation/dislocation performed. The wrist can be brought into ulnar deviation with supination to increase the sensitivity for subluxation.

Thumb CMC Arthritis

Thumb carpometacarpal (CMC) arthritis is the most common arthritic condition of the hand, affecting women six times more frequently than men, with a prevalence of 25-33% in post-menopausal women (16, 17). While diagnosis and severity grading are more commonly performed using radiographs, ultrasound guidance for injections has recently gained popularity. In a cadaver model, To and colleagues noted 75% accuracy with ultrasound guidance compared to 50% accuracy using a landmark based technique (18). Pollard et al. found an accuracy of 100% for ultrasound guided injections compared to 82% for landmark based injections (19).

The patient is seated across from the examiner with the elbow flexed to approximately 90 degrees, and the ulnar border of the forearm resting on the examination table. The wrist is in neutral and fingers in the normal resting cascade. The forearm is placed perpendicular to the line between the examiner and patient. A small footprint probe is then placed parallel to the longitudinal axis of the thumb metacarpal at the level of the CMC joint (Fig. 31a). The base of the metacarpal and trapezium are identified. In the setting of CMC arthritis, there is often radial subluxation of the base of the metacarpal, osteophyte formation, and a joint effusion (Fig. 32b). After sterile skin prep, a 25-gauge needle is inserted from proximal to distal and the needle is guided into the CMC joint (Figure 16b).

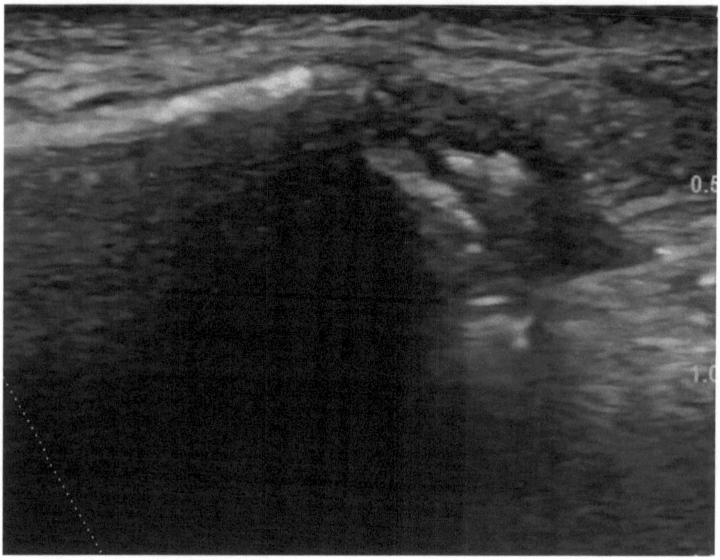

Figure 4-31a

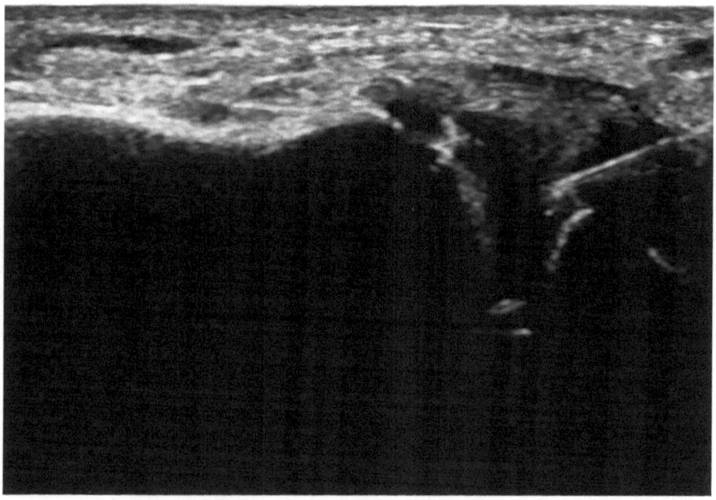

Figure 4-31a and b: Figure 31a Visual representation of the correct geographic location of the ultrasound probe demonstrating metacarpal base and trapezium at the level of the CMC joint. Figure 31b As the medication is injected, the joint will expand and trapezium translate away from the thumb metacarpal base. The mean volume capacity of the thumb CMC joint is approximately 1 ml (20).

Radiocarpal Injections

A number of conditions may benefit from an intra-articular radiocarpal injection, including a triangular fibrocartilage complex (TFCC) tear, crystalline arthropathy, radiocarpal arthritis, and wrist synovitis. In addition, aspiration of the radiocarpal joint under ultrasound guidance may give increased confidence that a "dry tap" was not actually just secondary to inability to penetrate of joint capsule and aspirate synovial fluid. In wrists without significant soft tissue swelling, palpation of bony landmarks and intervals is usually straightforward. However, the presence of soft tissue swelling may preclude examiners' ability to identify bony landmarks. Several studies have shown no difference in accuracy between ultrasound-guided and landmark-based radiocarpal injections (18, 21).

The patient is seated across from the examiner. The volar forearm is rested on the examination table with the wrist in neutral pronation/supination, the elbow flexed to 70-80 degrees, and fingers flat on the table. The probe is then placed in line with the longitudinal axis of the forearm at the level of Lister's tubercle. Scanning is performed in a proximal to distal fashion to identify the radius, lunate, and capitate. After sterile skin prep, the needle is inserted from a distal to proximal direction, in line with the probe, into the radiocarpal joint (Fig. 32).

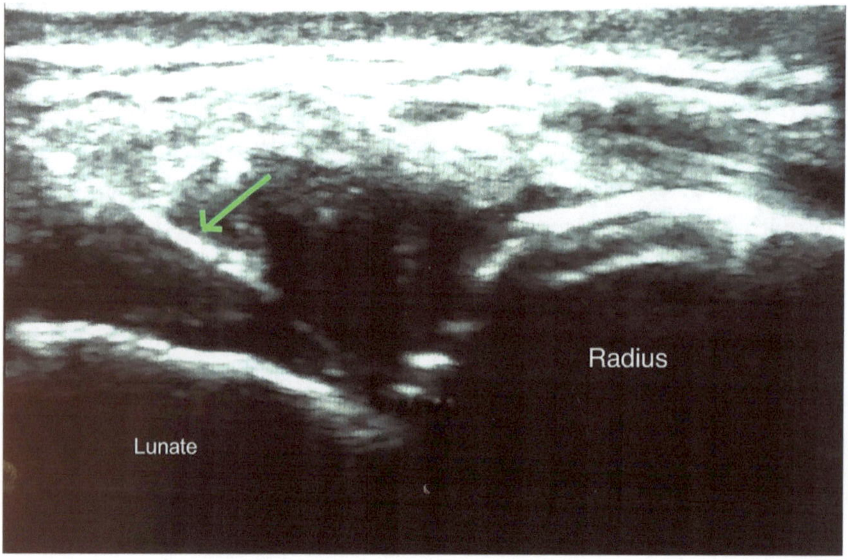

Figure 4-32: Long axis view of the radiocarpal joint demonstrating insertion a 25-gauge needle into the radiocarpal joint.

Intra-articular location is confirmed by easy flow of the medication into the joint with corresponding expansion of the joint on imaging.

Finger

Foreign Bodies in the Finger

Non-metallic foreign bodies are difficult, or even impossible, to visualize on plain radiographs, but can be easily identified with ultrasound. Bray and colleagues noted an incredible sensitivity of 94% and specificity of 99% for identification of foreign bodies in cadaver hands (22). Ultrasound can be helpful in planning incisions for foreign body removal and guiding surgical dissection.

For volar foreign bodies in the distal upper extremity, the finger is typically held by the examiner to stabilize the digit and allow manipulation during the examination. When examining fingers for foreign bodies, it is essential to use a large amount of ultrasound gel and a small footprint probe. This will allow better conduction and deeper propagation of the ultrasound waves, ultimately corresponding to better visualization of the foreign bodies on irregular surfaces such as a finger. The finger is scanned in both the long and short axis, slowly sliding the probe over the area of interest (Fig. 33). The patient is often very helpful in pointing out areas of maximal tenderness, allowing the examiner to focus his/her exam in this area.

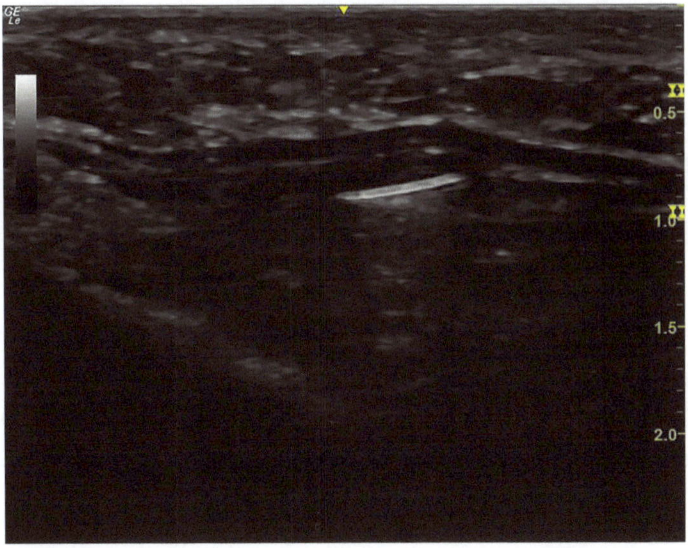

Figure 4-33a

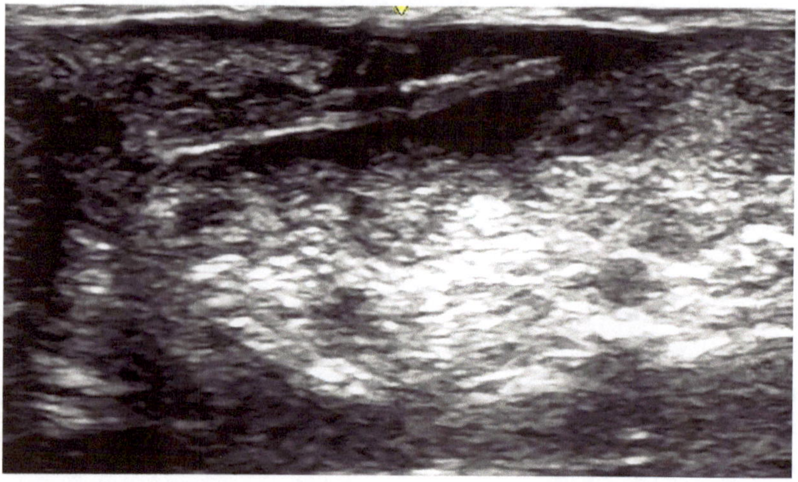

Figure 4-33b

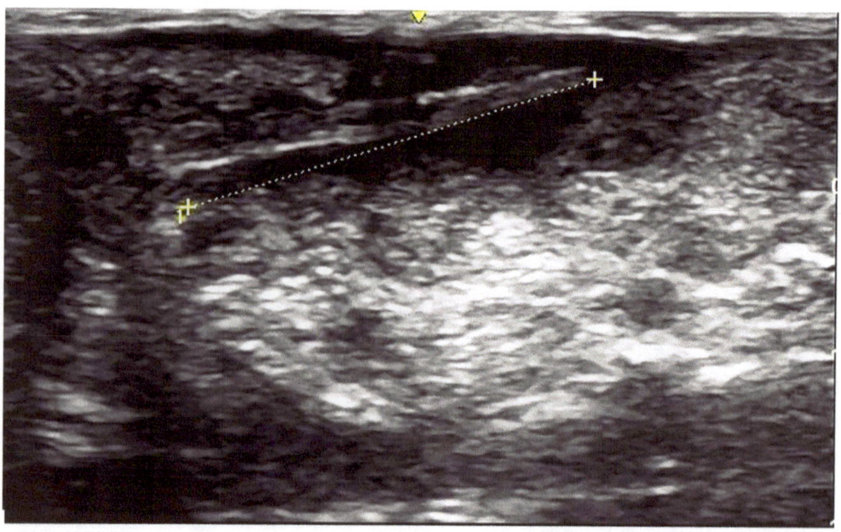

Figure 4-33c

Figure 4-33 a-c: Figure 33a: Long axis ultrasound image demonstrating a foreign body (a piece of glass) in the finger. Figure 33b and c. A piece of wood. The size of the piece of wood can be measured.

Ultrasound may have a role in the pre-operative evaluation of finger lacerations where there is concern of flexor tendon laceration. Clearly, physical examination is adequate in the vast majority of cases. However, ultrasound examination may supplement the physical examination, particularly in patients who may be fearful to move an injured finger. Lee et al. found a 90% accuracy when using ultrasound to pre-operatively evaluate the degree and location of presumed flexor tendon lacerations (23). The authors were able to identify the level of retraction of the proximal stump in the majority of complete flexor tendon lacerations, potentially altering the surgical plan by focusing the level of proximal dissection. In addition, ultrasound was able to determine the percentage of tendon injured in partial tendon lacerations. This could be useful information to the surgeon as a 25% partial laceration can likely be managed non-operatively, whereas a 75% partial laceration would represent an indication for surgical exploration and repair. In the post-operative period, ultrasound is also helpful to determine if lack of motion is due to adhesions or re-rupture. Jeyapalan and colleagues utilized ultrasound in 18 patients with lack of motion after flexor tendon repair and found that 15 of 18 tendons were intact (24). Surgery was avoided in those cases and the 3 with flexor tendon rupture confirmed on ultrasound examination were offered revision surgery.

When examining finger lacerations for flexor tendon lacerations, the dorsal forearm and dorsal hand are rested on the examination table (Fig. 34).

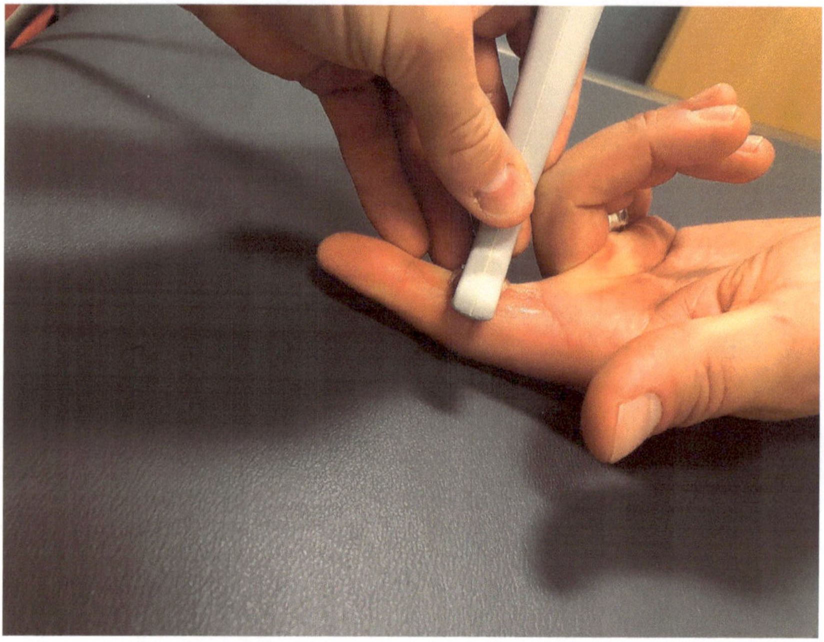

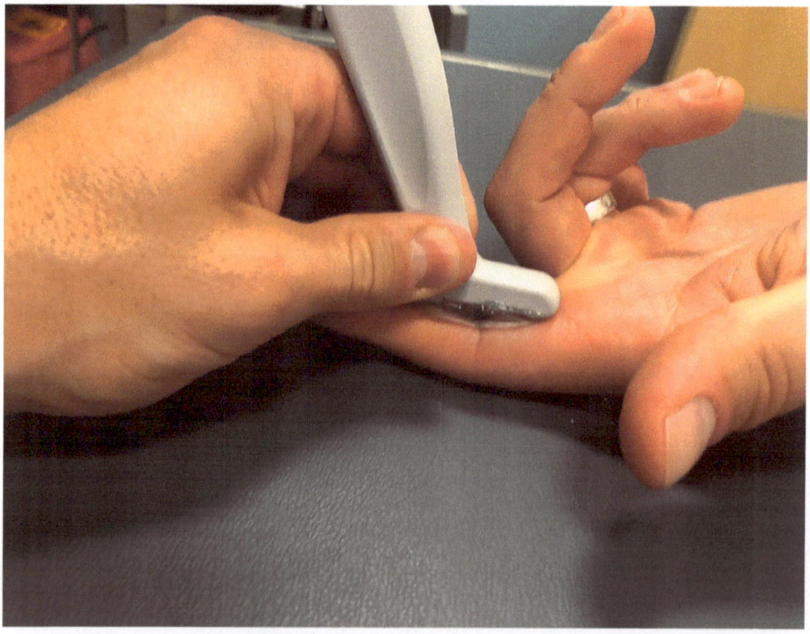

Figure 4-34a and b: Positioning for short axis (Figure 34a) and long axis (Figure 34b) flexor tendon evaluation (respectively).

The fingers are placed in extension to allow placement of the probe on the volar surface of the digit. A large amount of ultrasound gel is utilized and a small footprint probe used for the examination. Scanning is performed in both the short and long axis to visualize the flexor digitorum profundus (FDP) and flexor digitorum superficialis (FDS) (Figure 35 – image showing flexor tendon laceration).

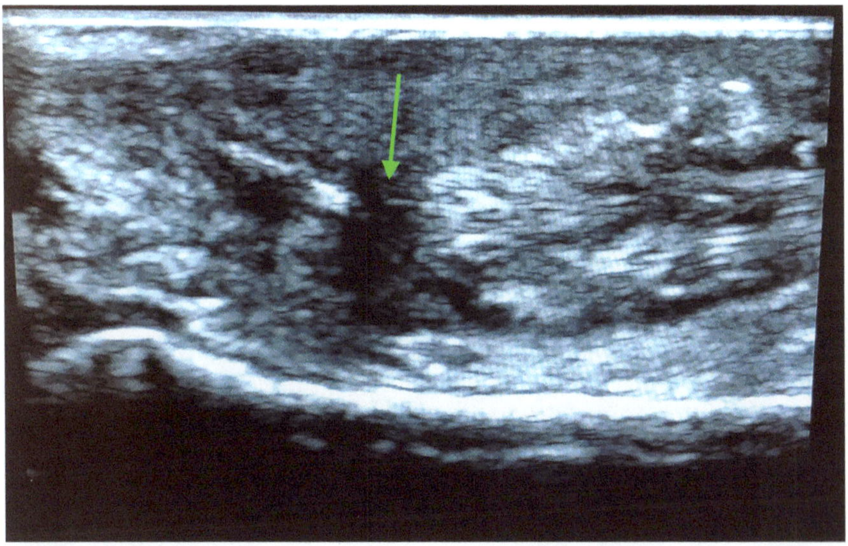

Figure 4-35: Long axis ultrasound evaluation of the finger demonstrating a laceration of the flexor digitorum profundus and flexor digitorum superficialis. Green arrow points to the location of the discontinuity.

The patient can be asked to flex the FDP and FDS, and competence of the flexor tendon can be dynamically evaluated. Adjacent fingers are used as an internal control. The flexor tendon sheath is also evaluated by examining the distance of the flexor tendon from the proximal phalanx on the long axis view. An increased distance from the proximal phalanx or middle phalanx may suggest an A2 or A4 pulley rupture.

Trigger Finger

Stenosing flexor tenosynovitis, more commonly referred to as trigger finger, results in clicking and "triggering" of the flexor tendons at the level of the A1 pulley. Clinical presentation ranges from absence of locking with painful movement to frank locking of the proximal interphalangeal joint in flexion. There can be an audible or palpable snap with "unlocking" of the tendon. Ultrasound examination of stenosing flexor tenosynovitis often shows hypoechogenic signal around the flexor tendons consistent with tenosynovitis with thickening of the A1 pulley (Fig. 36).

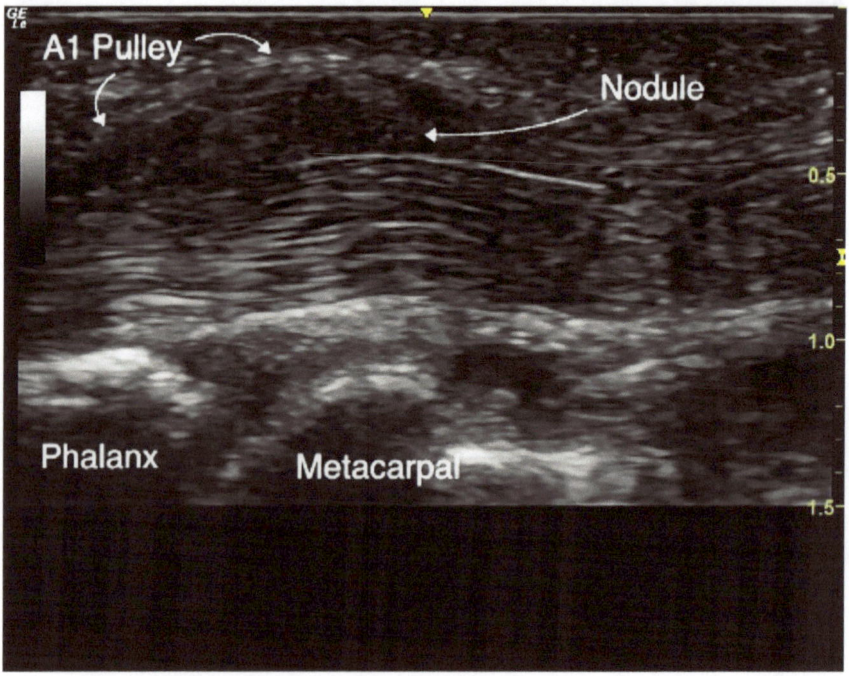

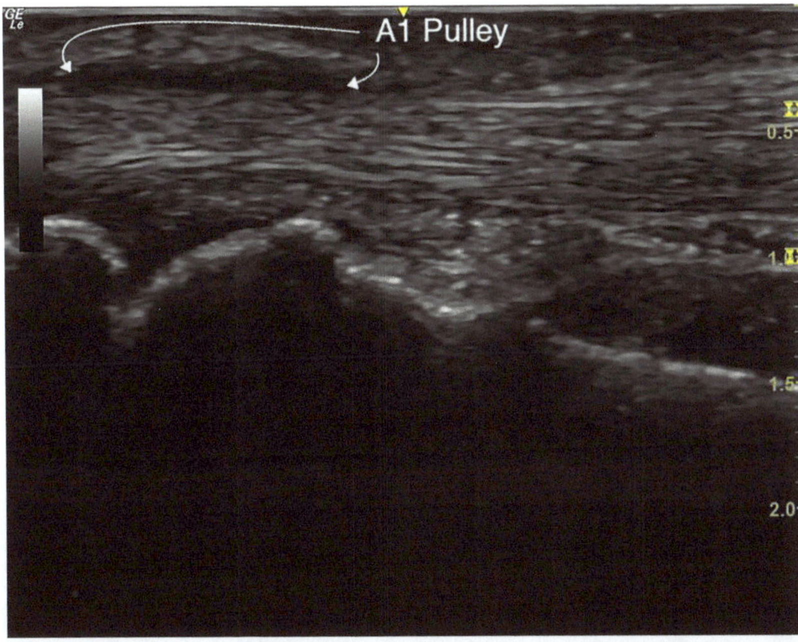

Figure 4-36a and b: Figure 36a Finger in the locked position but as extension is attempted. The tendon nodule and the overlying pulley are so similar that distinguishing them is difficult without dynamic testing. Figure 36b After the digit is dynamically ranged, the pulley is visualized by itself after a palpable "snap".

If the finger is examined in a "locked" position, the flexor tendons will be coiled/folded on itself proximal to the A1 pulley. On dynamic examination, the tendon can be visualized to spring back into the flexor tendon sheath when the finger is extended, which corresponds with a palpable "pop" or "snap"(Fig. 36a and b). Injection of the corticosteroids into the flexor tendon sheath provides equivocal therapeutic relief. Taras and colleagues demonstrated that injection of steroids outside the flexor tendon sheath was superior to intra-sheath injection with respect to recurrence of triggering (25). An escape of liquid from the tendon sheath is also possible, leading us to believe that true intra-sheath injection is not the goal.

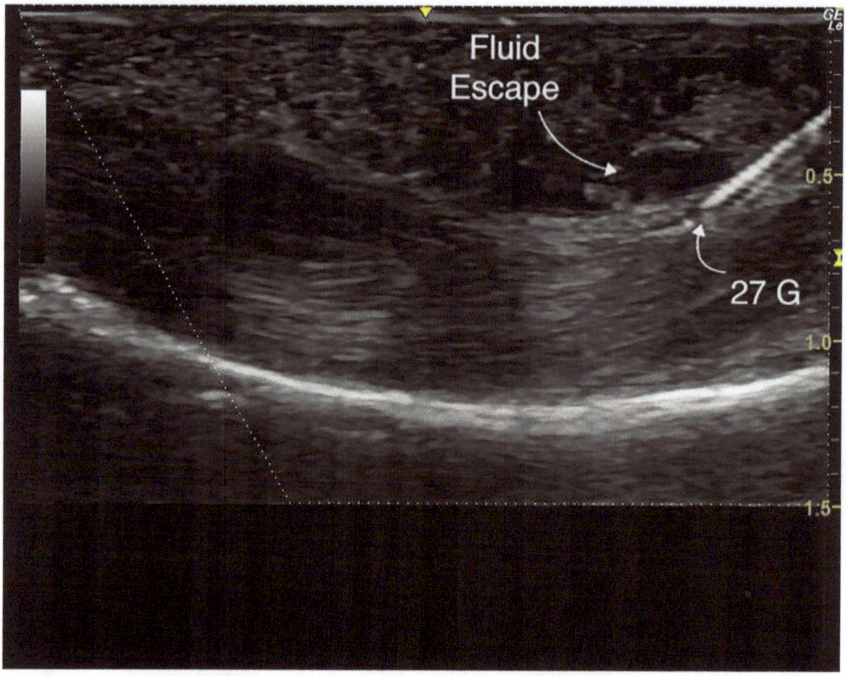

Figure 4-37: Injection of tendon sheath shows fluid outside of the sheath.

Ultrasound-assisted percutaneous trigger finger techniques have been described. Rajeswaran et al. performed ultrasound-assisted percutaneous trigger release in 35 patients, and noted complete resolution in 91% of cases with attenuation to pain levels, amelioration of patient-reported functional scores, and no statistically significant increased risk of complications (26). A local digital block is performed with 5-10 mL of 1% lidocaine with or without epinephrine. A small footprint probe is utilized and the A1 pulley is visualized in the long axis over the metacarpophlangeal joint. An 18-gauge needle is inserted from proximal to distal, and its location within the tendon sheath superficial to the flexor tendons is confirmed on both the short and long axes. The bevel of the needle is then used to transect the A1 pulley by levering the needle superficially and working from proximal to distal. The patient is asked to flex and extend the finger, and the finger is evaluated for crepitus and/or triggering. The process is repeated until complete release is obtained.

Clinical evaluation of the finger extensor mechanism can be challenging due to soft tissue swelling and the chronicity of the injury. In particular, clinical examination of the central slip is vexing as it is often hard to confidently identify the source of extension deficits. For example, etiologic agents for functional deficits following a traumatic injury (for example, a jammed digit) may be due to soft tissue swelling, a mild joint contracture secondary to delayed presentation, or even a central slip avulsion, amongst other pathologies. Westerheide et al. evaluated the central slip in a cadaver model and found 100% sensitivity and specificity for discontinuity of the central slip (27). The terminal tendon can also be evaluated with ultrasound, although the clinical significance is unclear, as the vast majority of mallet injuries are treated non-surgically, regardless of the appearance of the terminal tendon. However, confirming avulsion of the terminal tendon in cases without bony involvement on radiographs may reassure/educate some patients.

Evaluation of the finger extensor tendons is performed by placing the patient's hand flat on the examination table with the elbow extended and pronated as needed for patient positioning and comfort. A small footprint probe and a generous amount of ultrasound gel is often needed and utilized. The probe is then placed in the long axis and the extensor mechanism visualized at both the PIP and DIP joints. The examiner inspects for tendinous discontinuity and can subsequently measure the amount of retraction if present. For terminal tendon injuries, the examiner can confirm that DIP extension in a mallet-type splint by bringing the terminal tendon into apposition with the distal phalanx. For central slip injuries, the examiner can confirm that PIP extension splinting reduces the central slip within closer proximity to its anatomical location over the base of the middle phalanx.

Dupuytren's contracture

Dupuytren's contracture (Fig. 38a) is often complicated by its confluence of fibrotic tissue amongst nerves. Ultrasound represents a cheap and effective imaging modality to characterize pattern of pathologic tissue distribution and interposition to facilitate surgical fasciectomy. Indeed, in the early stages, one can easily differentiate normal from abnormal (Fig. 38b and c). However, in these early stages, patients may not require resection, or can be aided by minimal treatment/collagenase. In more severe cases, the relationship of tendon and fascia becomes more complex. You can still differentiate some structures (for example, tendon from overlying fascia) on long axis, but distinguishing nerves from cord on short axis can be difficult. As ultrasound technology improves, higher frequency probes may be able to better delineate this finely detailed anatomy and guide treatment (Fig. 38d).

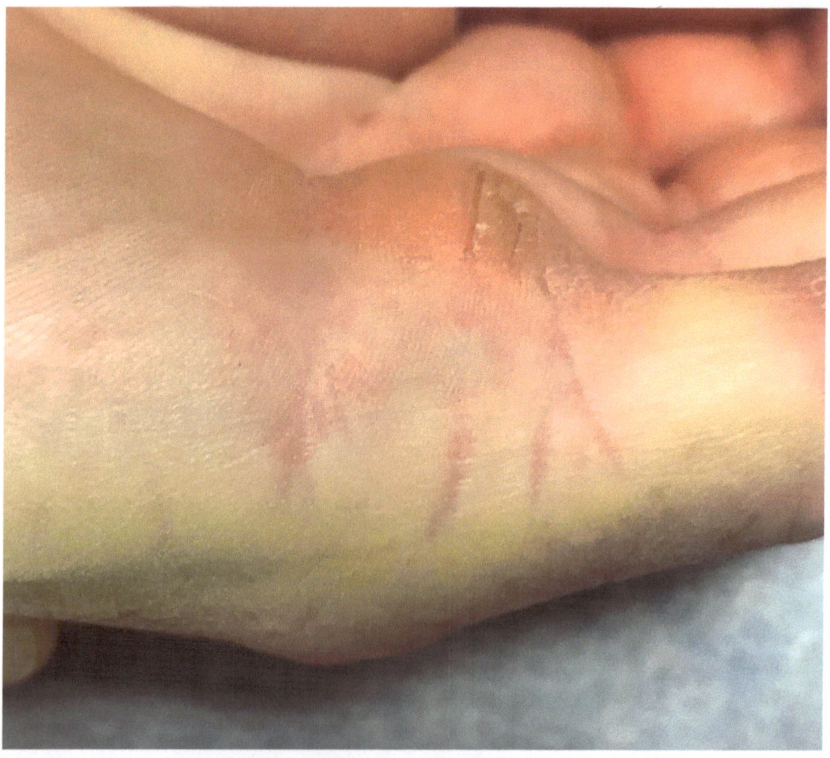

Figure 4-38a: An ulnar sided view of a little finger contraction. This picture was taken in the clinic and demonstrates early Dupuytren's contracture.

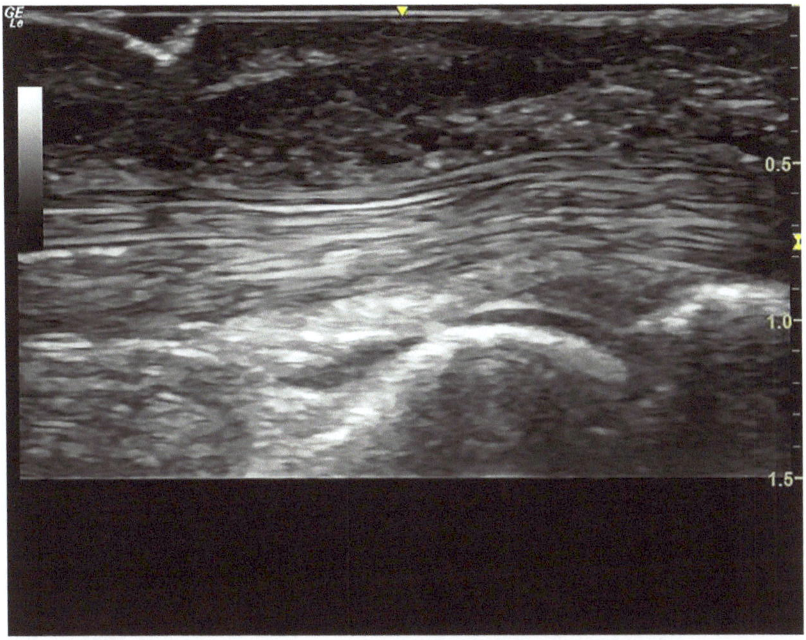

Figure 4-38b: Ultrasound visualization of early Dupuyten's, which is demonstrated by thickening of the palmar fascia and is easily distinguished from the underlying tendon.

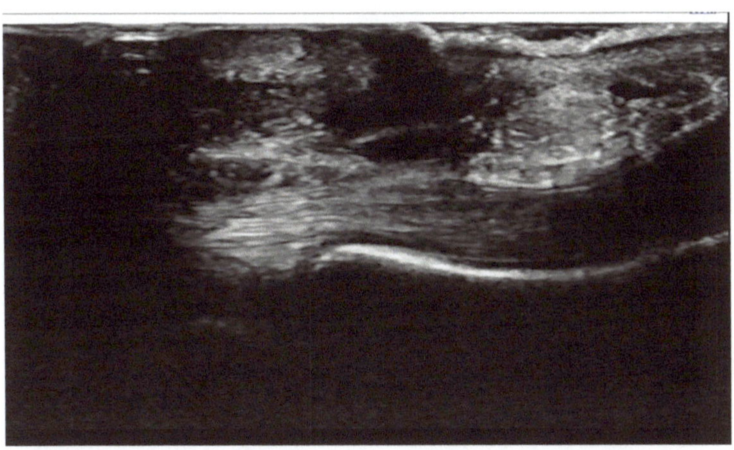

Figure 4-38c: In the long axis, the contracture can still be differentiated from the tendon even in a later stage.

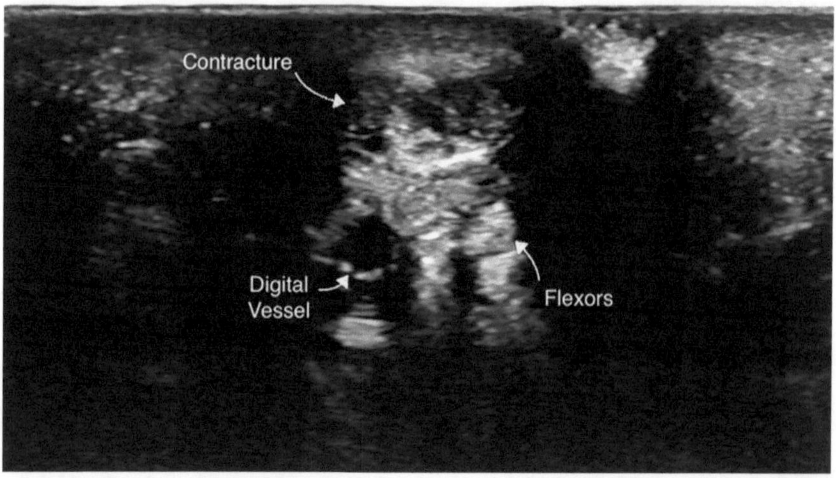

Figure 38d: In the short axis, we are able to visualize vessels (which may be aided by Doppler as well, but not shown here) and tendon/contracture, but not well enough to precisely localize digital nerves.

Finger Masses

Ultrasound may be helpful for diagnosis of finger masses (28). The vast majority of finger masses along the volar surface of the finger will be volar retinacular ganglia. A volar retinacular ganglion is a fluid-filled mass that emanates from the flexor tendon sheath (Fig. 39a and b).

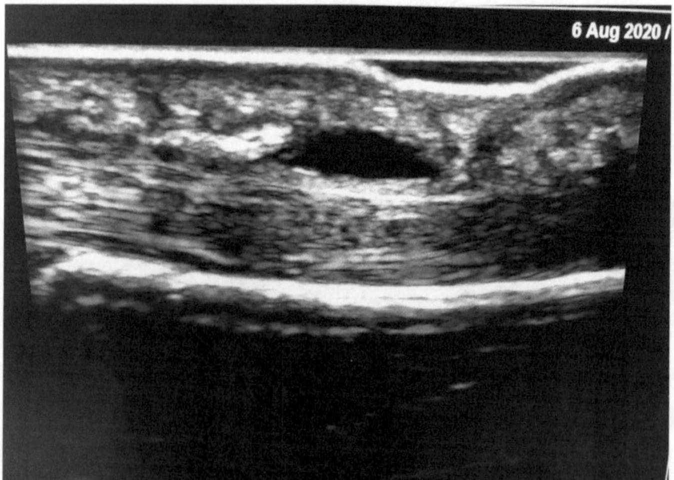

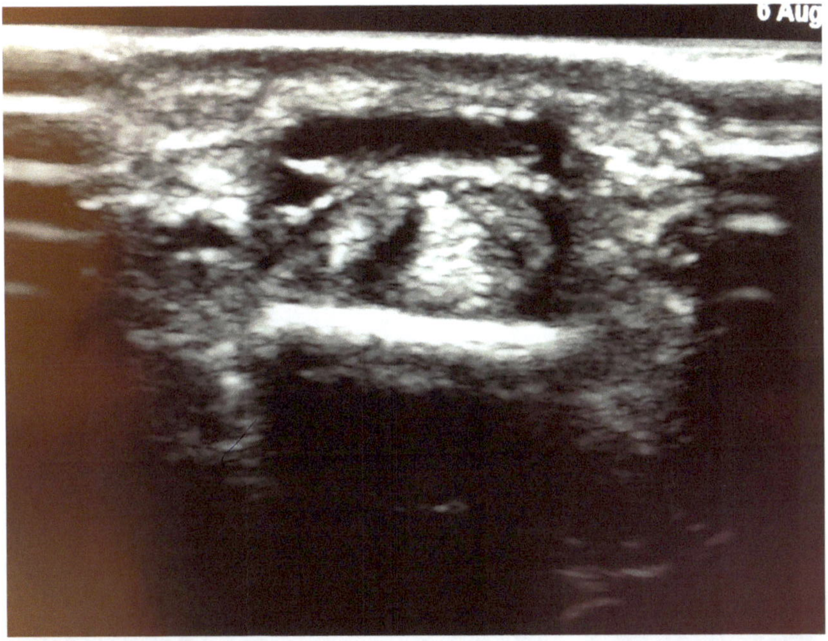

Figure 34-9a and b: Figure 39a Long axis ultrasound demonstrating a volar retinacular ganglion emanating from the flexor tendon sheath; Figure 39b Short axis ultrasound re-demonstrating the same volar retinacular ganglion.

The ultrasound findings will mirror those of wrist dorsal ganglions with a homogenous hypoechogenic mass and a connection to the flexor tendon sheath. This is in contrast to a heterogeneous, non-fluid-filled mass originating from the flexor tendon sheath or joint that would be more consistent with a giant cell tumor of tendon sheath.

Giant Cell Tumor

A man in his late 40s was referred with a diagnosis of Dupuytren's contracture.

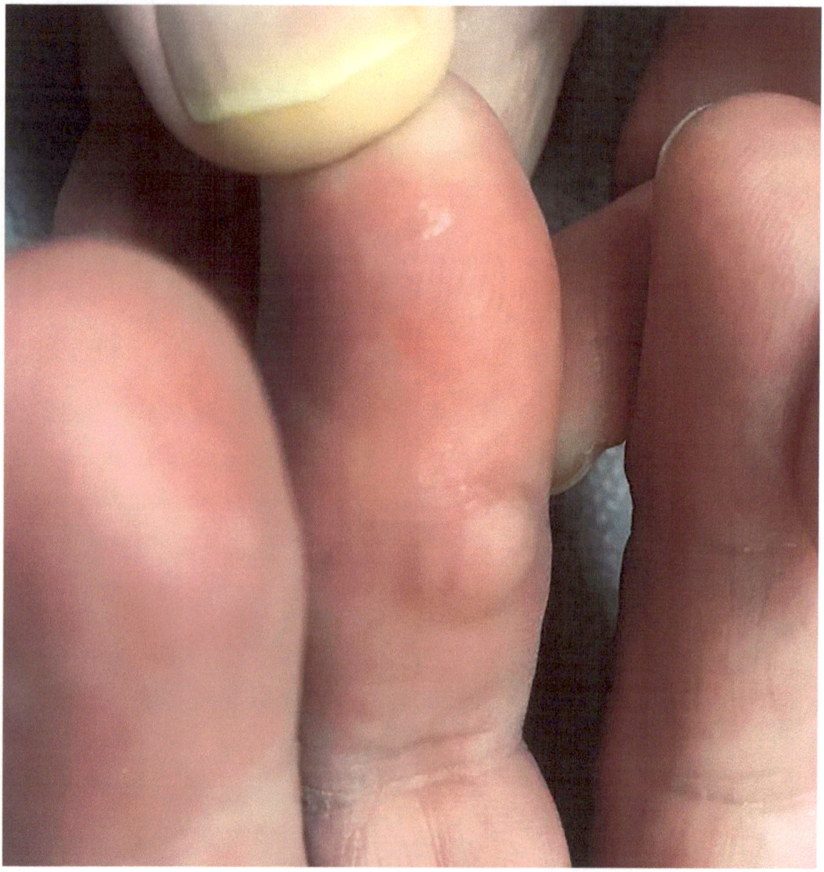

Figure 4-40a: A small mass at the DIP producing some limitation in flexion and associated with mild tenderness to palpation and ROM.

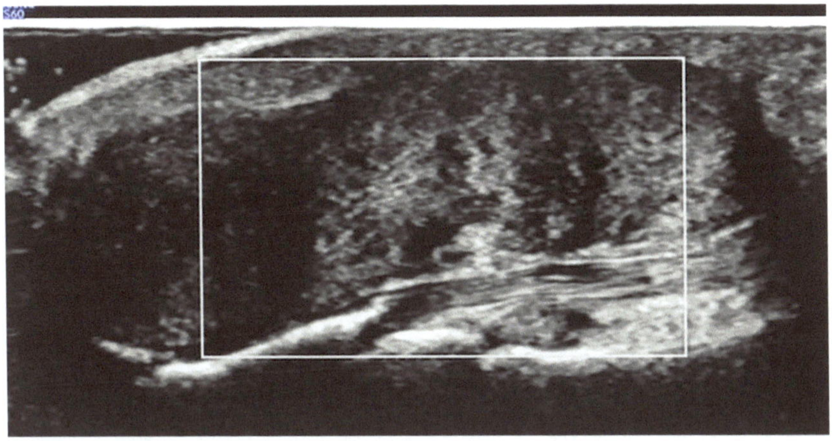

Figure 4-40b: Long axis view of the tumor on the volar side of the DIP centered near the insertion of the FDP (visualized on the inferior aspect of the image). There was no neovascularity, and the margins were demonstrated to be sharp.

Ultrasound may also identify digital nerve tumors such as schwannomas or neurofibromas. Other diagnoses in the differential diagnosis include foreign bodies, fibromas, and epidermal inclusion cysts. For masses that are atypical, or where the diagnosis is unclear based on ultrasound examination, magnetic resonance imaging (MRI) is recommended. Ultrasound examination of finger masses is similar to that for foreign bodies in that the digit is typically held by the examiner to stabilize the finger and allow manipulation during the examination. A large amount of ultrasound gel and small footprint probe aids in the examination. In addition, comparison of anatomy to adjacent digits provides utility as an internal control.

Cartilage Tumor
Over proximal phalanx

A middle-aged man presented with several months of an atraumatic, painful mas on the volar aspect of the left ring finger proximal phalanx. It was moderately tender to palpation but without overlying skin changes. There were no bony changes on x-ray, and, on ultrasound, the mass was noted to be a multi-loculated hypoechoic mass.

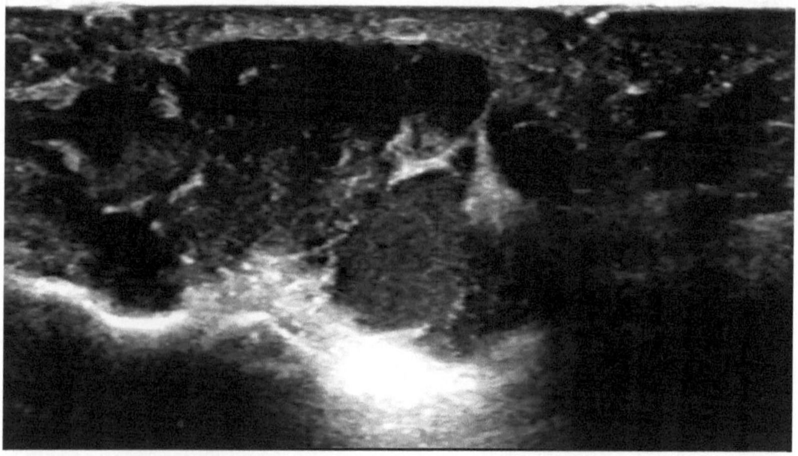

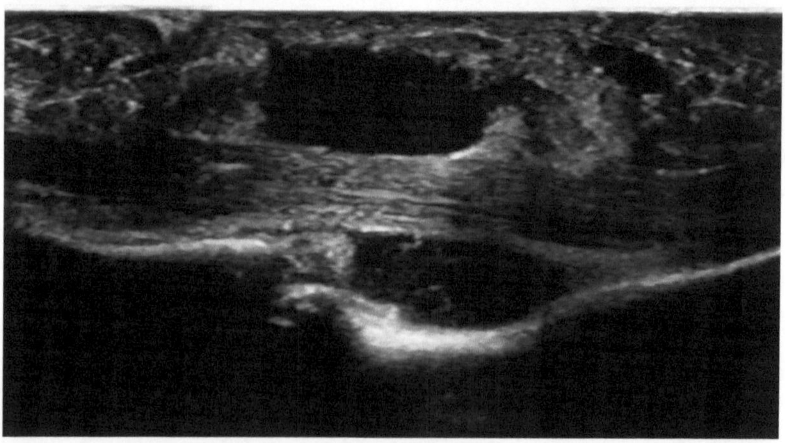

Figure 4-41a and b: Short axis (Figure 41a) and long axis (Figure 41b) views of a pre-operative cartilaginous tumor with the flexor tendons in profile.

Note the lobules were more anechoic than expected for a mass, and it was interpreted as a multiloculated cyst. Authors have increased the brightness to show that this was not merely clear fluid.

The pre-op diagnosis was that this was a benign process, probably a cyst. Ultrasound, particularly the color Doppler or power Doppler, was useful in facilitating a pre-operative resection plan.

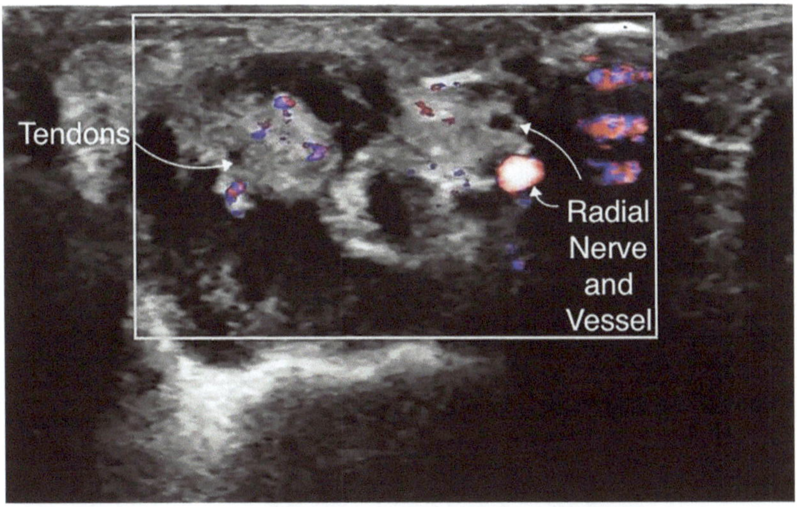

Figure 4-41c: Anatomical relationship of patient's cartilaginous tumor to local nerves and vessels on the radial side of the digit.

Color Doppler demonstrated that the radial digital artery and nerve would be easier to find and protect than the ulnar digital nerve and vessel. Consequently, a zig-zag (Bruner) incision was planned accordingly to expose the radial aspect.

The tumor turned out to be a soft-tissue chondroma, which is benign but has a 30% recurrence rate. In turn, he will be followed with serial ultrasonographical evaluations.

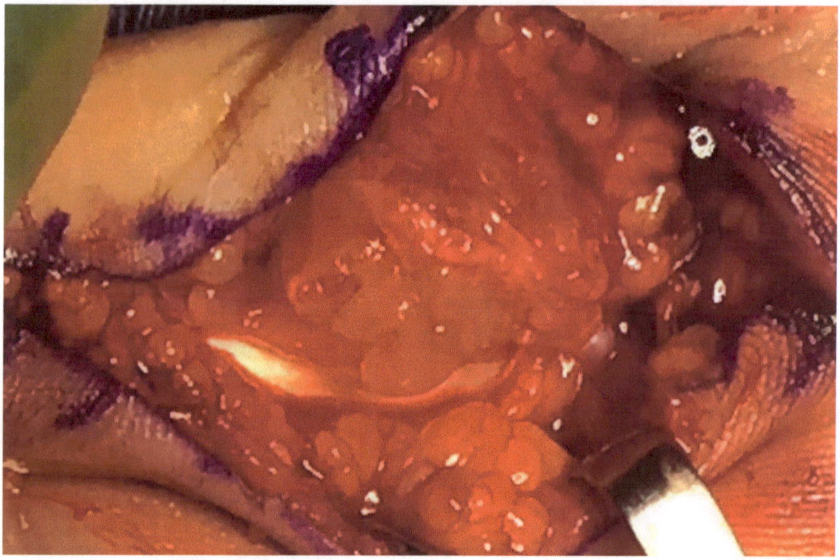

Figure 4-41d: Image demonstrating gross specimen of the cartilaginous tumor.

The radial digital nerve and artery were safely retracted, and the release allowed the tumor to fall towards the incision from the ulnar and deep aspects of the flexor tendons (compare with Fig. 41c). The learning point of this case was to increase gain on an anechoic mass to fully characterize its structures and distinguish whether it is truly cystic, or actually a hypoechoic solid mass.

Nailbed Tumor

Subungual tumors can also be assessed with ultrasound. This particular deformity is caused by a painful tumor of greater than six years duration.

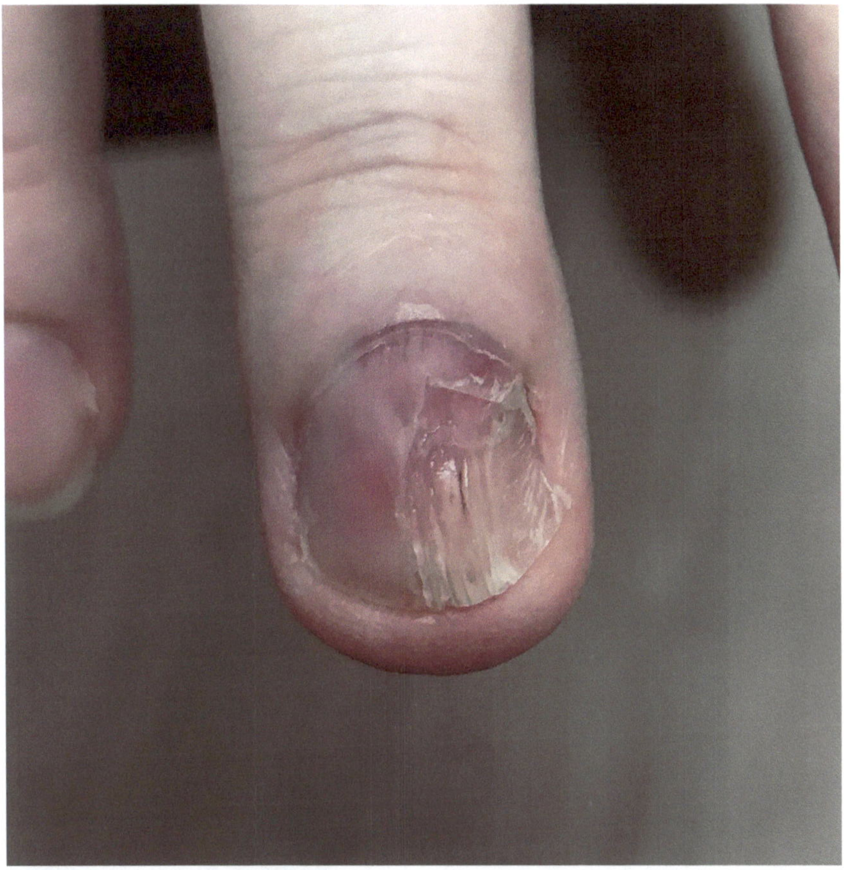

Figure 4-42a: The affected nail seen preoperatively.

On ultrasound, one can see the increased vascularity of the tumor, as well as the concavity in the underlying phalanx. This was confirmed to be a glomus tumor on histology.

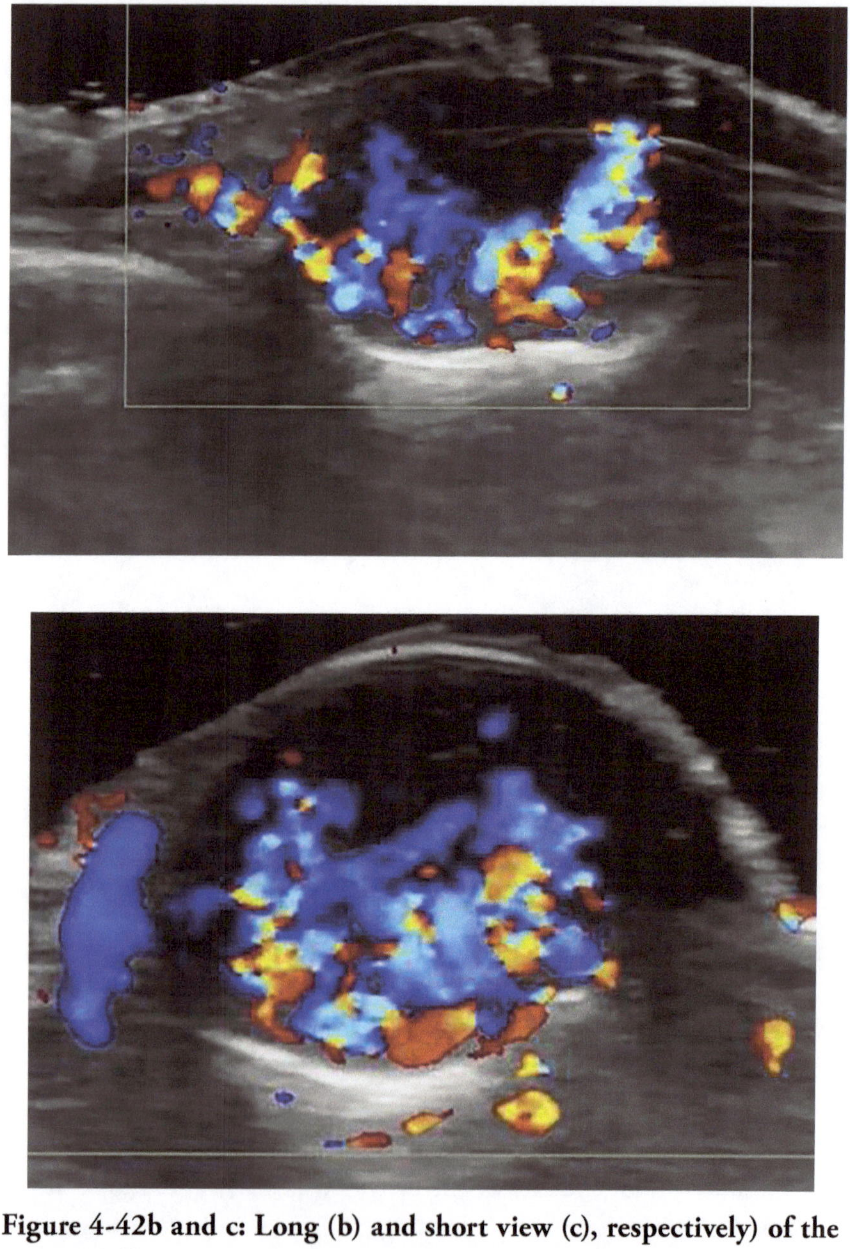

Figure 4-42b and c: Long (b) and short view (c), respectively) of the tumor, demonstrating its internal vascularity along with the concavity produced in the surrounding bone.

Small Joint (MCP/PIP) Injections

While metacarpophalangeal (MCP) and proximal interphalangeal (PIP) joint arthritis is less common than thumb CMC arthritis, therapeutic corticosteroid injections into these joints may provide symptomatic relief in patients with both inflammatory and osteoarthritis. In the "boggy" MCP joint, ultrasound may provide information regarding the location of the synovitis (for example, from the extensor mechanism or actual joint). In the non-swollen and non-arthritic hand, palpation of the joint and bony landmarks is usually straightforward. However, in the setting of joint space narrowing and soft tissue swelling, this physical exam maneuver proves more challenging. Raza and colleagues noted that the accuracy of intra-articular injection of the PIP and MCP joints was 59% using a landmark-based technique, and 96% using ultrasound guidance (29).

Ultrasound examination and/or injection of the MCP and PIP joints may be challenging for several reasons, including the nature of a small working space along with difficulty maintaining a flat surface and/or perpendicular angle of the probe to the structure of interest. A small footprint probe is essential. For MCP injections, I prefer to sit across from the patient and position his/her hand on a box of gloves. The wrist is extended and the MCP joint is flexed to 80-90 degrees over the edge of the box. The ultrasound probe is placed in the long axis over the metacarpal head (Figure 43). Both the proximal phalangeal base and metacarpal head are identified, and the needle is introduced and subsequently advanced intra-articularly in a distal to proximal orientation (Figure 43).

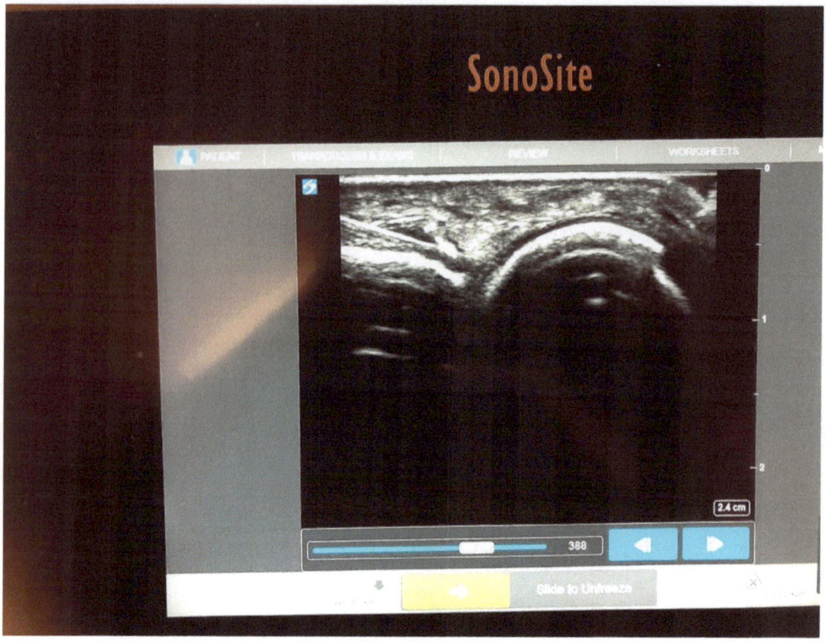

Figure 4-43: Ultrasound examination of the MCP joint and ultrasound guided long axis injection of the MCP joint.

For PIP injections, I prefer to introduce the needle from proximal to distal. Therefore, the examiner sits perpendicular to the digit, and a rolled towel is used to introduce 20-30 degrees of flexion to the joint.

Flexor tenosynovitis
Placement of the distal angiocath

Flexor tenosynovitis (FTS) is a rapidly progressing infection of the digit associated with devastatingly morbid complications if not urgently surgically released, and subsequently medically managed with antibiotics. While severe infections often require an extensile Bruner incision, early cases can be treated with irrigation and drainage of the tendon sheath through two portals for drainage: the first includes a palmar incision, while the second is a distal angiocath through which the irrigation is supplied. Ultrasound guidance allows precise placement of the distal angiocath without an additional incision.

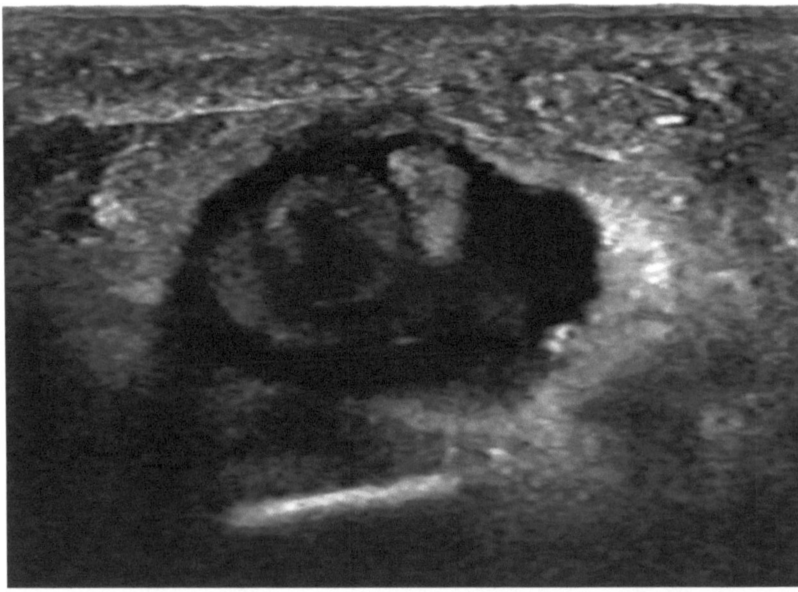

Figure 4-44a: A short-axis view of the involved sheath. The FDP is in the center with a slip of FDS on either side. Turbid fluid can be visualized surrounding the tendons.

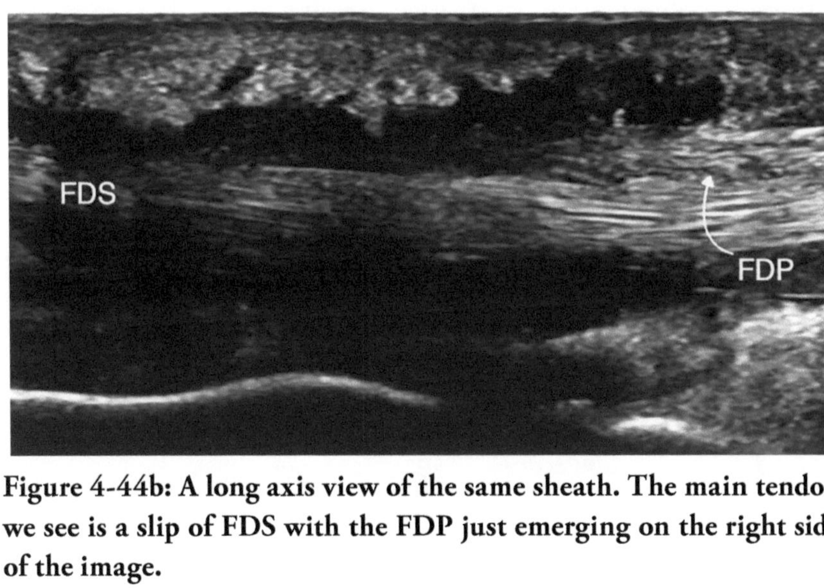

Figure 4-44b: A long axis view of the same sheath. The main tendon we see is a slip of FDS with the FDP just emerging on the right side of the image.

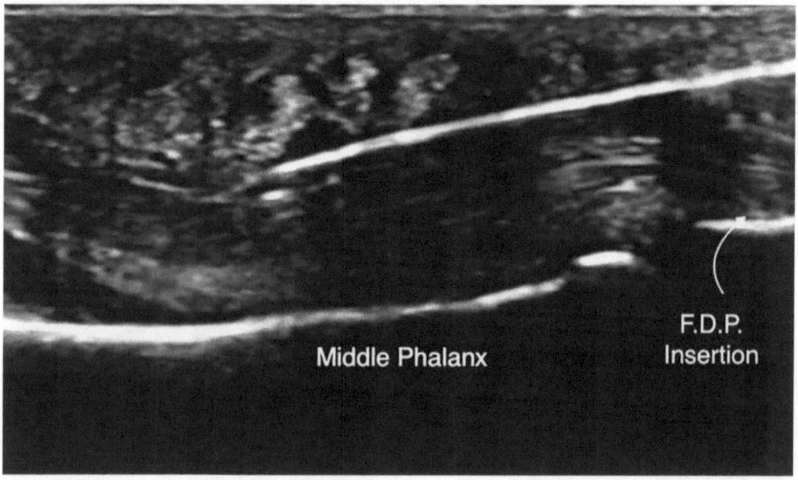

Figure 4-44c: Angiocath in sheath. An 18G angiocath is placed under ultrasound guidance through the center of the distal pad, and just inside the sheath as one would do when entering a vein.

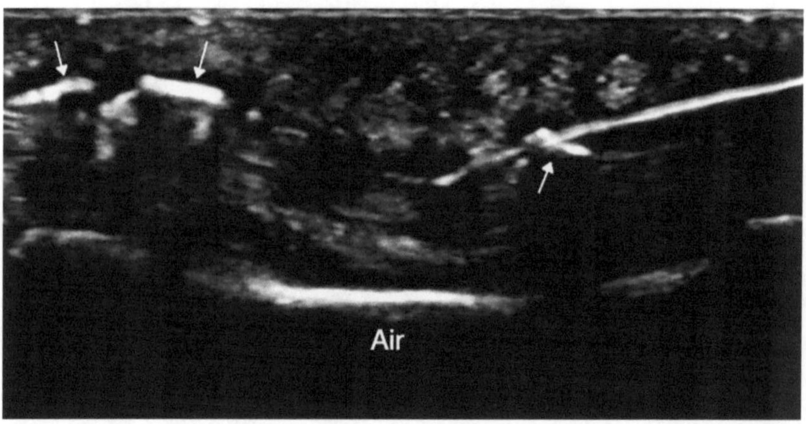

Figure 4-44d: Air in sheath. Ease of flow can be checked with air (arrows) to be sure the angiocath is not in the tendon. Then irrigation flow through the proximal incision is observed visually

Lacerations

3-week-old FDP laceration

In a moderately late FDP laceration, the end of the tendon can be localized, and both the FDP and the FDS can be observed.

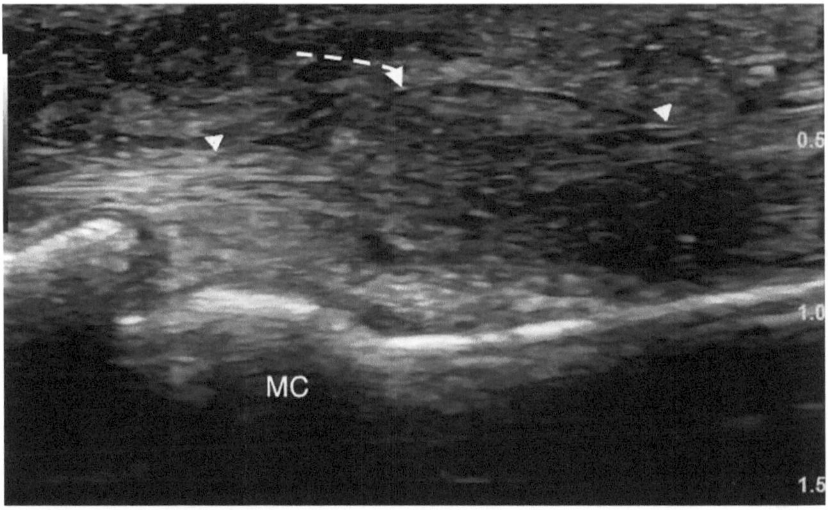

Figure 4-45a: The intact FDS (arrow heads) can be seen traversing directly over the MP joint and volar plate as it continues distally towards its insertion on the middle phalanx. The dashed arrow points to the lacerated aspect of the FDP tendon protruding through the split in the FDS.

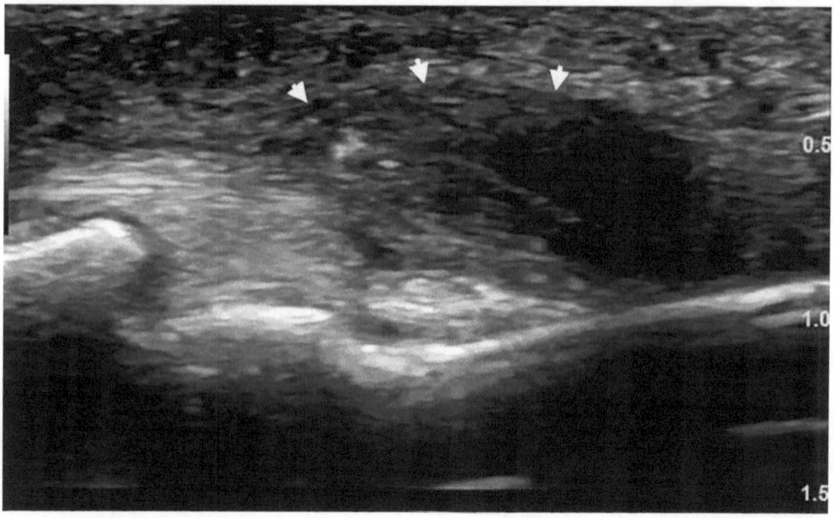

Figure 4-45b: In this view, the lacerated end of the FDP, rendered hypoechoic by swelling and anisotropy, is observed just proximal to the MCP joint.

Screwdriver injury to palm

A workman in his late 20s suffered a small stab wound to the palm from a screwdriver. The wound seemed minor, so he did not immediately seek medical attention. However, over the next two days, the patient began to develop insidious onset, progressive, and unremitting numbness along the ulnar aspect of the index finger and the radial aspect of the long finger. He subsequently presented to clinic for evaluation, where an ultrasound was utilized to confirm that the second common digital and its two proper digital branches were structurally sound. He was treated by observation, and most of the numbness went away over a short period.

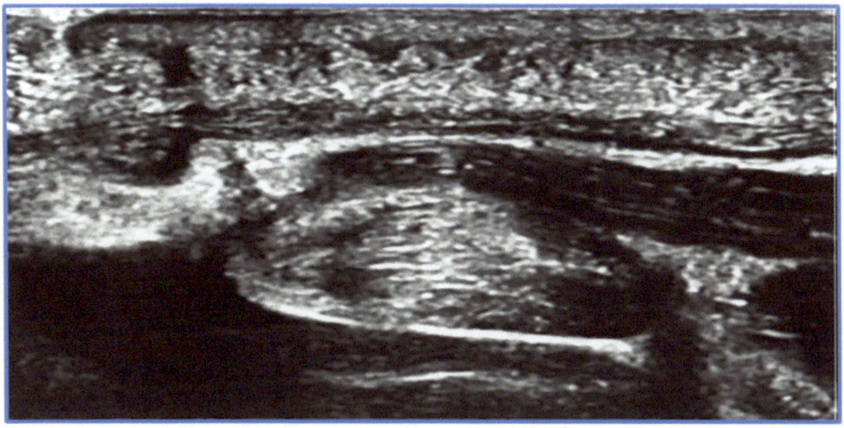

Figure 4-46: Long axis view of the second common digital nerve. The solid line indicates the approximate trajectory of the entry wound. The nerve appeared structurally intact without apparent laceration or surrounding infection, so no intervention was required

Assist in Fractures

Checking screw lengths: Radius ORIF

Protruding hardware on the dorsal side of the radius can interfere with tendon function. Ultrasonography can be utilized to perform a cheap, efficient, and safe evaluation for dorsally protruding screws. This is especially useful distally, where Lister's tubercle can obscure the lateral view on x-ray. Screw identification and localized can be determined by rotating individual screws and observing movement on ultrasound.

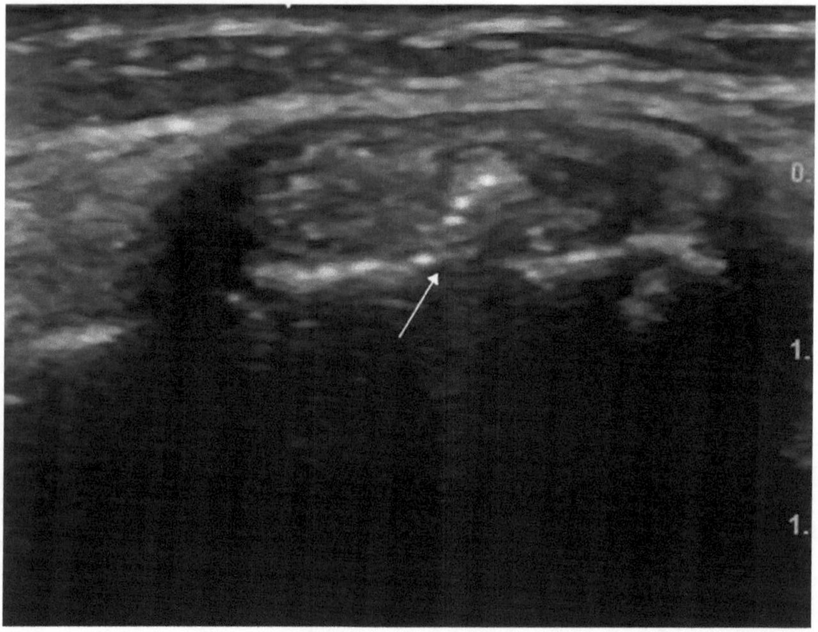

Figure 4-47: Dorsally protruding distal screws during ORIF of a distal radius. Screws protruding into the radial wrist extensor compartment (compartment II). On a lateral x-ray, the protrusion of a screw tip is often obscured by Lister's tubercle.

Evaluation of Volar Radial Plate for Post-op Complications

US can also be used to evaluate the status of hardware in the post-operative period. This patient was 6 weeks status post-ORIF of a distal radius fracture who presented to post-operative appointment with new complaints of a "loosening" sensation on the volar wrist (Fig. 48). We first assessed a common post-op complication (mechanical irritation of the FCR), and confirmed the FCR tendon was of normal appearance and free of lacerations or contact with the plate. Once this complication was ruled out, we proceeded with a more comprehensive evaluation and noticed that one of the distal screws had backed out, and was prominent under the radial artery. The screw was subsequently removed a few days later.

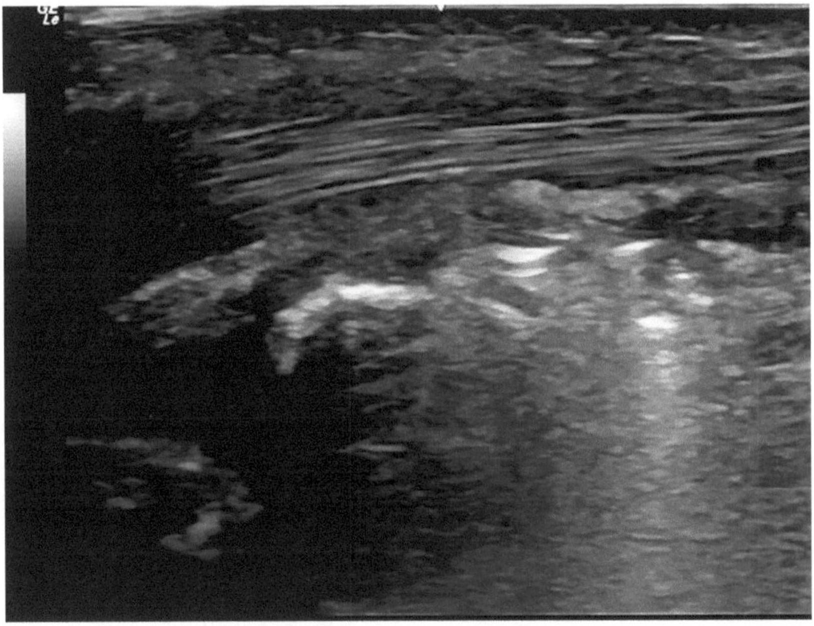

Figure 4-48a:The FCR tendon is not touching the plate (bright echogenic segments). There is no decrease in echogenicity, or a brake in the fibrillar pattern of the FCR.

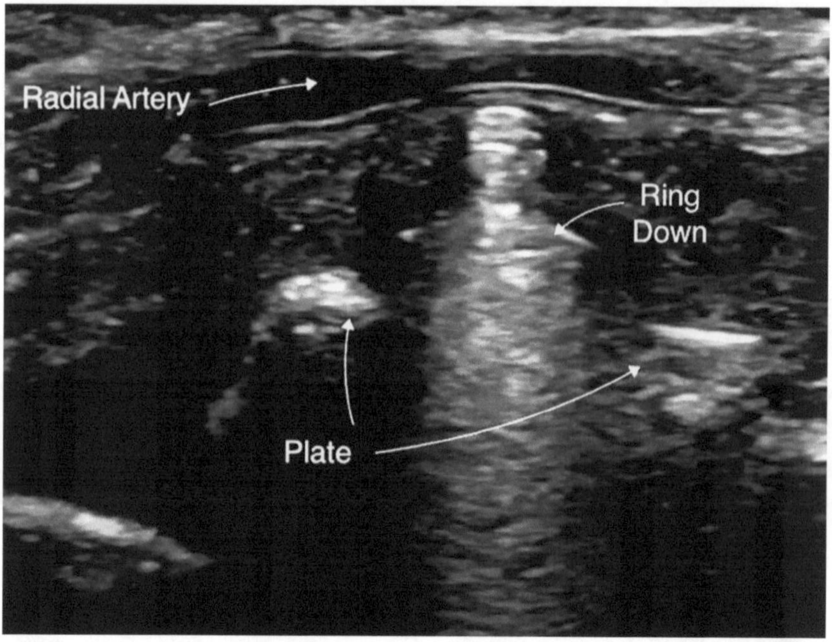

Figure 4-48b: The amount of screw back-out was best seen in the long axis. The radial artery is visualized draped over the screw head.

In-Office Ulnar Nerve Block
For facilitating reduction of ulnar digit fractures
(median block is in the giant cell tumor section)

There are certain (usually traumatic) conditions which we may wish to treat in the clinic, however, they may be precluded by patients' tolerance secondary to pain associated with the treatment. Among these are metacarpal and phalangeal fractures, which often may have an unacceptable alignment, but do not require surgical treatment.

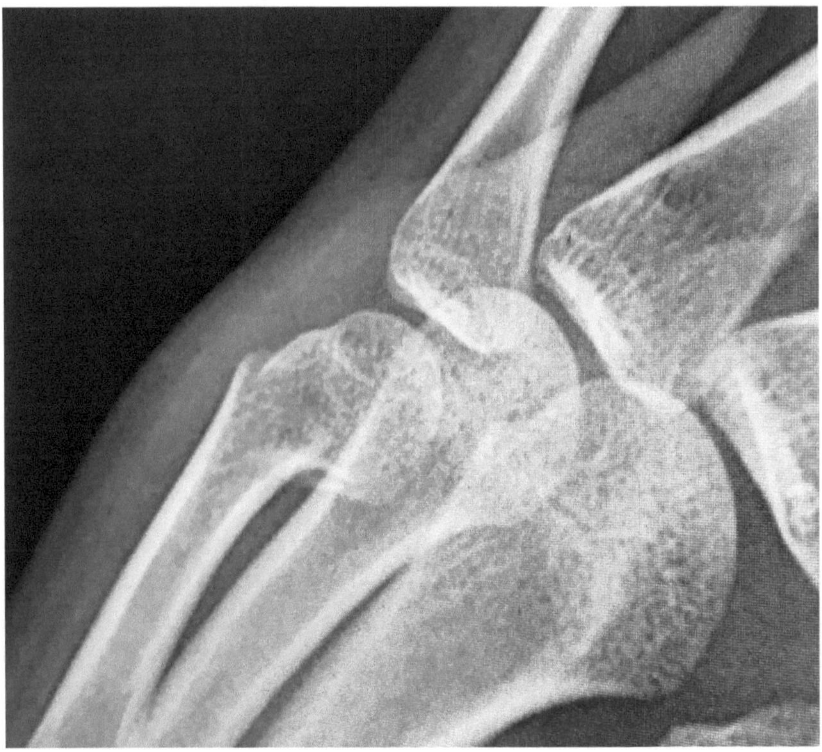

Figure 4-49a: Boxer's Fractures of the right hand. This fifth metacarpal fracture was felt to be angulated beyond the acceptable limits.

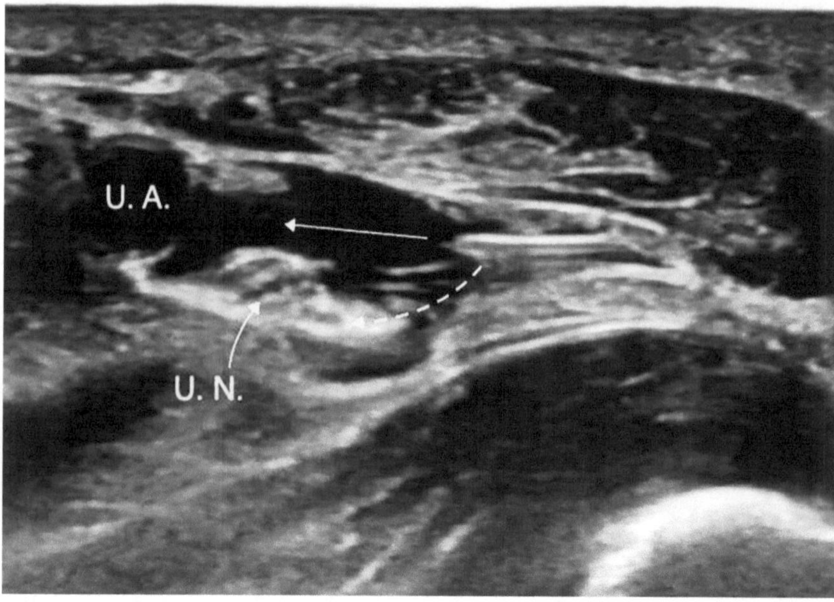

Fig. 4-49b: Hydro-dissection from local anesthetic administration to the ulnar nerve. With an ulnar approach, a superficial hydro-dissection (solid arrow) can first be administered, then followed by a deep hydro-dissection (broken arrow) through the same needle stick and trajectory.

Future Studies and Advanced Techniques:

Ultrasound technologies continue to improve, and image resolution seems to become augmented with each new generation of ultrasound system. Ultrasonography is even being revolutionized by the ability to connect to one's smart phone, and perform ultrasounds with unparalleled efficiency, and without physical constraints/restrictions. This is an exciting time, and technical improvements allow us to answer more and more questions with ultrasound that otherwise may have been difficult to answer. We have been able to utilize ultrasonography to improve our clinical diagnosis (for example, carpal tunnel syndrome), and we can improve our accuracy with injections. Ultrasound has even been able to improve diagnosis of tendon injuries; however, there remain improvements to be made and areas of future study. Post-operative stiffness following flexor tendon repair may occur, and it can be difficult to determine whether a loss of motion is secondary to adhesions or a re-rupture of the tendon. Renfree et al. (30) showed in a cadaver model that, even with a dynamic exam, it is difficult identify whether a partial re-rupture or gap formation in the repair is the source of stiffness. This is likely due to the surgical changes and suture material, however ,as technology and our understanding improves, this would be a great clinical question to answer that could ultimately vastly improve outcomes, whether they require a rapid return to the operating room, or can engage in something as simple as more vigorous therapy. The TFCC can also be evaluated on ultrasound. This is not an easy exam as it is a small and deep structure, but a thorough systematic evaluation of the ulnar side of the wrist can help to illuminate other pathologies of this structure as well.

References

1. Nakamichi K, Tachibana S. Ultrasonographic measurement of median nerve cross-sectional area in idiopathic carpal tunnel syndrome: Diagnostic accuracy. *Muscle Nerve.* 2002;26(6):798-803.

2. Hobson-Webb LD, Massey JM, Juel VC, Sanders DB. The ultrasonographic wrist-to-forearm median nerve area ratio in carpal tunnel syndrome. *Clin Neurophysiol.* 2008;119(6):1353-7.

3. Mallouhi A, Pulzl P, Trieb T, Piza H, Bodner G. Predictors of carpal tunnel syndrome: accuracy of gray-scale and color Doppler sonography. *AJR Am J Roentgenol.* 2006;186(5):1240-5.

4. Fowler JR, Gaughan JP, Ilyas AM. The sensitivity and specificity of ultrasound for the diagnosis of carpal tunnel syndrome: a meta-analysis. *Clinical orthopaedics and related research.* 2011;469(4):1089-94.

5. Green DP, MacKay BJ, Seiler SJ, Fry MT. Accuracy of carpal tunnel Injection: A prospective evaluation of 756 patients. *Hand (NY).* 2020;15(1):54-8.

6. Wolf JM, Sturdivant RX, Owens BD. Incidence of de Quervain's tenosynovitis in a young, active population. *The Journal of Hand Surgery.* 2009;34(1):112-5.

7. Gonzalez MH, Sohlberg R, Brown A, Weinzweig N. The first dorsal extensor compartment: an anatomic study. *The Journal of Hand Surgery.* 1995;20(4):657-60.

8. Witt J, Pess G, Gelberman RH. Treatment of de Quervain tenosynovitis. A prospective study of the results of injection of steroids and immobilization in a splint. *The Journal of Bone and Joint Surgery American Volume.* 1991;73(2):219-22.

9. Kutsikovich J, Merrell G. Accuracy of injection into the first dorsal compartment: a cadaveric ultrasound study. *The Journal of Hand Surgery.* 2018;43(8):777 e1- e5.

10. Cooper HJ, Shevchuk MM, Li X, Yang SS. Proliferative extensor tenosynovitis of the wrist in the absence of rheumatoid arthritis. *The Journal of Hand Surgery.* 2009;34(10):1827-31.

11. VanHeest AE, Luger NM, House JH, Vener M. Extensor retinaculum impingement in the athlete: a new diagnosis. *Am J Sports Med.* 2007;35(12):2126-30.

12. Wang Y, Tang J, Luo Y. The value of sonography in diagnosing giant cell tumors of the tendon sheath. *J Ultrasound Med.* 2007;26(10):1333-40.

13. Sole JS, Wisniewski SJ, Newcomer KL, Maida E, Smith J. Sonographic evaluation of the extensor carpi ulnaris in asymptomatic tennis players. *PM R.* 2015;7(3):255-63.

14. Erickson J, Kwart A, Steven Yang S. Extensor carpi ulnaris tendon anatomy may mimic tears. *J Hand Surg Asian Pac Vol.* 2019;24(2):175-9.

15. Inoue G, Tamura Y. Surgical treatment for recurrent dislocation of the extensor carpi ulnaris tendon. *J Hand Surg Br.* 2001;26(6):556-9.

16. Armstrong AL, Hunter JB, Davis TR. The prevalence of degenerative arthritis of the base of the thumb in post-menopausal women. *J Hand Surg Br.* 1994;19(3):340-1.

17. Yao J, Park MJ. Early treatment of degenerative arthritis of the thumb carpometacarpal joint. *Hand Clinics.* 2008;24(3):251-61, v-vi.

18. To P, McClary KN, Sinclair MK, Stout BA, Foad M, Hiratzka S, et al. The accuracy of common hand injections with and without ultrasound: an anatomical study. *Hand (NY)*. 2017;12(6):591-6.

19. Pollard MA, Cermak MB, Buck WR, Williams DP. Accuracy of injection into the basal joint of the thumb. *Am J Orthop* (Belle Mead NJ). 2007;36(4):204-6.

20. Lutsky KF, Liss F, Graham J, Beredjiklian PK. Volume of the thumb carpometacarpal joint. *J Wrist Surg*. 2020;9(1):19-21.

21. Cunnington J, Marshall N, Hide G, Bracewell C, Isaacs J, Platt P, et al. A randomized, double-blind, controlled study of ultrasound-guided corticosteroid injection into the joint of patients with inflammatory arthritis. *Arthritis Rheum*. 2010;62(7):1862-9.

22. Bray PW, Mahoney JL, Campbell JP. Sensitivity and specificity of ultrasound in the diagnosis of foreign bodies in the hand. *The Journal of Hand Surgery*. 1995;20(4):661-6.

23. Lee DH, Robbin ML, Galliott R, Graveman VA. Ultrasound evaluation of flexor tendon lacerations. *The Journal of Hand Surgery*. 2000;25(2):236-41.

24. Jeyapalan K, Bisson MA, Dias JJ, Griffin Y, Bhatt R. The role of ultrasound in the management of flexor tendon injuries. *J Hand Surg Eur Vol*. 2008;33(4):430-4.

25. Taras JS, Raphael JS, Pan WT, Movagharnia F, Sotereanos DG. Corticosteroid injections for trigger digits: is intrasheath injection necessary? *The Journal of Hand Surgery*. 1998;23(4):717-22.

26. Rajeswaran G, Lee JC, Eckersley R, Katsarma E, Healy JC. Ultrasound-guided percutaneous release of the annular pulley in trigger digit. *Eur Radiol.* 2009;19(9):2232-7.

27. Westerheide E, Failla JM, van Holsbeeck M, Ceulemans R. Ultrasound visualization of central slip injuries of the finger extensor mechanism. *The Journal of Hand Surgery.* 2003;28(6):1009-13.

28. Guerini H, Morvan G, Vuillemin V, Campagna R, Thevenin F, Larousserie F, et al. Ultrasound of wrist and hand masses. *Diagn Interv Imaging.* 2015;96(12):1247-60.

29. Raza K, Lee CY, Pilling D, Heaton S, Situnayake RD, Carruthers DM, et al. Ultrasound guidance allows accurate needle placement and aspiration from small joints in patients with early inflammatory arthritis. *Rheumatology* (Oxford). 2003;42(8):976-9.

30. Renfree K, Dahiye N, Zhang N. Comparative sensitivity and specificity of static and dynamic high-resolution ultrasound in diagnosis of small gaps in repaired flexor tendons: a cadaveric study. *The Journal of Hand Surgery.* 2020;46(3):247e1-247e7

Chapter 5 Hip and Thigh

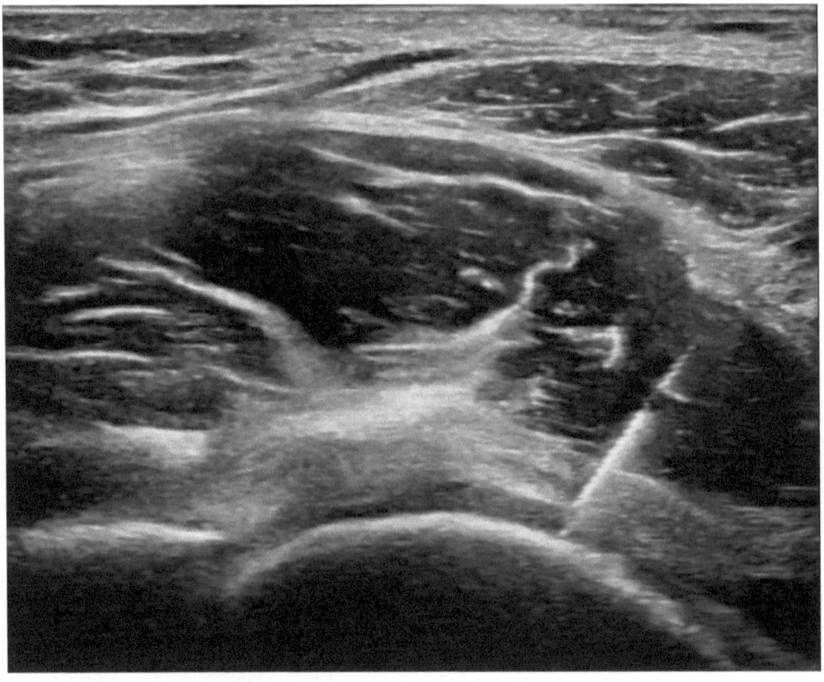

- Alexander M. Riordan, MD;
- Christopher M. Jobe, MD, RMSK

Introduction:

Given the depth of the structures in and surrounding the hip, ultrasonographic analysis is commonly (and incorrectly) believed to provide limited clinical utility. In actuality, the hip joint is very amenable to ultrasound (US) in diagnosis, procedures, surgical planning, and as an aid in surgery. For example, numerous osseous and soft tissue structures are frequently evaluated with US, and intra-articular injections are facilitated by its use. This ease with ultrasound is related to the relatively large size of the structures of the hip, the high muscle content, which provides concomitant conductivity as well as contrast. In addition, dynamic problems, such as a snapping iliotibial band syndrome, are also easily visualized for the same reasons. As in most other regions of the body, the hip ultrasound exam tends to be problem-focused, rather than complete, as it is in the shoulder.

Diagnostic Exam

Positioning, Draping, Probe Use, and Image Optimization

As with any orthopaedic procedure, set-up and positioning are paramount to success. We highly recommend the learning orthopaedic ultrasonographer reference section of the book as a general guide that can be adapted to the abilities of one's own office setting. For ultrasonographic evaluation of the hip and pelvis, there are four general patient positions that can help provide a 360° evaluation: supine (anterior), lateral decubitus (lateral), prone (posterior) and frog leg (medial). All positions and evaluations can be performed on a standard examination table. A seated position for the examiner is recommended, as it allows for improved probe handling and stability. An examination table that allows for height adjustment is desirable, but not required. The screen of the ultrasound machine should be placed so that it can be viewed by the examiner by simply looking upwards from the patient without twisting or rotating the neck (see Figure 5-1). During technically challenging approaches, a small secondary monitor can be placed to facilitate the operator's visualization of the probe, screen, andprocedure-specific instruments in the same field of view. (See small secondary screen in the Intro chapter.)

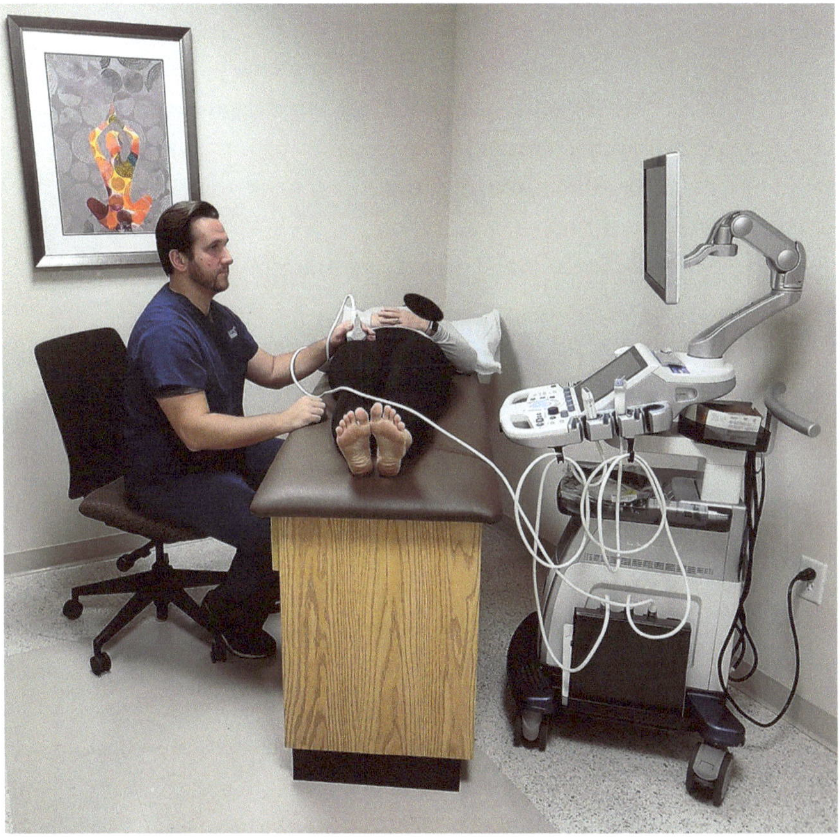

Figure 5-1

Room set up for anterior hip evaluation. Note the examiner's ability to comfortably look from the screen to the probe and back, without significant neck or body repositioning. The cord is wrapped around the examiner's wrist for added probe control and stability.

Various draping methods are described and generally accepted . Since the orthopaedic surgeon will typically be performing a localized examination, loose- fitting shorts with undergarments still in place are recommended. Baggy shorts allow for simple, efficient, and stable coverage of the groin and gluteal cleft. Additionally, they are easily adjusted for targeted exposure of the region being examined and simultaneously allow for maintenance of undergarments, which augments patient comfort and overall office efficiency. Occasionally, undergarments will need to be adjusted, or held in specific positions by the patient while a region is evaluated; however, allowing the patient to control the exposure further facilitates comfort during the evaluation.

The large curvilinear is the preferred ultrasound probe for almost all regions of the hip. This curved probe provides a wide field of view, and its low-frequency sound waves are capable of reaching the deep tissues that are commonly being evaluated. While the scope of focus is large, one limitation of the large curvilinear probe is diminished resolution secondary to the relatively lower frequency of the ultrasound waves transmitted by this probe. Still, since the structures of the hip are large relative to other regions of the body, the curvilinear probe provides enough resolution to visualize sufficient detail in this region.

When handling the probe, it is recommended to allow plenty of cord slack, as this allows the examiner to wrap the cord once around his/her wrist and provide a fixed point for stability (see Figure 5-1). It is recommended that the orthopaedic ultrasonographer gain comfort and skill in holding the probe with the non-dominant hand, regardless of the hip laterality being evaluated. In turn, this mediates easy progression to procedures, in which the syringe is liable to be held in the surgeon's dominant hand. The probe should be grasped with the surgeon's thumb, index finger, middle finger, and radial side of the ring finger. The ulnar side of the ring finger, small finger, and sometimes palm should rest on the patient's skin for added control and image stabilization (see Figure 5-2).

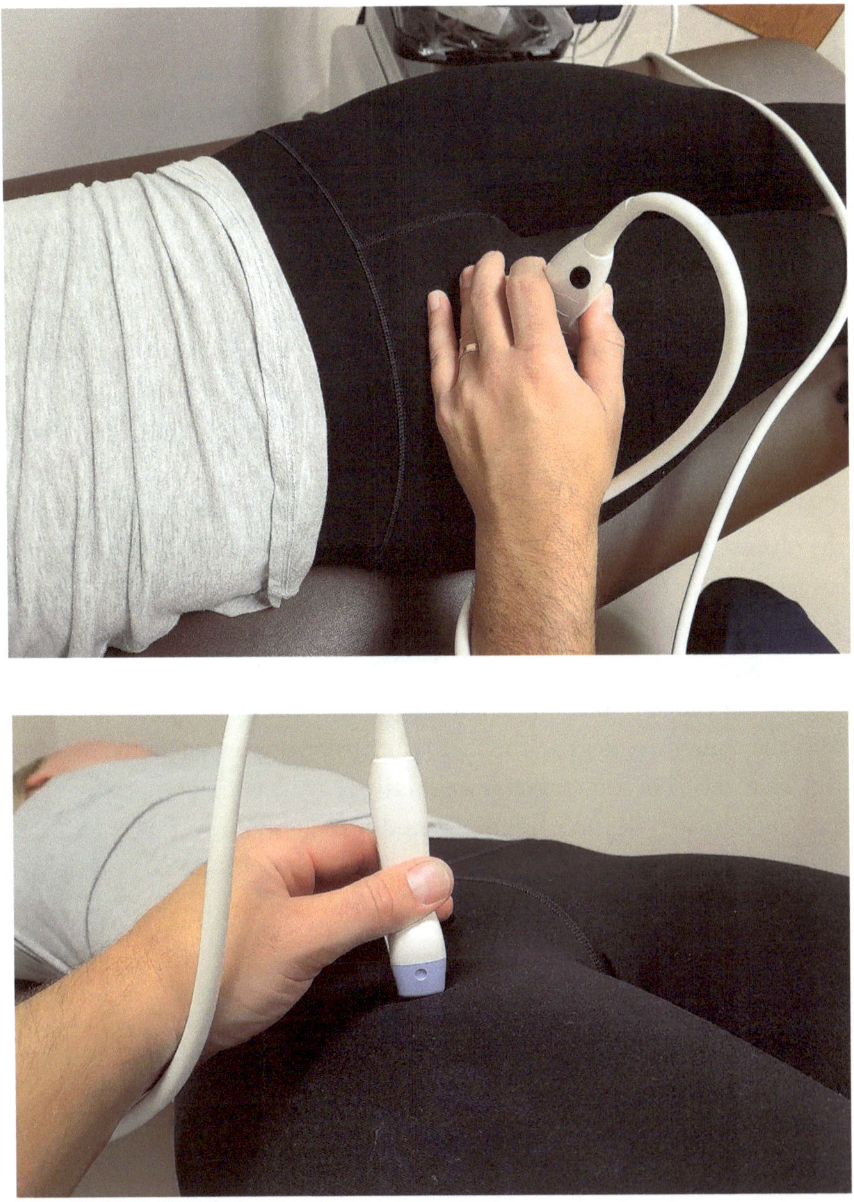

Figure 5-2a and b

Figure 5-2.

a. **A secure and stable probe hold. Note the radial side of the ring finger is on the side of the probe, while the ulnar side of the ring finger rests on the patient. The small finger and ulnar palm may also rest on the patient for further control and tactile feedback during the exam.**
b. **Probe view from the examiner's perspective. This is called an in-line view and is lined up with the long axis of the femoral neck, allowing for simple imaging and needle intervention if indicated.**

One should pay particular attention to a typically raised or etched reference marker (dot or line) on the probe which matches up to one side of the ultrasound screen (see Figure 5-3. It is most natural for the orthopaedic surgeon to have the movement of the probe on the patient match the direction of movement on the ultrasound screen. This is analogous to simple arthroscopy of the knee, for example. The probe can easily be flipped to ensure that the movement direction matches. Forming this habit will assist with the ability to integrate the three-dimensional gross anatomic location and ease the transition into procedural use by having the gross needle movement match the needle movement direction on the screen.

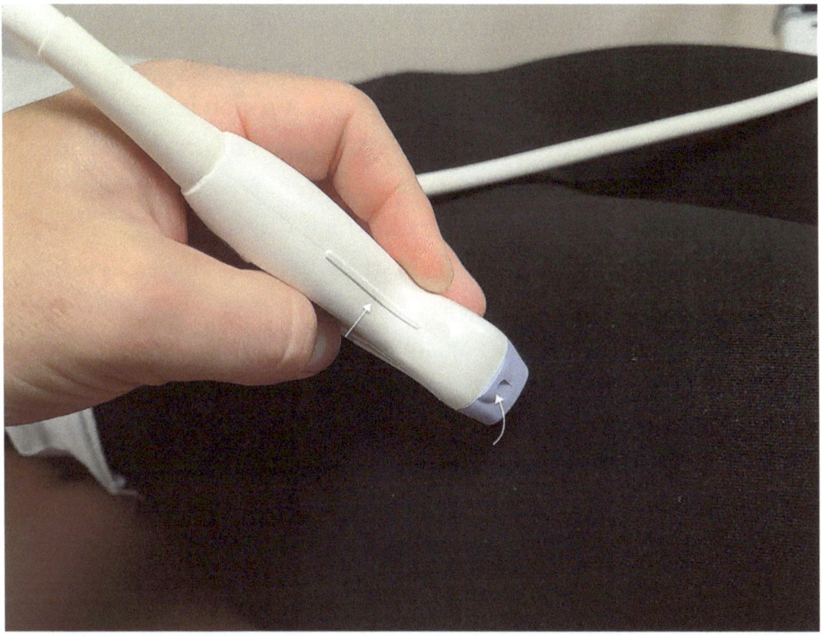

Figure 5-3

In this example, the raised line on the side of the probe (arrow) shown is the indicator line, which corresponds to the left side of the screen on this machine. Note that in Figure 5-2(b) the examiner orients the indicator line proximally toward the femoral head (far side), which allows both the image to and probe to synchronously move in the same direction. The paralleling movement of both the probe on the patient and the image on the screen is always desirable and proves especially useful for needle intervention.

Most modern ultrasound machines can automatically optimize for the region being examined, and selecting the hip region setting typically provides the correct frequency. Once the correct region is selected and the probe is overlying the structure of interest, the examiner should attempt to center the structure on the ultrasound screen. Many times, the depth of the image will need to be adjusted, which can usually be performed by the simple turning of a knob. Brightness (gain) is also easily adjusted in a similar manner. For average-size patients, it's uncommon to need to consistently make additional adjustments throughout the examination. For larger patients, however, the depth will typically have to be increased, and the gain decreased to darken the image. Darkening the image helps minimize the reflective-type effect that excess adipose tissue imposes on the image. Conversely, the depth may need to decreased for thinner patients, or even utilize the linear probe if desired (especially for evaluation of more superficial pelvic structures).

The use of an assistant for diagnostic, and even procedural ultrasonography, of the hip is optional, but certainly useful in the early phases of the learning curve. Some ultrasound machines perform continuous video capture automatically in the background, thereby allowing you to freeze the image upon termination of the exam, and then to subsequently scroll backwards to obtain time-specific screen shots of different structures as needed. Alternatively, some machines employ image capture buttons directly on the probe. Yet another option is to position the ultrasound machine close enough to the examiner so that the image capture button can be pushed with one hand, while the other hand is holding the probe evaluating the structures of interest. This last option is technically more challenging, and recommended after there is a high level of comfort with using the probe and machine.

Anterior Hip

Positioning

The anterior hip evaluation is done with the patient in the supine position. As an option for improved patient comfort, the ipsilateral knee, or both knees, may be placed on a pillow to allow slight hip flexion, which does not interfere with nor affect the image quality. The ideal ultrasound screen position is across the table at the patient's waist level (see Figure 5-1). If spatial limitations in clinic preclude this position, one can place the screen at the patient's head or foot as an alternative. The waistband of the shorts is pulled down to expose the anterior hip. Bringing the waistband about one and a half hand breaths below the tip of the greater trochanter is typically sufficient. The patient is asked to pull their undergarment slightly upwards from the inguinal crease if needed. If helpful, additional draping covering the medial groin can be added using a bed sheet or disposable paper sheet.

Hip joint proper.

The workhorse position of anterior hip ultrasonography for the orthopaedic surgeon involves viewing the anterior femoral neck, femoral head, and acetabulum. Obtaining an anterior image in line with the long axis of the femoral neck centered at the base of the femoral head will prove useful for injection and/or aspiration of the hip joint proper. Additionally, it provides a reproducible image location with easy-to-visualize landmarks, whilst simultaneously facilitating identification of common intra-articular pathologies, such as effusions or osteophytes.

The image can be obtained reliably and quickly by placing the large curvilinear probe so that the entire surface sits just distal to the inguinal skin fold at an angle in line with the femoral neck (see Figure 5-2). For example, when viewing a right hip, the probe can be rotated clockwise 50° from the vertical/longitudinal position. As always, ensure that the probe movement corresponds with the directionality of the movement on the ultrasound screen. That is, for a right hip when the examiner slides his or her hand to the left on the patient (proximally in line with the femoral neck) the image should move left on the screen. Once the appropriate image orientation, quality, depth, and gain are ensured, the positioning of the probe should be optimized. The optimal image for the anterior hip joint region is produced when the base of the femoral head centered within the screen and the probe is held longitudinally and parallel to the middle of the femoral neck (see Figure 5-4).

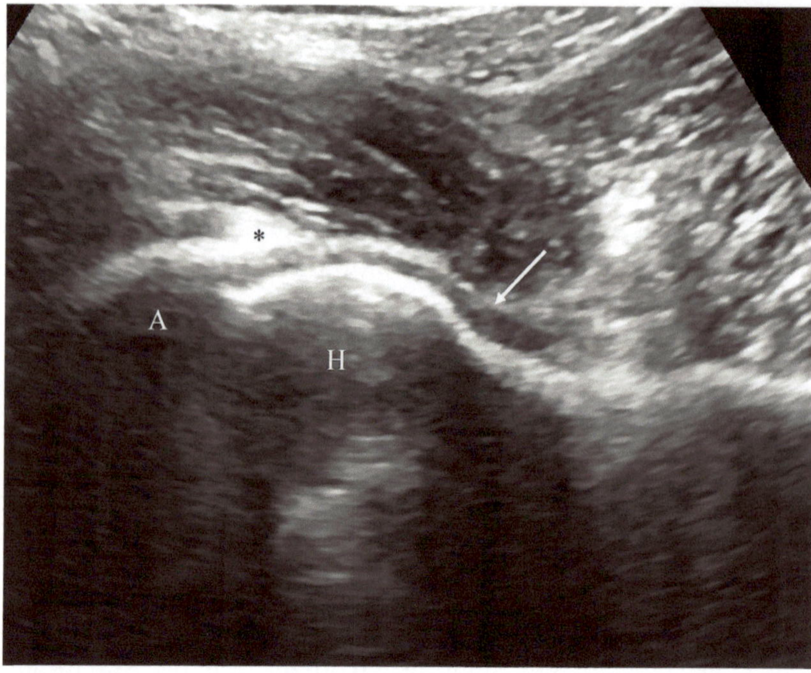

Figure 5-4a

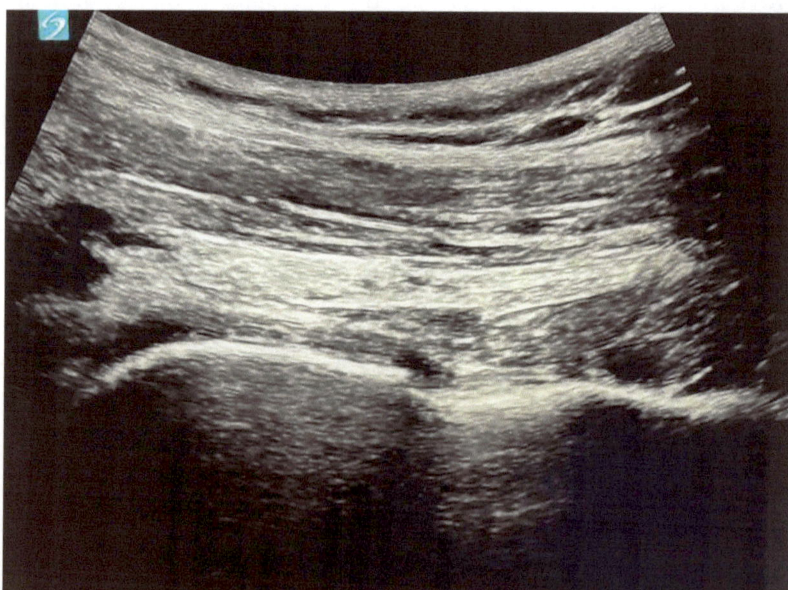

Figure 5-4b

Figure 5-4a and b

a. **The articulation of the anterior acetabulum (A) and femoral head (H) is shown. In this "workhorse" view, note a well-defined hyperechoic femoral neck nearly parallel to the sound waves and the base of the femoral head in the center of the image. Normal- appearing, cloudy, heterogenous, and hypoechoic synovium is seen directly beneath the joint capsule (arrow). The intensely hyperechoic labrum (*) is more easily visualized in thin patients.**
b. **In addition, in this same view, the contour of the anterior head and neck junction can be observed, and structural abnormality, including femoroacetabular impingement (FAI), may be visualized. This image depicts a "cam lesion" of FAI: observe the flattened contour of the head-neck junction seen in B compared with the normal rounded view of that in A.**

Mastering these skills in the hip region provides a strong foundation for developing further ultrasonographic concepts, and these techniques can be used as a paradigm for many other areas of evaluation. First, ensure that the femoral neck is perpendicular to the probe (the anterior cortical line will therefore be horizontal and parallel to the floor on the screen). The bone is most hyperechoic when the probe is completely perpendicular. Soft tissues are usually draped over the bone and should be most echogenic in that same position of the probe. If the hip is flexed with the knee on a pillow, then you will need to alter your probe orientation accordingly to obtain the ideal image, whilst also accounting for the natural anteversion of the femoral neck. To simplify, however, maintaining the probe perpendicular to the patient's skin is typically the best starting position to obtain the desired image.

If the examiner experiences difficulty positioning the femoral neck horizontal and parallel to the floor, the image may be adjusted accordingly with small rocking, rotating, and sweeping movements to the probe. First, the utility of rocking will be described, using the right hip as an example. If the distal end of the neck is lower on the image screen than the proximal end (neck is somewhat diagonal, instead of horizontal), then rocking your probe towards the heel (examiner's thumb end) will correct the image. The concept is that the distal end of the femoral neck projected lower on the screen (deeper) than the proximal end of the femoral neck, and rocking the probe towards the heel (grossly closer to the deeper structure) brought that distal region of the femoral neck up into a more parallel orientation. Alternatively, the hip could be internally rotated, thereby removing the anteversion in the femoral neck and allowing your probe to stay parallel to the floor. Second, rotating the probe around its center axis may be necessary to view the entire neck, head, and acetabulum together in one view. Typically, this is easily resolved with trial and error when obtaining the image. Sweeping superolateral to the superior femoral neck and inferomedial to the calcar means keeping the base of the femoral head in the center of the image but sliding/translating the probe on the skin without tilting or rotating the probe. Sweeping the probe from the inferior to the superior neck provides a reliable way to ensure that the probe is parallel to, and centered on, the femoral neck. For example, if the examiner slides the probe towards the superior neck, but the femoral head disappears on the image prior to the neck disappearing, then the probe is oriented too vertically on the patient. Trial and error along with sweeping along the neck while simultaneously maintaining visualization of the femoral head and hip joint will allow you to construct mental borders of the anatomical landmarks. Confirmation of appropriate probe placement at the hip joint proper is done by having the patient point and rotate their toe inward and outward to internally and externally rotate the hip, respectively. Movement of the femoral head within the acetabulum will be easily visualized. Alternatively, gentle flexion at the knee from the supine position will show the femoral head dive into the acetabulum. These concepts and motions can be applied to every ultrasound exam region or structure.

The most practical anatomy visualized in this position is the anterior labrum, femoral head, hip joint capsule, and any associated joint effusion. Normally, no fluid is visible within the hip joint capsule (see Figure 5-4) and is diagnosed upon visualizing a homogenous anechoic region surrounding the femoral head and neck with distention of the overlying thin hyperechoic capsular layer. It can also be measured and monitored in this position if desired. The femoral head should be visualized as a smooth, round structure. In contrast, straight or oval appearing structures are atypical, and may clue the evaluator into a pathology like femoroacetabular impingement or osteophyte impingement, for example. The arthritic hip will be visualized as an irregular-appearing femoral head with variable amounts of osteophytes and bony hypertrophy most commonly occurring at the anterior and lateral aspects of the base of the femoral head (see Figure 5-5). Inflammatory arthritis is typically associated with less osteophyte formation, a tendency towards larger effusions, and erosions that resemble destructive arthropathy. Synovium can appear mostly hypoechoic, and hypertrophy of the synovium (synovitis) can distend the capsule. The hip labrum can be visualized from this position as well, especially in thin patients which will appear as a homogenous, hyperechoic, triangular structure adjacent to the acetabulum without separation or irregularity. If abnormality is indeed visualized, a labral tear is a possible etiologic mediator. However complete evaluation of the labrum is difficult, especially medially, laterally, and posteriorly. Therefore, MR arthrogram remains the gold standard diagnostic test for labral pathology.

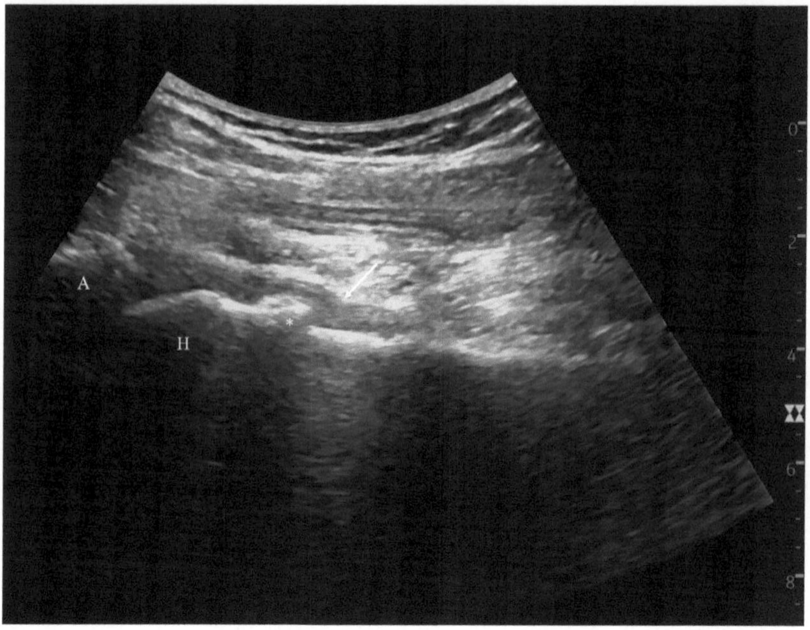

Figure 5-5

Figure 5-5
Image with the acetabulum (A) and femoral head (H) articulation in view, while centering on the base of the femoral head where an osteophyte (*) is seen. Directly superficial lies heterogenous, hypoechoic synovium and a more linear hyperechoic capsule is seen extending down towards the intertrochanteric region to the right on the image. Some capsular distention is noted from underlying inflamed, hypertrophic, boggy synovium.

Iliopsoas and Neurovascular Bundle

Imaging the iliopsoas tendon is typically most useful for interventional and/or postoperative scenarios. In the native hip, it is frequently utilized for tendonitis and snapping hip pathology (coxa saltans interna). The image is obtained with the patient supine (position seen in Figure 5-2). If the probe is first positioned in line with the femoral neck as described previously, the curved probe can be rotated to a transverse orientation, and slowly slid medially to visualize the structure. The iliopsoas tendon is most frequently located just proximal to the base of the femoral head level as the tendon begins to transverse the pelvis (see Figure 5-6). Beginners will be often surprised by the large muscle belly of the iliacus at this level; however, it serves as an important landmark as the tendon will appear dense and hyperechoic at the inferomedial aspect of the muscle.

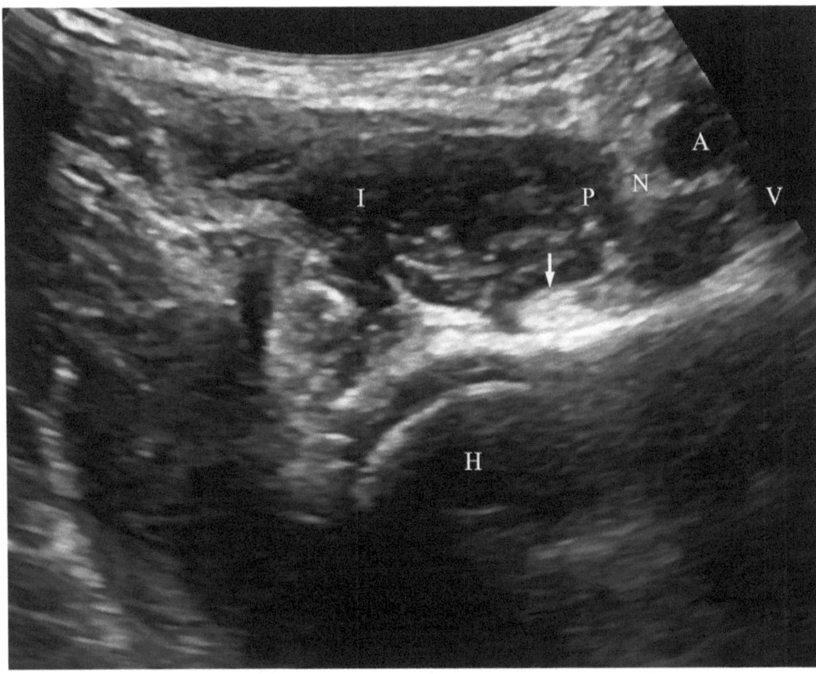

Figure 5-6

A utilitarian short-axis view of a normal iliopsoas tendon (arrow) is shown at the level of the most proximal portion of the femoral head (H). Tendon fibers organize densely at the deep portion of the muscular contributions from the iliacus (I) and psoas (P). The femoral nerve (N), external iliac artery (A), and external iliac vein (V) can be visualized as the structures just medial the muscular junction.

The iliopsoas tendon will disappear due to anisotropy as you translate the probe distally beyond the femoral head since it dives posterior to insert on the lesser trochanter at the very posteromedial aspect of the base of the intertrochanteric region. Confirming location by sliding further medially to identify the femoral neurovascular bundle is recommended. Color Doppler may be used, or the pulsating femoral artery can be used as a landmark to facilitate identification of the adjacent femoral nerve (lateral to the artery) and femoral vein (medial to the artery and compressible with probe pressure) (see Figure 5-7).

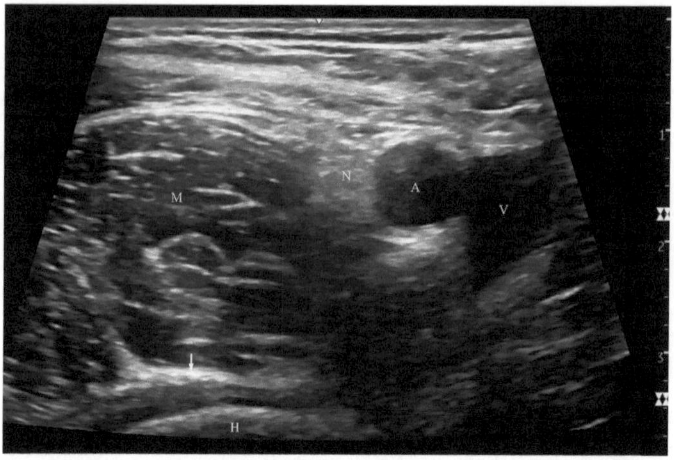

Figure 5-7a

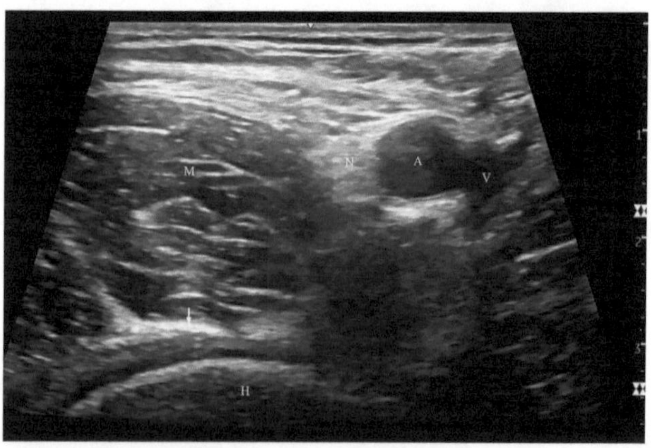

Figure 5-7b

Figure 5-7.

a. Short-axis, close-up view of the femoral nerve (N), external iliac artery (A), and external iliac vein (V). Note the honeycomb appearance to the nerve. Iliopsoas muscle (M) and tendon (arrow) are seen at the level of the superior femoral head (H).

b. Note the significant decrease in lumen size as downward probe pressure allows compression of the external iliac vein (V). This maneuver helps confirm the local anatomy being visualized.

Localization can also be confirmed by sliding up proximally into the pelvis and following the tendon and muscle belly (see Figure 5-8). Back at the level of the pelvic brim and acetabulum, the iliopsoas tendon can be visualized in long axis by centering the probe on the tendon transversely (similar to Figure 5-6), and then rotating the probe parallel to the longitudinal view (see Figure 5-9).

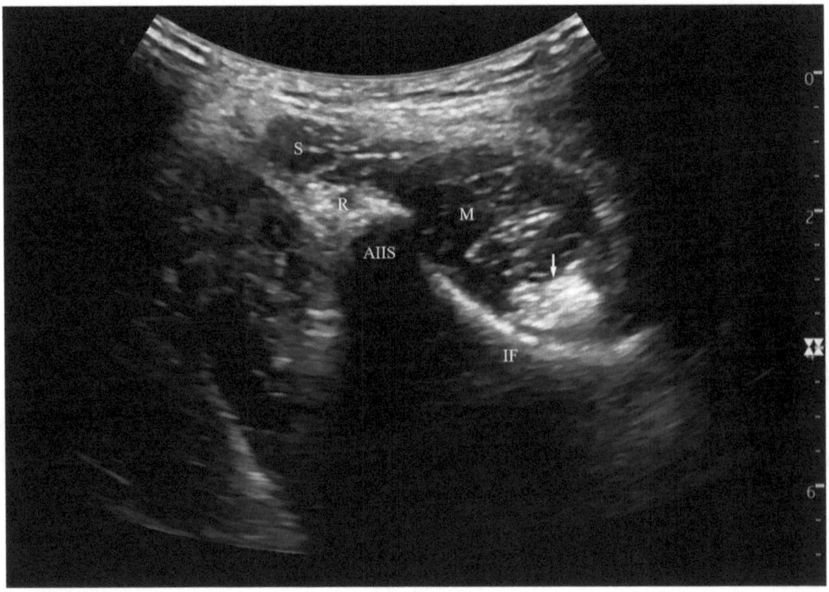

Figure 5-8a

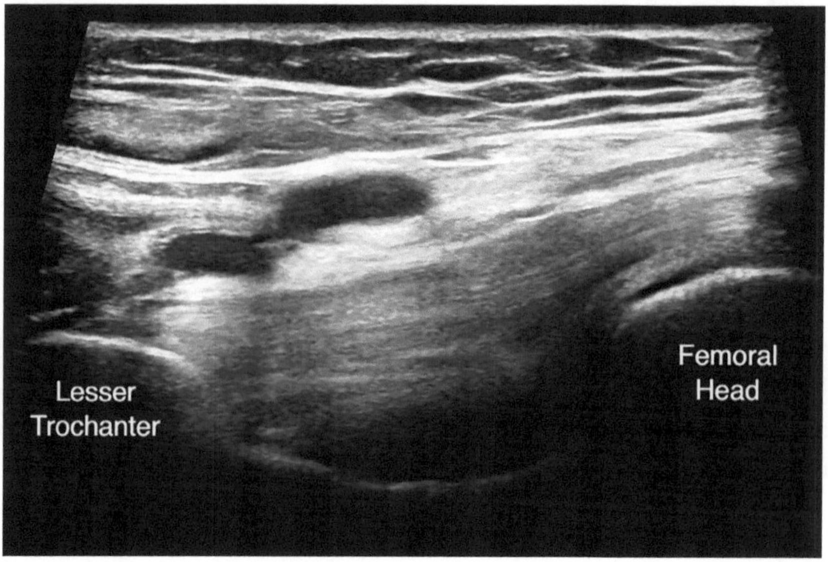

Figure 5-8b

Figure 5-8.

a. Short-axis view at the level of the anterior inferior iliac spine (AIIS). Clear visualization of the iliopsoas muscle (M) and tendon (arrow) are seen lying on the iliac fossa (IF). The origin of the direct head of the rectus femoris (R) and the sartorius (S) are also seen well at this level. The iliacus (M) is separated into medial and lateral heads by a thin fascia. The medial head, next to the psoas, is involved in one form of snapping hip.

b. Placing the hip in a figure 4 position to fully externally rotate the femur allows a nice longitudinal view of the psoas tendon, here seen over the head and inserting into the lesser trochanter.

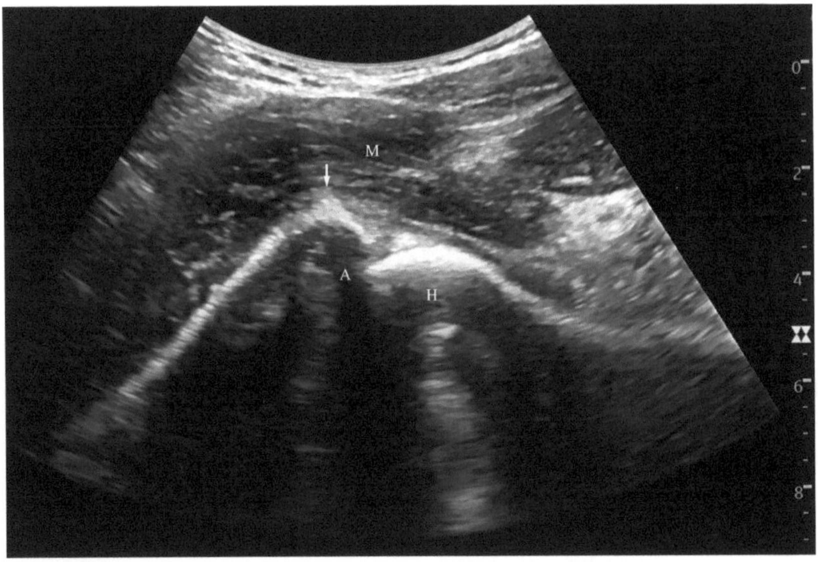

Figure 5-9

Figure 5-9
Long axis view of the iliopsoas muscle (M) and tendon (arrow) crossing over the pelvic brim, and diving downwards distally towards the lesser trochanter. The relationship and course of the tendon with both the acetabulum (A) and femoral head (H) is easily appreciated on this view, which can be utilized to dynamically assess isometric hip flexor contraction and demonstrate irregular tendon movement over the pelvic brim.

At the level of the pelvic brim, the normal psoas tendon is a slightly flattened, oval, homogenous, and hyperechoic structure directly cephalad. The muscle belly extends superolaterally from the tendon (the lateral iliacus muscle is broader than the more medial psoas muscle portion) and is typically hypoechoic due to relative attenuated density of the tendon fibrils adjacent to the denser main tendon deep on the pelvic brim. Tendinopathy will present as a thickened, rounded, less echoic major tendon. It may have irregular borders and hypoechoic regions within the tendon itself. Dynamic exam is done most practically by having the patient perform hip flexor isokinetic contraction so that the tendon can be seen sliding over the pelvic brim. Pathologic snapping of the iliopsoas can occur when the hip goes from full flexion, abduction, and external rotation back down to a neutral resting supine position. The snapping action can be difficult to visualize initially due to tendon anisotropy, and maintenance of probe position during this maneuver can prove impractical. The snap is thought to be produced by the sudden re-emergence of the medial iliacus from inside the pelvis colliding with the psoas tendon on the rim of the pelvis.

AIIS

Visualizing the tendon of the direct head of the rectus femoris is utilized for cases of tendinopathy, or more rarely, tendinous tearing from its origin, which is a common source of postoperative pain after arthroplasty. The image of the tendon is obtained with the patient supine. The anterior superior iliac spine (ASIS) is an easily palpable landmark: the probe is first placed over the ASIS in short axis (transverse), and then swept distally along the anterior pelvic border. During the sweep, once the bony cortical "valley" begins to become apparent and rises up to second "peak", which is the anterior inferior iliac spine (AIIS). The direct head of the rectus femoris tendon appears hyperechoic as the tendinous converge on their origin at the AIIS (see Figure 5-8). Rotating the probe 90 degrees will provide a long axis view of the tendon for better evaluation of tendon quality (see Figure 5-10). The indirect (reflected) head of the rectus femoris tendon lies deep to the direct head and is less often clinically implicated in snapping hip pathology. It is a relatively shorter tendon, and there is less of an actual dense hyperechoic tendon appearance until the very proximal aspect at its origin at the superolateral aspect of the acetabulum.

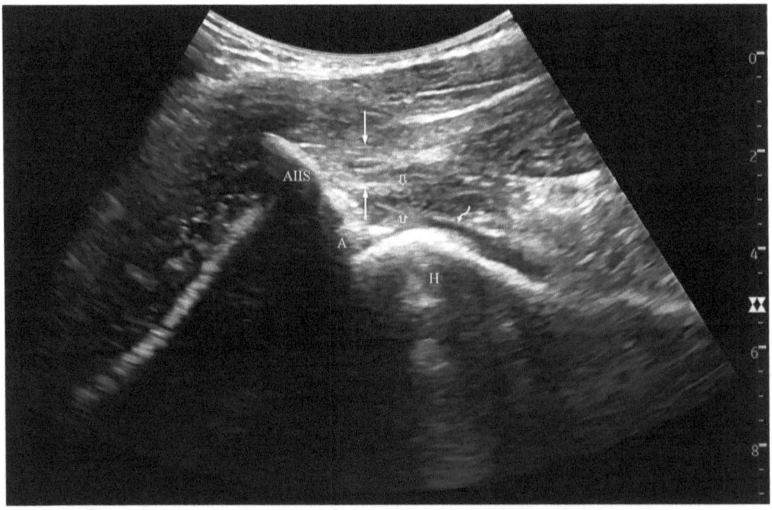

Figure 5-10

Figure 5-10

Long axis view of the tendon of the direct head of the rectus femoris (closed straight arrows) at its origin on the anterior inferior iliac spine (AIIS). The indirect head of the rectus femoris (open arrows) lies directly deep to the direct head, and immediately superficial to the thin, hyperechoic anterior hip capsule (curved arrow). It courses over superolateral femoral head (H) to its origin at the superolateral acetabulum (A).

Pathologies in this region include general tendinitis, tendon rupture, and calcific tendinitis. Tendinitis is visualized as a thickened tendon with areas of relative hypoechogenicity. Tendon tearing would present as a continuous purely hypoechoic area at the AIIS origin. Although rare, calcific tendinitis has been described to occur in the tendons surrounding the hip (Martinolli, 2008). When compared with shoulder tendinitis, that in the hip typically presents with a few days to weeks of severe, atraumatic pain that started with an insidious onset . Radiographs will typically show irregular calcifications near a tendon origin or insertion without surrounding mass or destructive characteristics (see Figure 5-11). Typically, calcified nodules will be visible on ultrasound directly adjacent to the tendon origin or insertion, (see Figure 5-12). These nodules can exhibit variable appearance: they tend to be purely hyperechoic early in the disease course due to immature calcium deposition. Later, these nodules develop a heterogeneous appearance with a hyperechoic exterior and hypoechoic interior secondary to increased calcium solidification and organization within the tendon. This appearance is similar to that of a bony cortex.

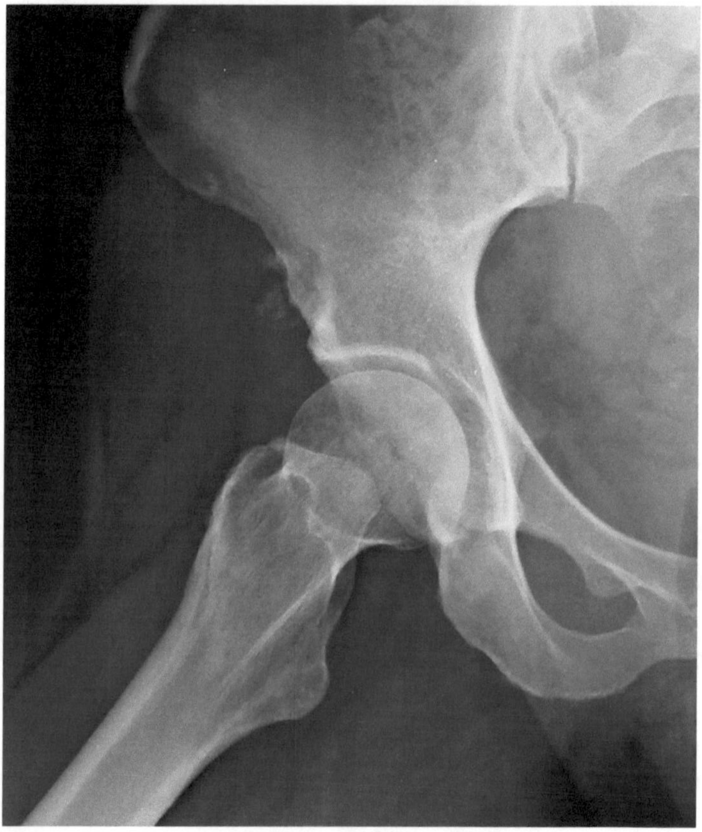

Figure 5-11

Figure 5-11
Frog Leg Lateral Radiograph of right hip demonstrating calcium nodules adjacent, and just distal to, the AIIS, consistent with calcific tendinitis of the direct head of the rectus femoris.

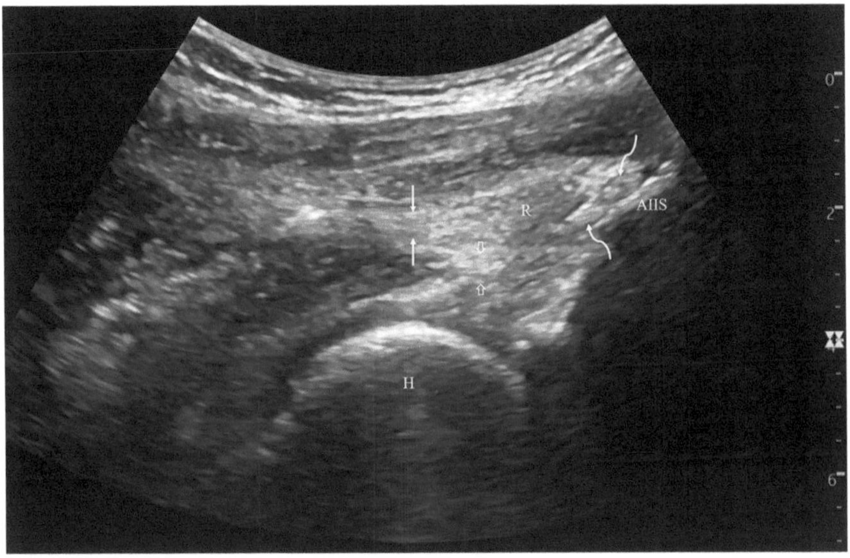

Figure 5-12

Figure 5-12.
Long axis view of the direct head of the rectus femoris tendon with femoral head (H) below. The tendon distally appears normal (closed straight arrows), but then becomes thickened and bulges with some relative hypoechogenicity proximally (R). Directly at the anterior inferior iliac spine (AIIS) origin itself the tendon has calcified nodules within its substance (curved arrows).

ASIS

The ASIS is the anatomic origin for the tensor fasciae latae (TFL) and sartorius (see Figure 5-13). It is an uncommon site for pathology, but tendinopathy and tearing are possible. The ASIS is simple to locate under ultrasound by using gross palpation to orient the probe location. When obtaining a long-axis view of the TFL, one must remember that the tendon courses laterally in the more distal region of the proximal aspect of the tendon. Therefore, instead of a straight longitudinal/vertical probe orientation, it must be oriented to aim towards the lateral aspect of the ipsilateral knee. Similarly, the sartorius enters the ASIS from the medial side at a 15-20-degree angle. At their origin, the tendons are typically flat, and directly superficial to the ASIS.

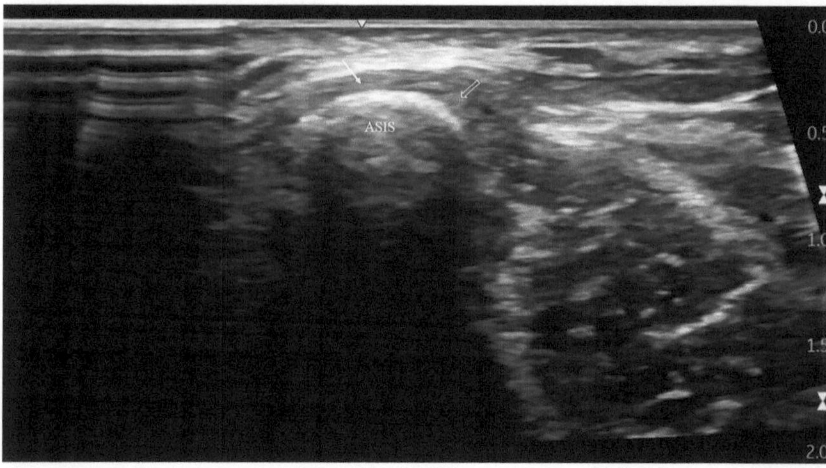

Figure 5-13

Figure 5-13
Short-axis view of the flat, superficial tendons of the tensor fasciae latae (closed arrow) and sartorius (open arrow) originating at the anterior superior iliac spine (ASIS).

Lateral Hip

Positioning

Lateral hip evaluation is most effectively performed with the patient in the lateral decubitus position. The examiner can comfortably align their view with the axis of the probe, and also see the screen easily without significant neck motion required (see Figure 5-14).

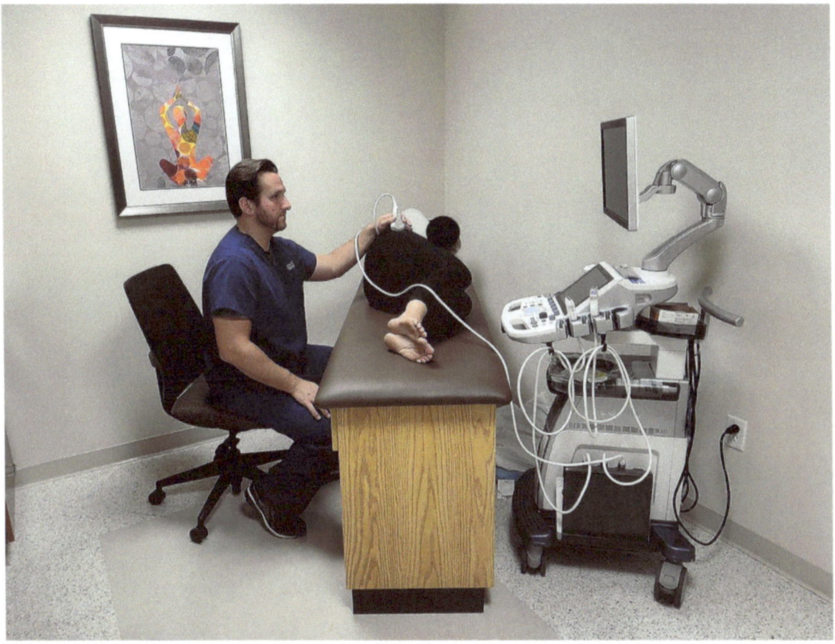

Figure 5-14

Figure 5-14.
The patient is positioned in the left lateral decubitus position for lateral hip evaluation. Note the examiner's in-line view with the long axis of the probe and simultaneous ease of viewing the screen with his position across the table.

The probe is initially placed transversely over the lateral hip to visualize the greater trochanter (GT). If the GT is not readily identified, the transducer is moved distal and transversely over the proximal femoral shaft. Moving the probe proximal while simultaneously maintaining the image of the femur facilitates fine visualization of the contours of the GT. Specifically, the apex of the GT between the anterior and lateral facets can be observed slightly anterior to the lateral hip. The gluteus minimus tendon inserts on the anterior facet, while the distal gluteus medius inserts on the posterior facet, and the gluteus maximus lies superficial to the posterior facet without inserting on it. (Figure 5-15).

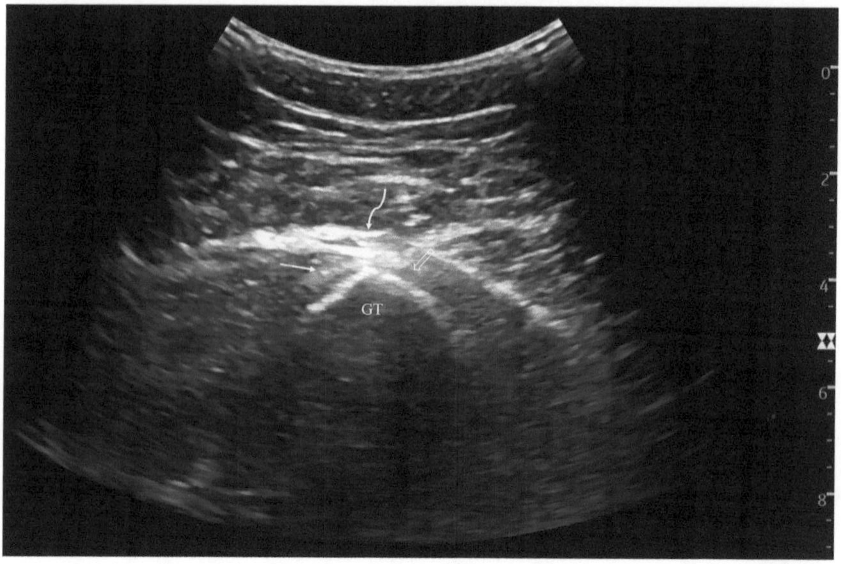

Figure 5-15: Short- axis view of the GT region displaying the peak of the lateral GT, which separates the anterior facet from the overlying gluteus minimus tendon (open arrow), and lateral and posterior facets with the overlying gluteus medius tendon (closed arrow). The curved arrow points at the gluteus maximus tendon and iliotibial band complex closely overlying the aforementioned deeper tendons .

The sub-gluteus minimus bursa lies directly deep to the gluteus minimus over the anterior facet while the hypoechoic muscle of the gluteus medius is superficial (Figure 5-16).

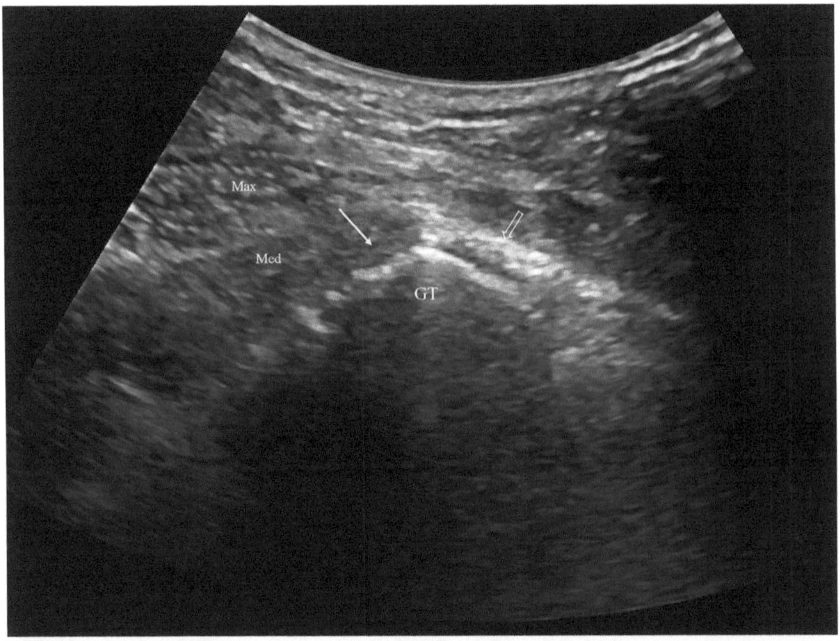

Figure 5-16: Short axis view focusing on the gluteus minimus insertion (open arrow) and the directly superficial sub-gluteus minimus bursa (dark area just above the anterior facet of the greater trochanter [GT]). Note the anisotropy of the gluteus medius tendon (closed arrow), gluteus medius (Med), and gluteus maximus (Max) with the probe oriented as such.

The iliotibial tract is observed even more superficial as a hyperechoic band of tissue and a continuation of the fascial layers enveloping the gluteus maximus posterior and tensor fascia latae anterior. The iliotibial tract is also visualized superficial to the gluteus medius tendon over the lateral facet. With external rotation of the hip, the gluteus maximus can also be observed superficial to the gluteus medius tendon. Each facet of the greater trochanter should be separately evaluated in the transverse orientation, adjusting the probe to make sure it is perpendicular to the cortex of the facet and eliminating any anisotropy of the overlying tendon. Any distended bursa can also be visualized with proper probe orientation, and of note, there are bursas present between each tendon and their respective trochanteric facet. The trochanteric bursa is between the gluteus maximus and posterior facet and, therefore, the probe must be positioned posterior to ensure any bursal distention in this area is not overlooked (Figure 5-17).

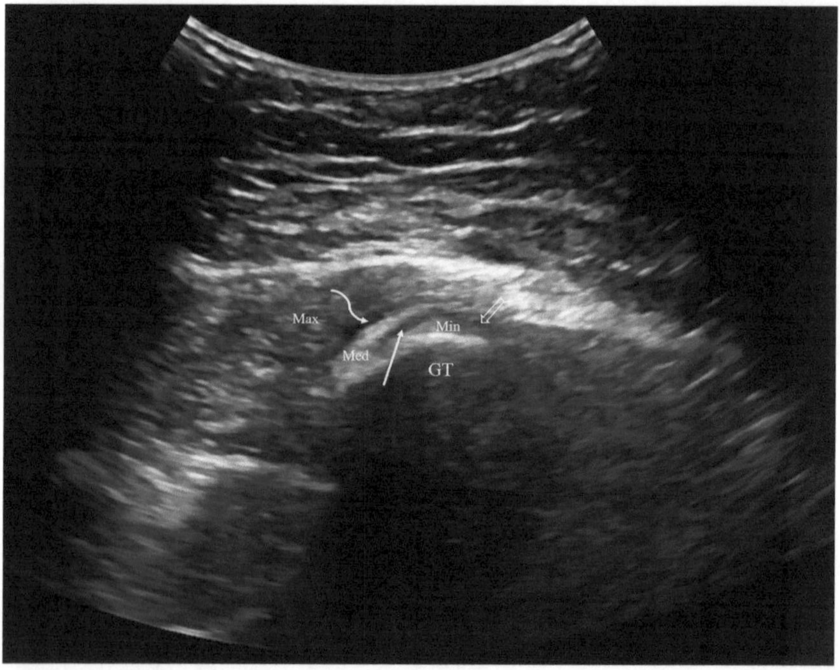

Figure 5-17: Short-axis view separately evaluating the lateral and posterior facets. This view allows the ultrasonographer to more distinctly visualize the insertion of the gluteus medius tendon (Med) with overlying gluteus maximus muscle (Max) and the greater trochanteric bursa (curved arrow). The sub-gluteus medius bursa (closed arrow) can be seen directly beneath the gluteus medius and superficial to the greater trochanteric (GT) cortex of the lateral facet. The posterior aspect of the gluteus minimus insertion (Min) can also be seen here, but only more anteriorly on the far anterior aspect of facet: the insertion is subject to anisotropy (open arrow) and cannot be reliably visualized unless the probe is translated more anteriorly, or the hip is externally rotated.

Distension of the trochanteric bursa can also extend laterally between the gluteus medius tendon and iliotibial tract.

The gluteus minimus tendon is imaged longitudinally by initially obtaining a short-axis view directly superficial and perpendicular to the anterior facet, visualizing the gluteus minimus tendon transversely. The probe is then rotated 90 degrees, and oriented slightly anterior. A similar technique is used to obtain a longitudinal view of the gluteus medius over the lateral facet, angling the probe slightly posterior (Figure 5-18).

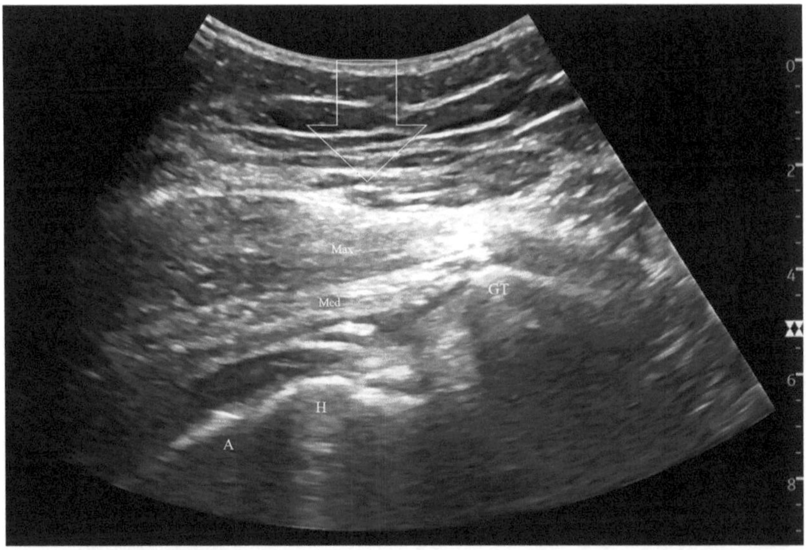

Figure 5-18: Long-axis view of the gluteus medius tendon (Med) and gluteus maximus (Max) musculotendinous junction focused ~2 cm proximal to the insertion on the greater trochanter (GT). The large open arrow notes the ultrasound beam direction; underlying structures are best visualized when the beam is projected perpendicularly to the structures of interest. Note, the anisotropy of the Med at its insertion at the GT. Additionally, this view facilitates a comprehensive view of the hip as both the posterior femoral head (H) and acetabulum (A) can be visualized as well.

Since the gluteus medius attaches to both the lateral and superoposterior facets, the probe should be moved proximal and posterior to visualize the full extent of this tendinous insertion. Pathology within the gluteus medius tendon can be seen on both short-axis (Figures 5-19 and 5-21) and long-axis (Figures 5-20 and 5-22) views.

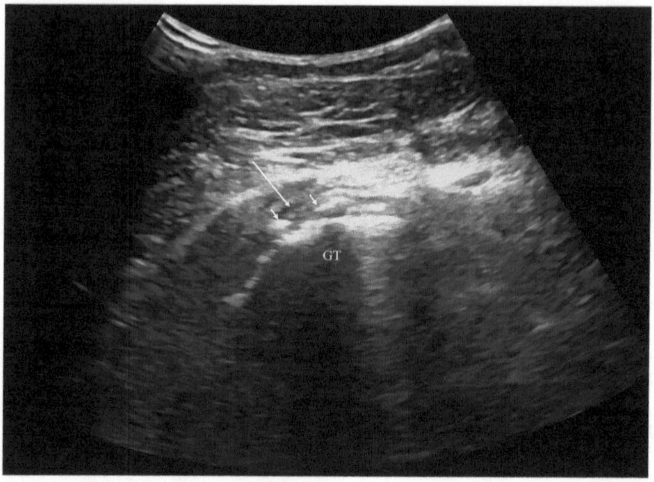

Figure 5-19: Short axis view of the lateral hip over the greater trochanter (GT) showing mulifocal, partial tearing of the gluteus medius tendon (closed arrows) near its insertion, as can be evidenced by the heterogeneously hypoechoic bursal-type tissues that has infiltrated the space surrounding the torn tendon strands.

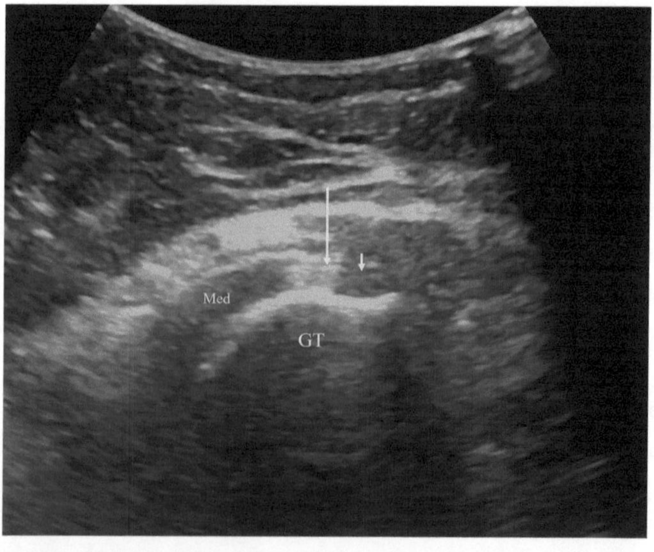

Figure 5-20: Long-axis view of the lateral hip over the greater trochanter (GT) showing significant insertional partial tearing (short, closed arrow) of the thickened, tendinotic insertion (long closed arrow) of the gluteus medius (Med).

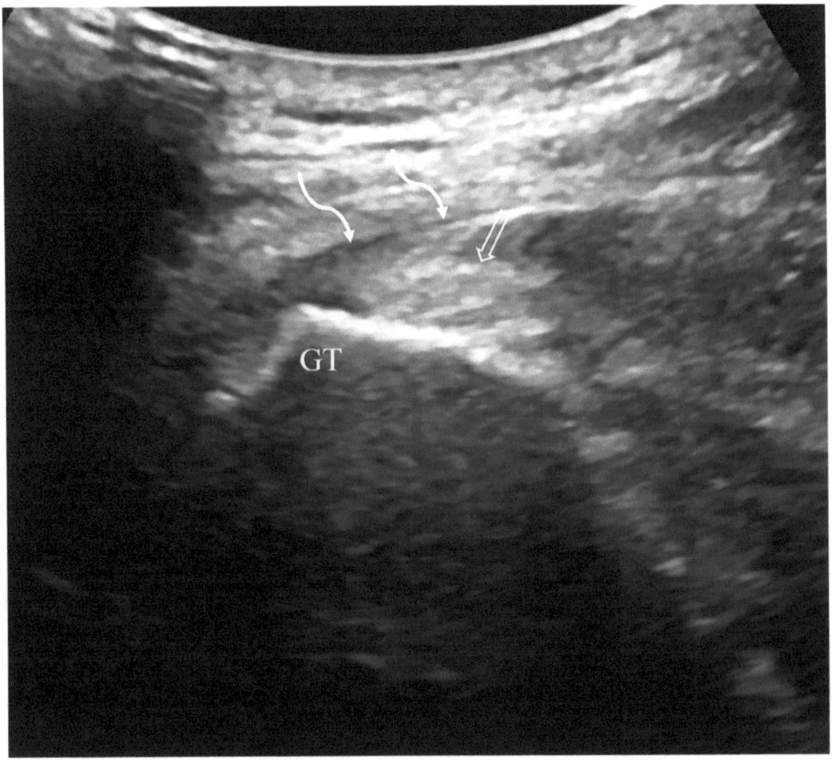

Figure 5-21: A magnified short-axis view of the lateral hip over the greater trochanter (GT). Here, significant thickening of the gluteus medius tendon with areas of heterogeneity and hypoechogenicity at and near its insertion on the lateral facet (large, hollowed arrow). No definitive partial tearing is observed. Note the hypoechoic fluid (curved arrows) within the greater trochanteric bursa directly superficial and deep to the gluteus medius and gluteus maximus, respectively.

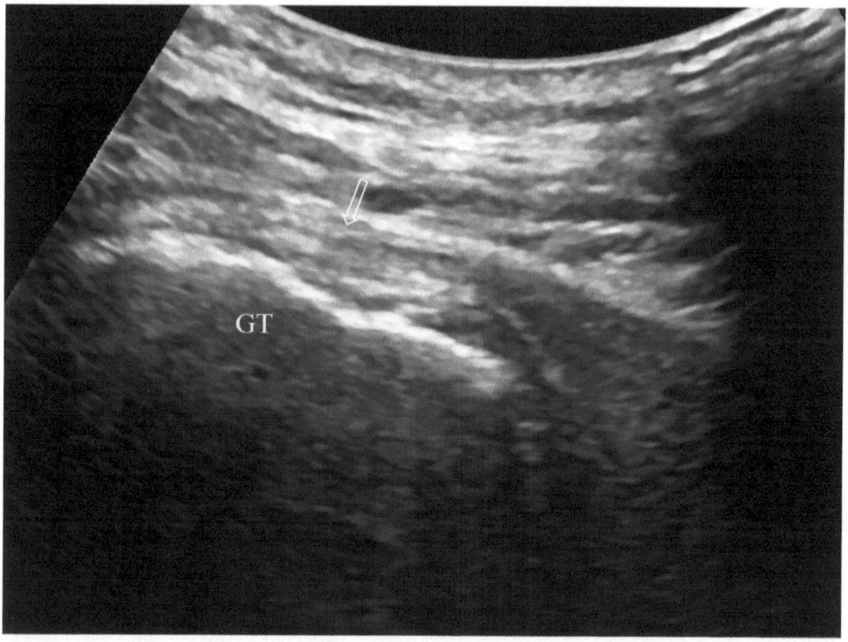

Figure 5-22: Magnified long-axis view of the lateral facet of the greater trochanter (GT) showing tendinosis with a slightly thickened gluteus medius tendon (open arrow) with distinctly longitudinal hypoechoic regions. Much like in MRI, small intra-substance tendon tearing cannot be reliably differentiated from severe tendinosis. However, the greater number and surface area of hypoechoic regions within the tendon, the more likely they are to represent regions of partial tearing.

Posterior Hip

Posterior hip examination

Ultrasound examination and treatment of the posterior hip region begins with the lumbar spine and works distally. Examination in this area is usually specific for a particular area (as in the hand, foot, or knee), but not quite as comprehensive as that in the shoulder. Orthopaedic ultrasound interventions are also rare in the posterior region of the hip for various reasons that we will discuss.

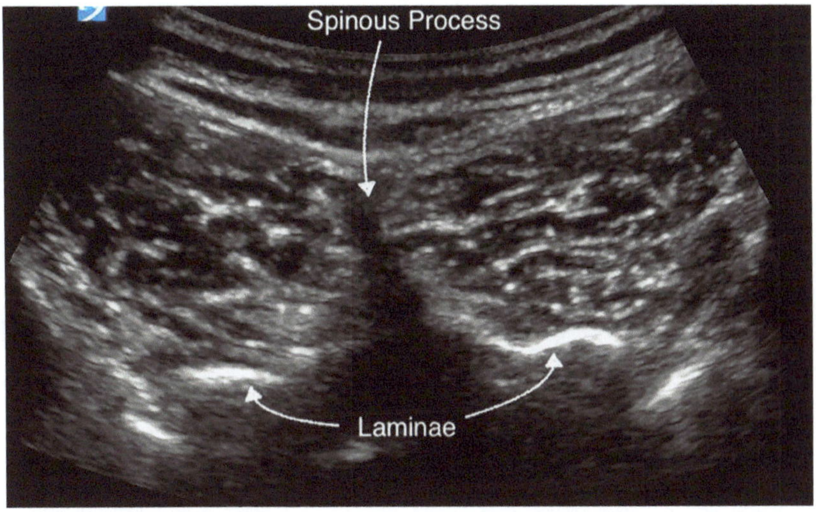

Figure 5-23: Posterior view of the L4 vertebra. An ultrasound shadow is cast deep to the spinous process between the hyperechoic laminae.

The most proximal evaluation begins with the L4 vertebra. This allows us to adjust depth and gain to develop an initial fundamental understanding of the patient's physiognomy. However, in general, interventions in this region are more accurately and routinely performed with CT (e.g., facet injection). The laminae are perpendicular to the beam, and are therefore the most echogenic (Figure 5-23), whereas the spinous process is reduced to a mere shadow.

Once examination is complete in this initial region, evaluation is then moved distally to both the sacrum and the sacroiliac joint. The probe should be positioned initially in the midline over the sacrum. The sacrum is then visualized from proximal to distal, initially identifying the posterior foramina (Fig. 5-24), the lateral sacral crests (Fig. 5-25), and the distal end (Fig. 5-26).

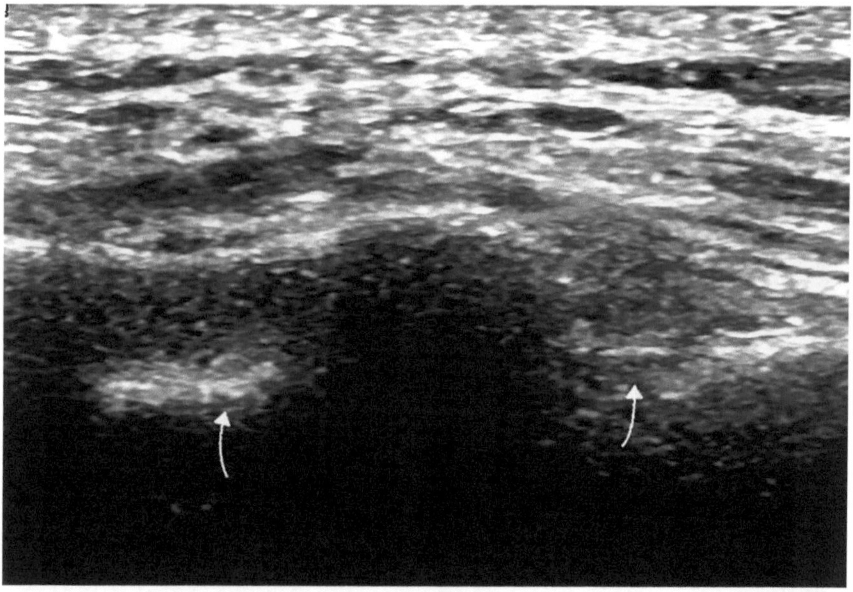

Figure 5-24: Image of the posterior foramina (arrows) with the probe oriented transversely over the sacrum.

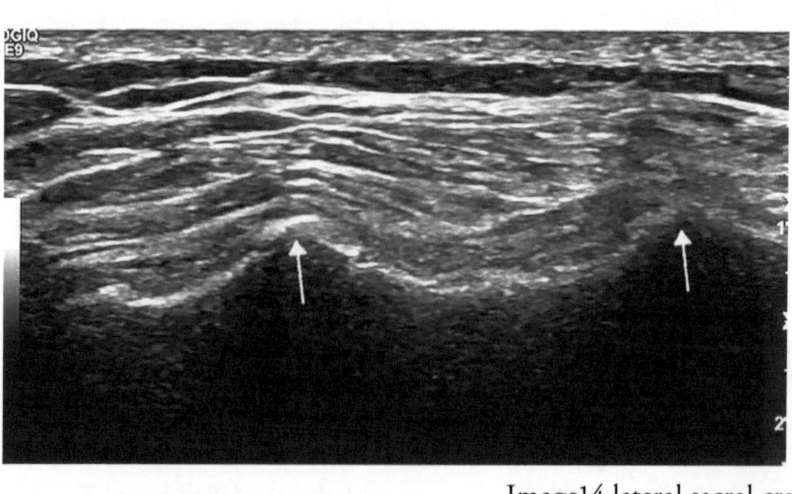

Image14 lateral sacral crest

Figure 5-25: The lateral sacral crests (arrows) seen on the short axis.

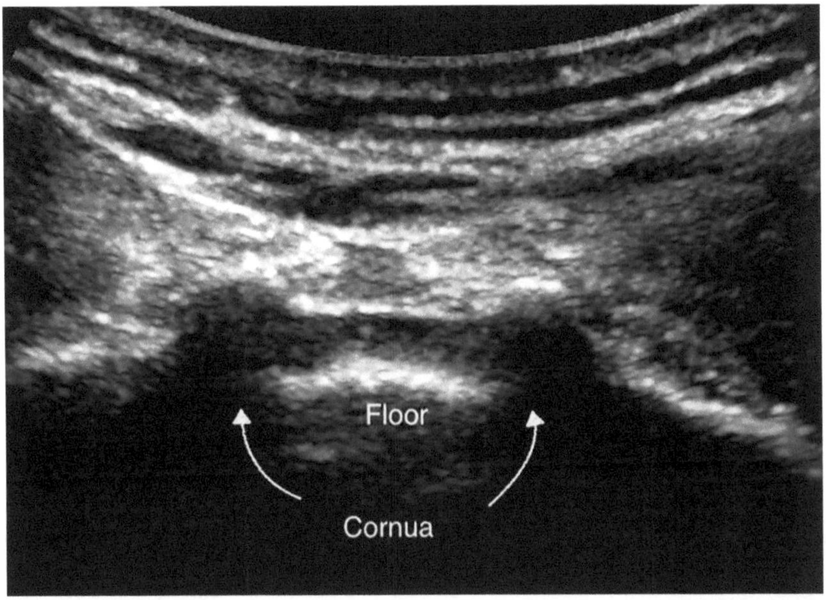

Figure 5-26. The distal sacrum. Note the gap in the roof of the canal, through which, the floor of the canal is visualized. Extending laterally, the sacrum has two small bony horns or cornua, and these gaps are frequently targeted and utilized by pain doctors and anesthesiologists.

The probe is then placed back on the proximal sacrum, before being moved laterally to visualize the posterior sacral foramina, the sacroiliac joint, and adjacent posterior ilium. The sacroiliac ligaments run distal from the ilium to the sacrum. The short ligaments are seen by orienting the probe in a slightly oblique and transverse view from superior/lateral on the ilium to inferior/medial on the sacrum (Fig. 5-27).

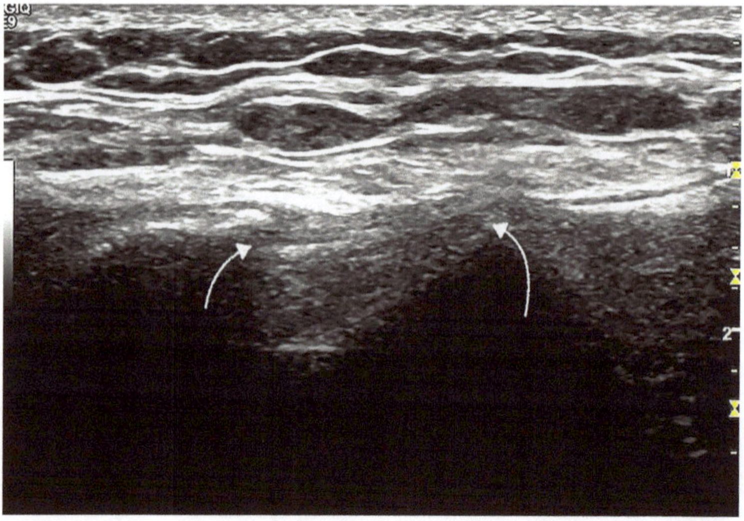

Figure 5-27: The sacroiliac ligaments (arrows) course distally from the ilium to the sacrum. Here the probe is positioned obliquely from the upper lateral (ilium) on the left, to lower medial (sacrum) on the right.

As the transducer is advanced to the distal aspect of the sacroiliac junction, the SI joint proper is visualized (Fig. 5-28). The ultrasonographer should look for the "U" shaped area between ilium and sacrum, as can be performed under direct visualization in this region.

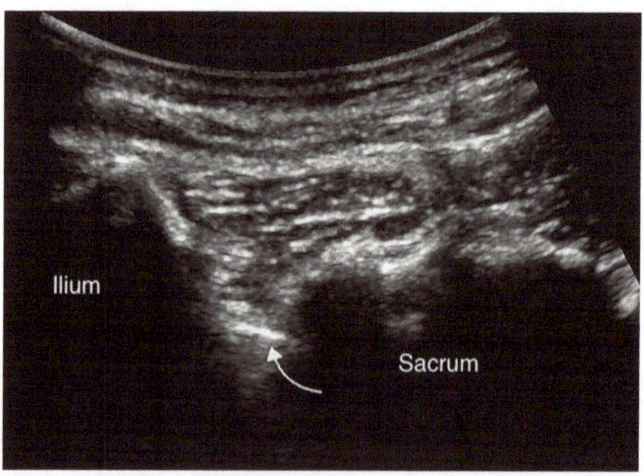

Figure 5-28. The SI joint proper (arrow) visualized at the lower end of the sacroiliac junction. Look for the "U" shaped area between ilium and sacrum.

Posterior Muscles

The piriformis is visualized by placing the linear or curvilinear probe at 45° to the long axis. The transducer is first positioned transversely over the SI joint, and then translated distally into the greater sciatic notch. Once there, the probe is rotated 45 degrees inferolateral towards the greater trochanter to obtain a longitudinal view of the piriformis (Fig. 5-29, 30).

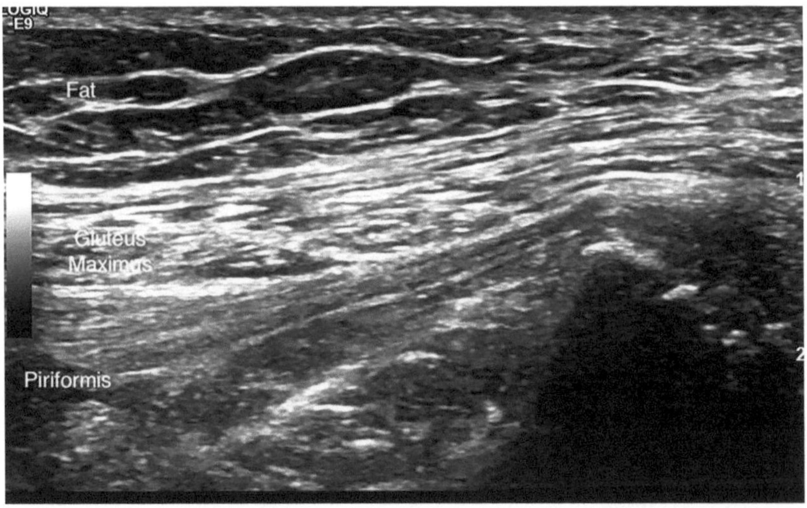

Image30 piriformis

Figure 5-29: Piriformis is visualized deep to the gluteus maximus.

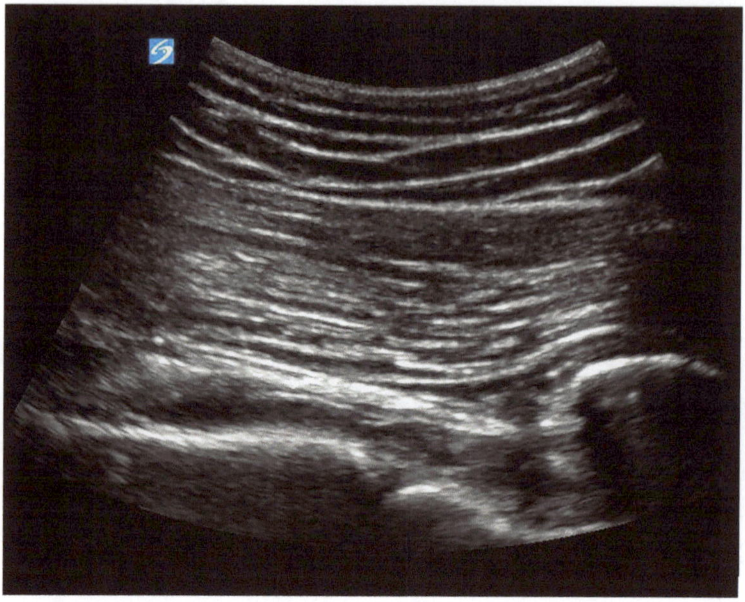

Figure 5-30: The upper portion of piriformis may traverse the ilium (left) followed by the femoral head as it approaches its insertion site on the greater trochanter (right).

The piriformis is the only muscle observed in that plane, as it lies under gluteus maximus, without the sciatic nerve between them. With a higher order machine, the sciatic nerve can be visualized underneath -- and exiting – below the muscle, however, this can be technically difficult even in the hands of the most experienced ultrasonographers.

Evaluation of the quadratus femoris, obturators, and gemelli begins by imaging the ischial tuberosity in the transverse plane at the hamstring origin. The obturator internus is a useful landmark as it is the only one of the lateral rotators to originate within the pelvis. It then crosses the ischium and the femoral head as it inserts on the greater trochanter, which is best identified dynamically (Fig. 5-31).

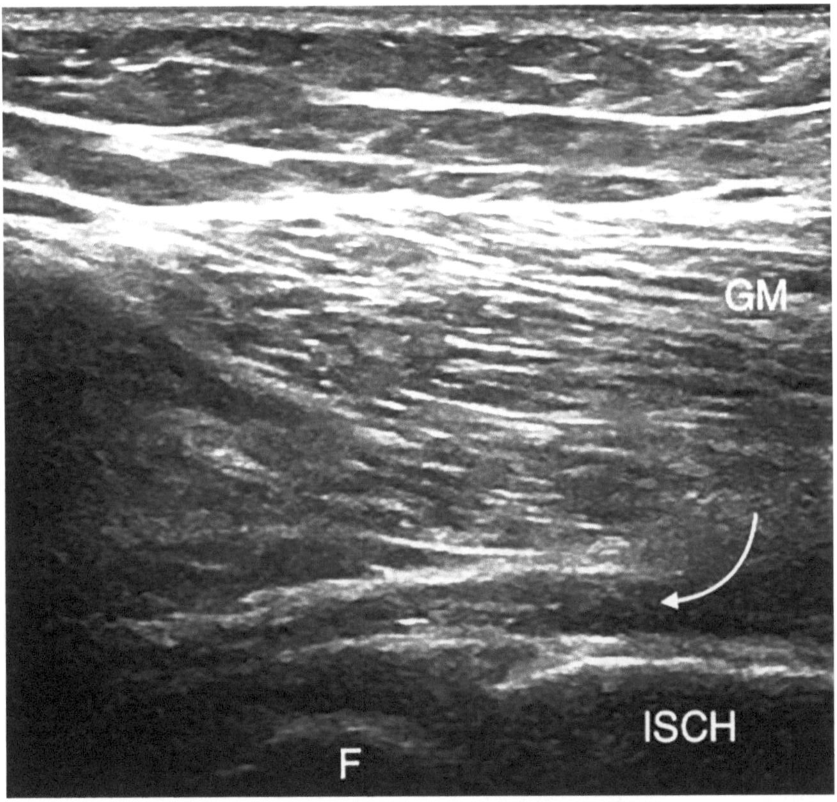

Image38 obturator internus copy

Figure 5-31: Obturator internus (arrow) originating within the pelvis (out of view to the right), and then crosses the ischium (ISCH) and the femoral head (F) on its way to the trochanter (off screen to the left).

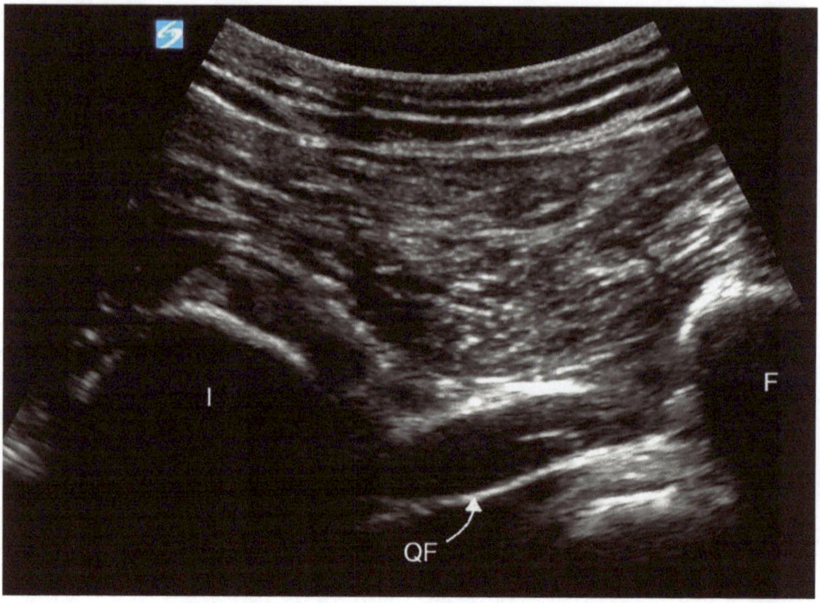

Figure 5-32: Quadratus femoris (QF) running between the ischium (I) and the femur (F), imaged here with the hip in internal rotation.

The quadratus femoris, also best identified dynamically, is the most caudal of the five lateral rotators, and is visualized lateral to the ischial tuberosity and deep to the sciatic nerve (Fig. 5-32). It represents a very helpful landmark as it divides the ischium and the femur. With the hip in external rotation, the quadratus femoris attachment on the greater tuberosity approaches that on the ischium, and the muscle thickens. The proximal hamstrings are imaged above close to their origin from the ischium on this view, as is the sciatic nerve (a little more visible over the quadratus than over the other lateral rotators) (Fig. 5-33).

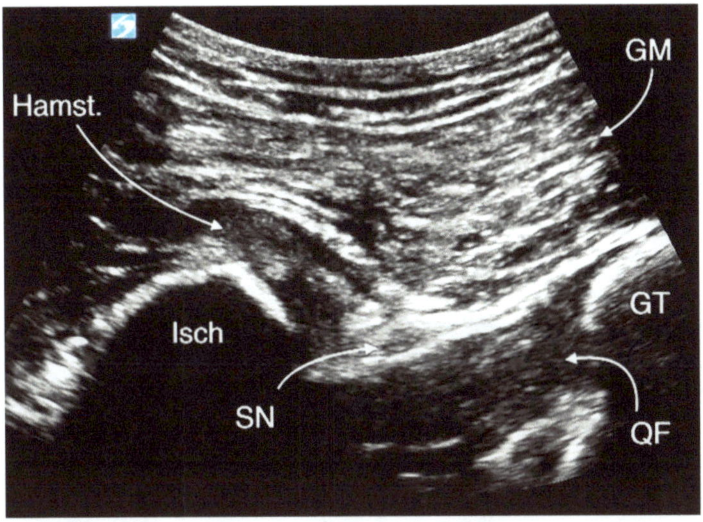

Figure 5-33: Quadratus femoris (QF) with the hip in external rotation. Its insertion on the greater trochanter (GT) approaches the ischium (Isch). The proximal hamstrings (Hamst.) and sciatic nerve (SN) are also visualized.

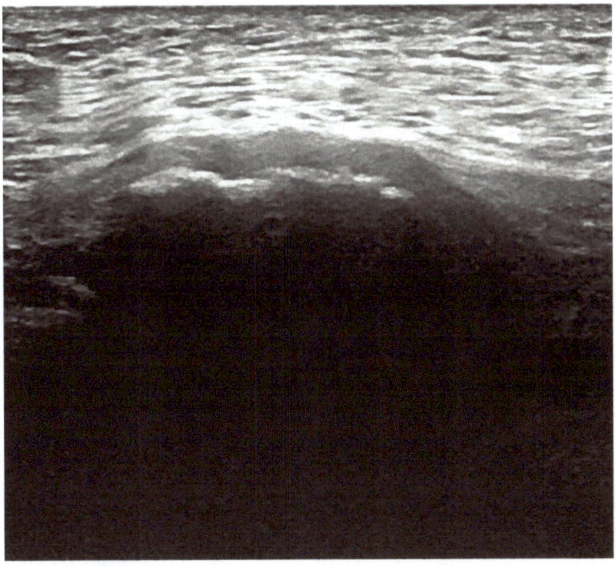

Image24 ischial tuberosity

Figure 5-34: Transverse view of the ischial tuberosity covered by the hamstring origin.

The ischial tuberosity is covered by the thick hamstring tendinous origin. With the hip in extension, the upper tendons may be rendered dark by anisotropy (Fig. 5-35). Placing a pillow under the pelvis will allow a little hip flexion to provide tension on the hamstring origin. In turn, this maneuver straightens the tendon, thereby improving echogenicity and eliminating the anisotropy artifact (Fig. 5-36).

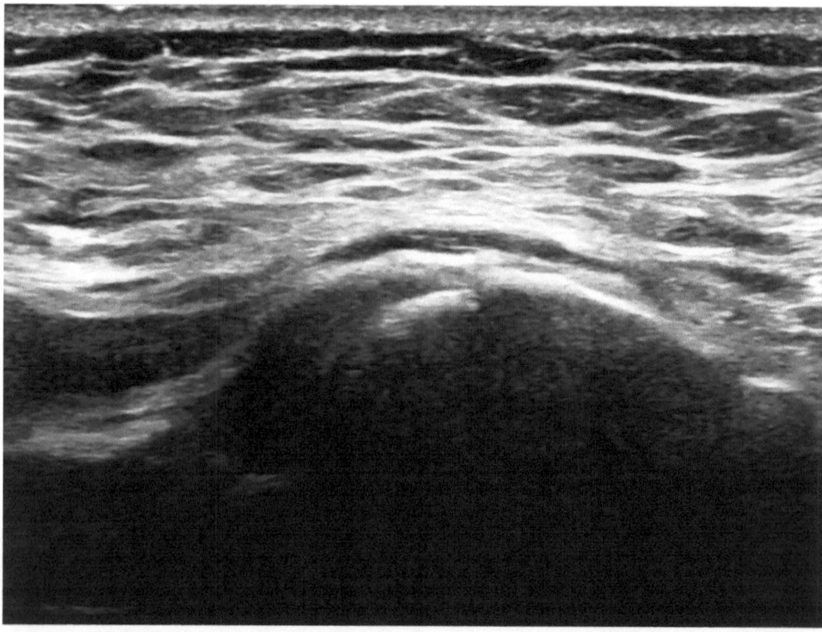

Figure 5-35: Ischial tuberosity with the hip in extension. Hamstring attachment seen as anechoic due to anisotropy.

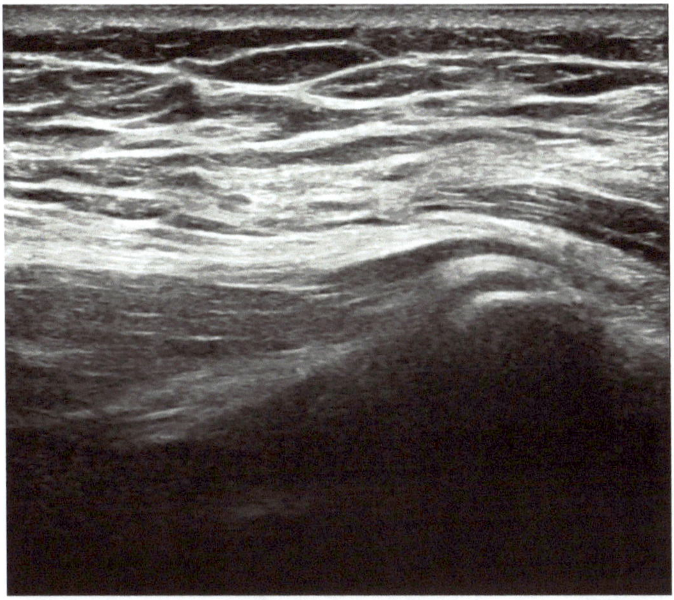

Figure 5-36: Hamstring origin from the ischium with the hip in some flexion, eliminating some of anisotropy artifact.

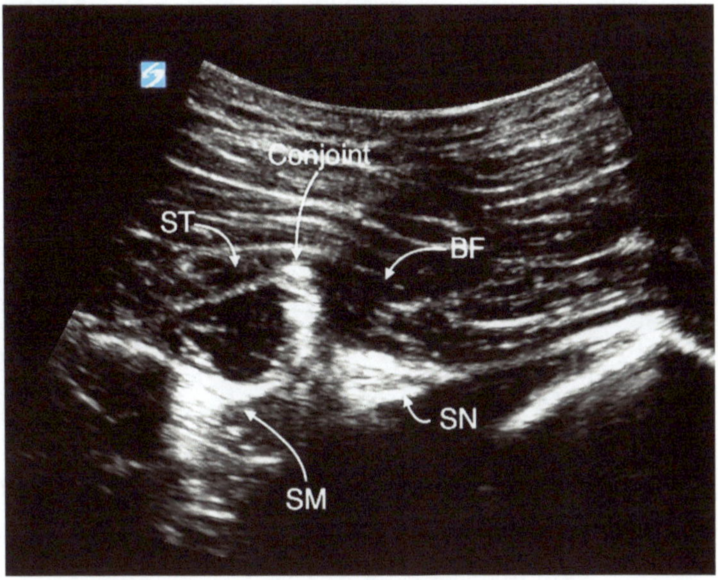

Figure 5-37: Short-axis view of proximal hamstrings, including the biceps femoris (BF), semitendinosus (ST), their conjoint tendon (Conjoint), the sciatic nerve (SN), and the deep semimembranosus (SM).

In the short axis, the upper hamstrings allow for good visualization of the nerve thanks to the muscles. The conjoint tendon of biceps femoris and semitendinosus runs between the two muscles. The sciatic nerve is usually located deep, or deep and lateral to the conjoint tendon. As the probe is moved proximally, the sciatic nerve appears more lateral since the tendons are moving medial to join the ischium. The semimembranosus lies deep to semitendinosus, while the gluteus maximus forms the roof, and the adductor magnus represents the floor (Fig. 5-37 & 38).

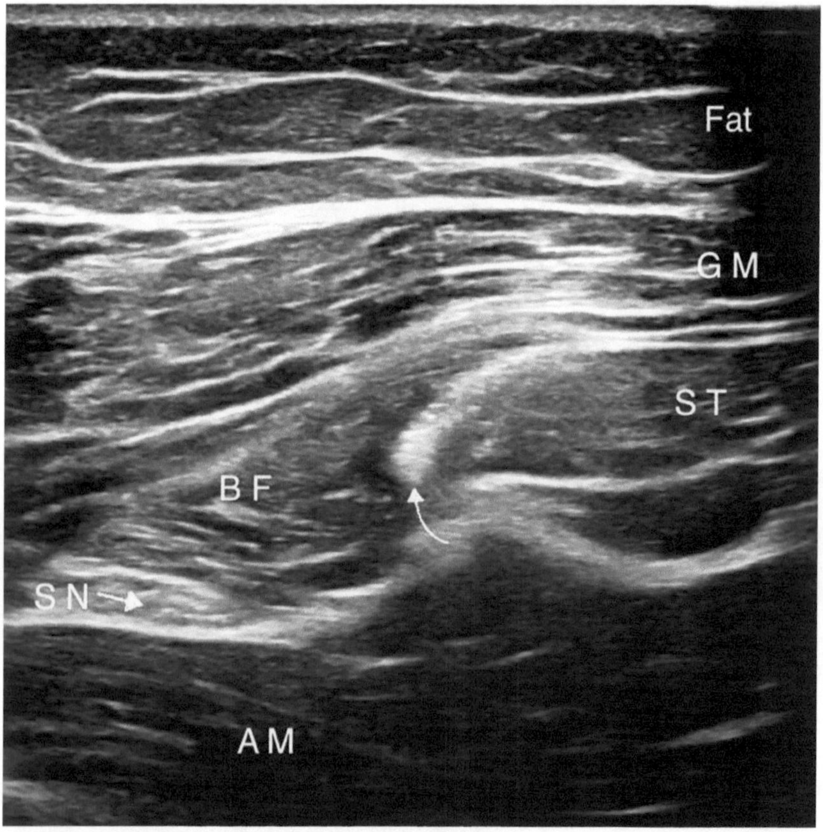

Figure 5-38: Proximal hamstrings in the short axis with higher frequency linear probe. Lateral is to the left, medial to the right.

Biceps femoris (BF) and the sciatic nerve (SN) are visualized laterally while the semitendinosus (ST) and the semimembranosus lie more medial. Gluteus maximus (GM) forms the roof while adductor magnus (AM) represents the floor. The arrow points to the deep end of the conjoint tendon.

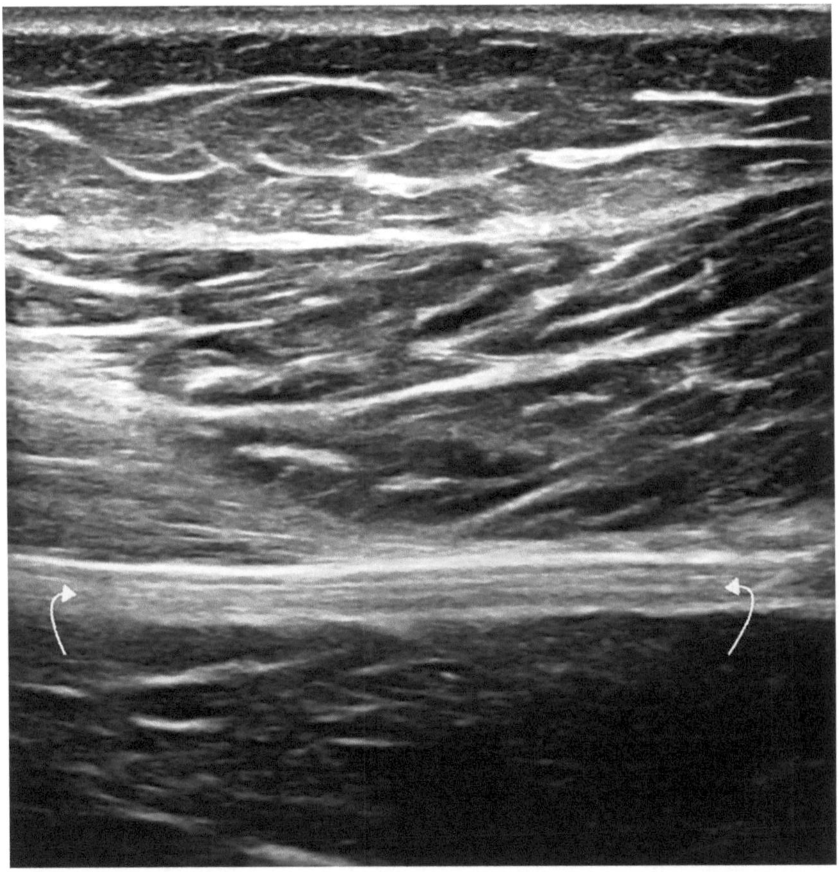

Figure 5-39: Longitudinal view of the sciatic nerve (arrows) in the thigh.

The sciatic nerve is also easier to see in its long axis in the thigh (Fig. 5-39) than it is in the posterior hip. It can be visualized running deep to the hamstring muscles, and superficial to the adductor magnus. In the short axis, the sciatic nerve is easier to find in the proximal thigh than it is directly behind the hip (Fig. 5-40). Therefore, it can be identified here, and the probe can be translated proximally to the posterior hip.

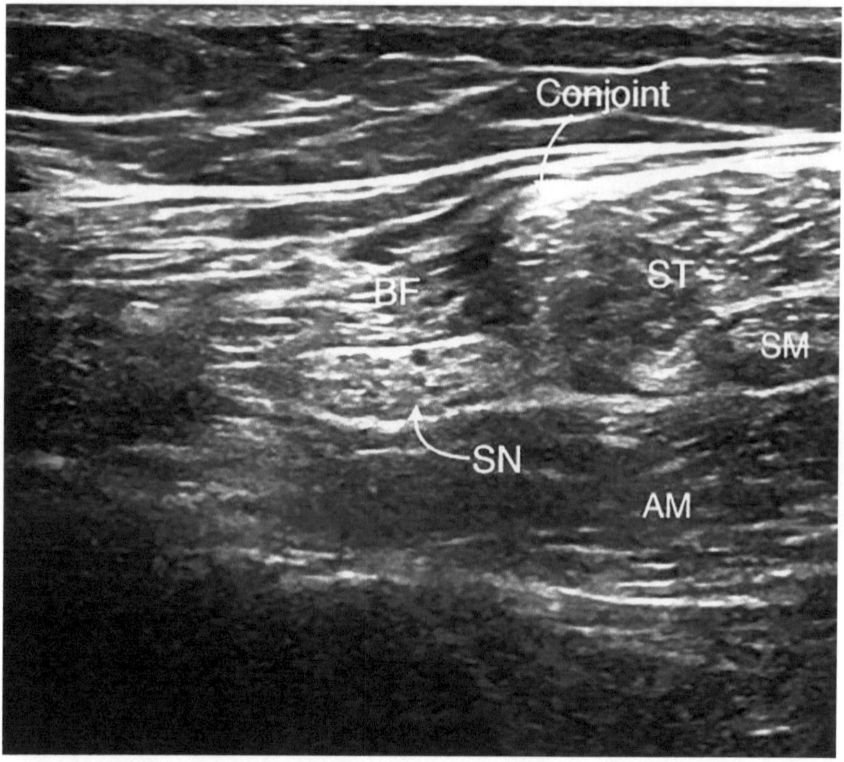

Figure 5-40 Short-axis image of the sciatic nerve (SN) in the upper thigh region easily visualized deep to the biceps femoris (BF), lateral to the conjoint tendon (Conjoint), semitendinosus (ST), and semimembranosus (SM), and superficial to the adductor magnus (AM).

In-office dynamic exams

Snapping psoas tendon

A snap with motion in the groin area is best evaluated dynamically. When the hip is in flexion/external rotation, the medial head of iliacus retracts into the pelvis. As the hip moves into extension the medial head emerges suddenly and pushes the psoas tendon against the brim of the pelvis. Although the re-emergence of the medial head is the etiologic agent, it is the sudden movement of the psoas tendon that is more apparent. This is a somewhat difficult exam to perform, as the probe must stay parallel to the brim of the pelvis during movement. It may take several attempts to appreciate the "snap." The images below illustrate the psoas just before and after the "snap." Temporary relief of pain can be obtained by injecting the iliopsoas bursa on the pelvic brim.

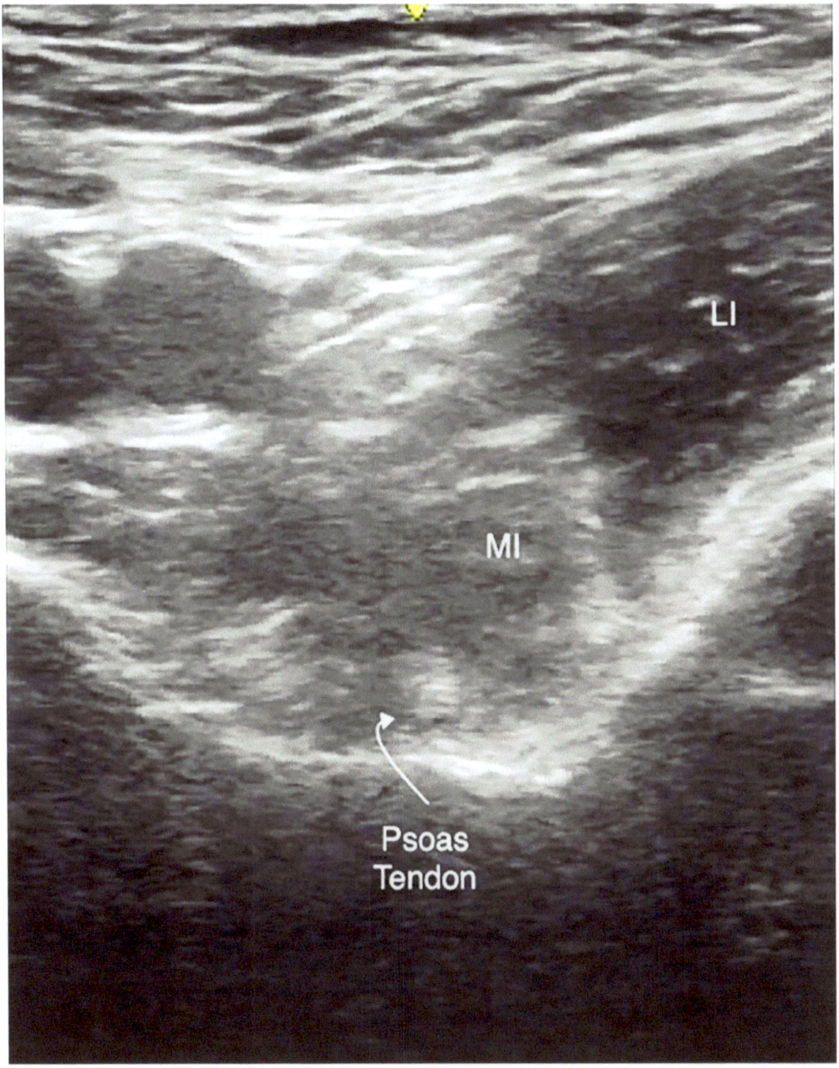

Figure 5-41a

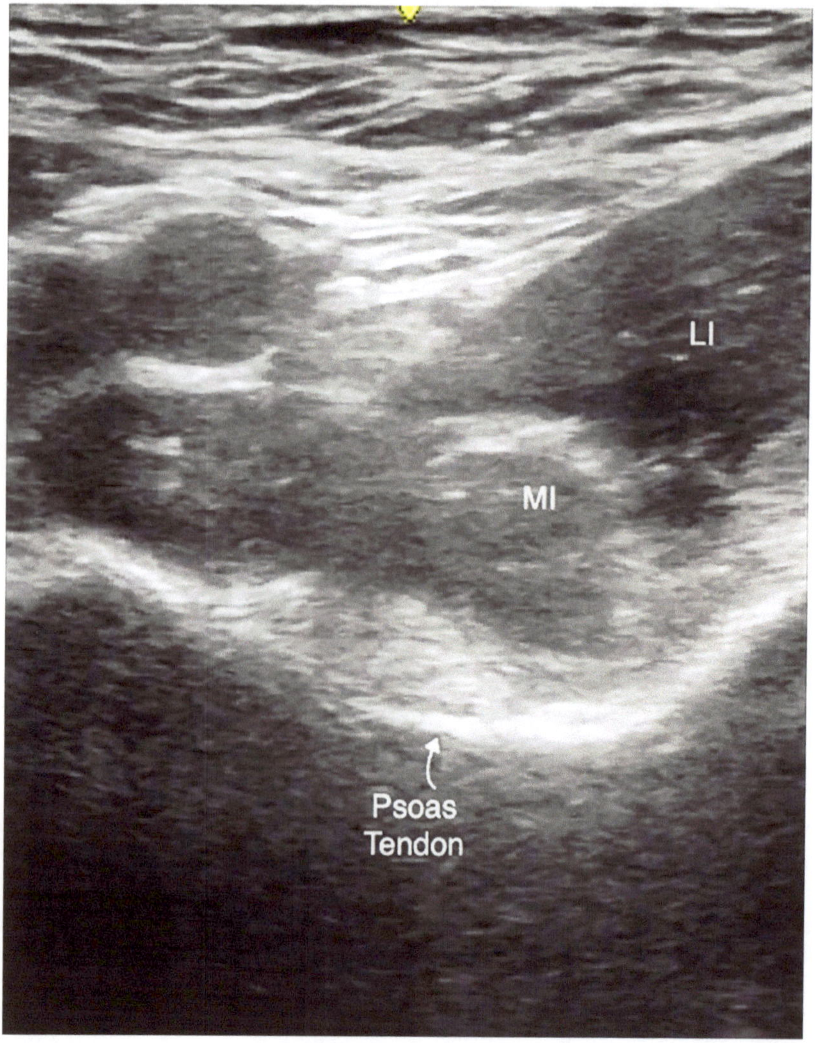

Figure 5-41b

Figure 5-41a and b. Snapping psoas tendon in 16 y.o. female athlete. Flexion-abduction-external rotation motion incarcerates the medial iliacus between psoas and inner pelvis. As the hip returns to its neutral position, the medial iliacus emerges and forces the psoas against the rim. These two views are stop-action views just before (Figure 5-41A), and just after (Figure 5-41B, the "snap." Note that after the "snap," the part of the psoas against the pelvis is thicker, less echogenic, and more medial.

Snapping Iliotibial Band

A lateral snap at the hip is produced by an amalgam of the tensor fasciae latae, gluteus maximus, and iliotibial band complex ascending and falling off of the greater trochanter. Like the other "snap," this is best observed dynamically. For positioning, the patient lies in the lateral decubitus position upon the uninvolved hip. The hip being examined is placed in slight adduction, and ranged between flexion and extension. The "snap" is appreciated and visualized during the dynamic motion.

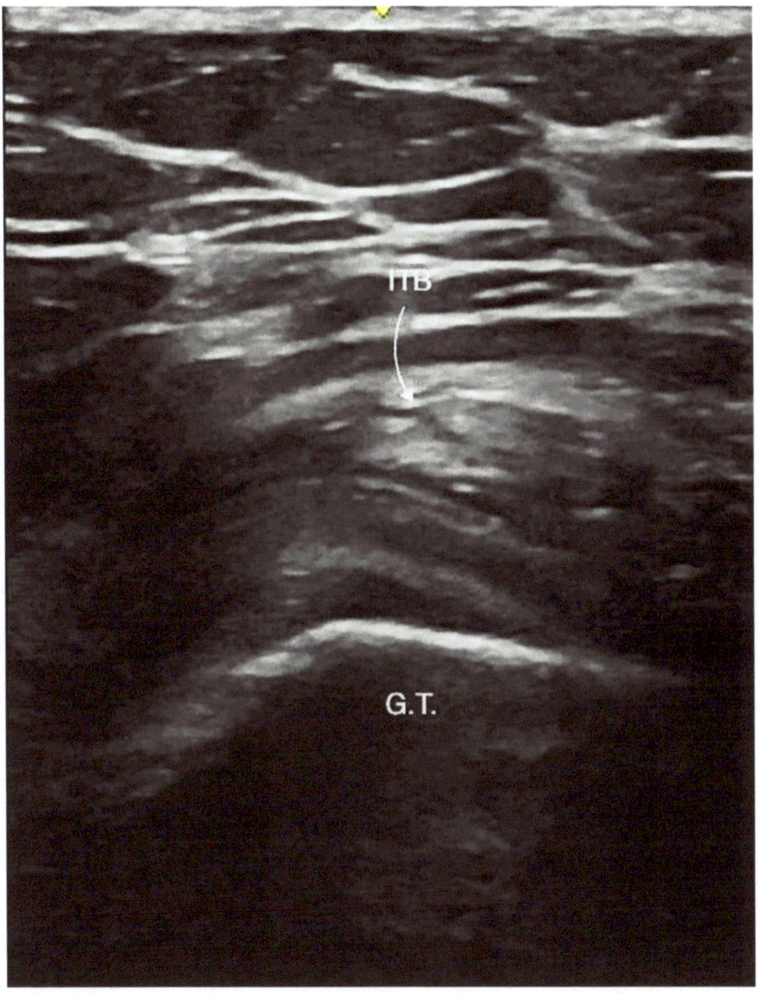

Figure 5-42a

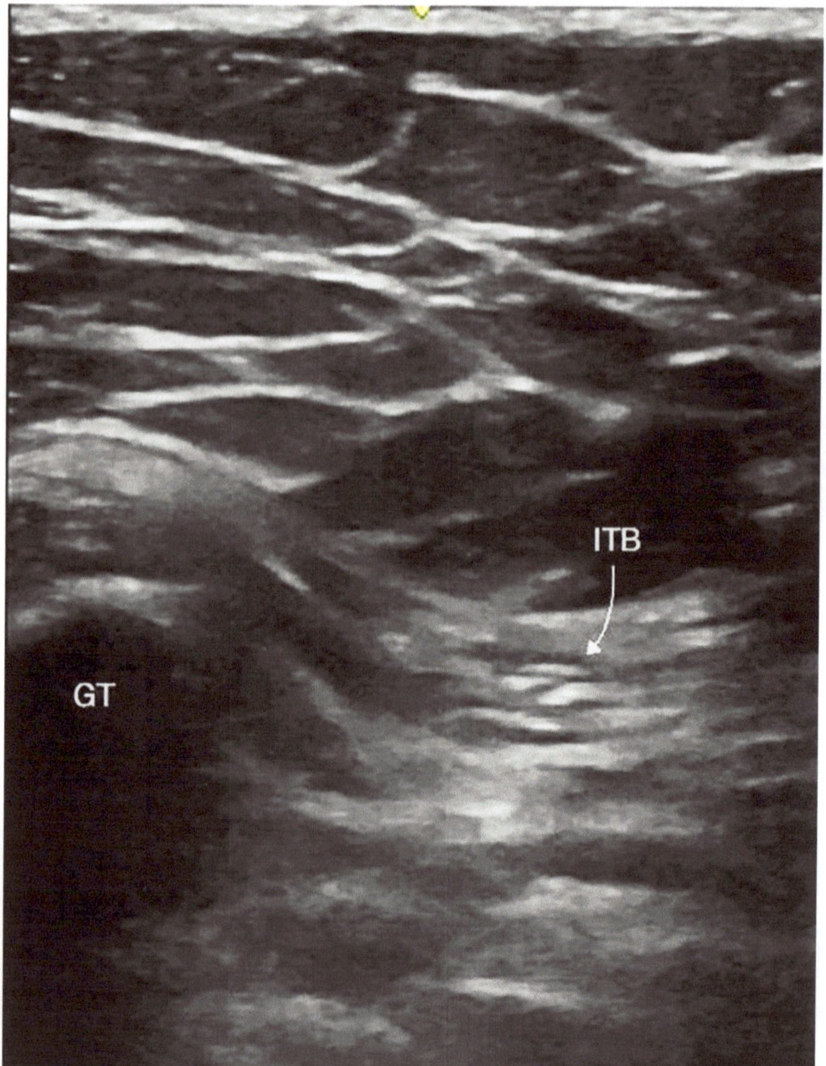

Figure 5-42b

Fig. 5-42a and b: Iliotibial band (ITB) in short axis on the greater trochanter (A) and anterior (B) to the trochanter. Note that the ITB appears pathologically thickened.

The Postoperative Hip

Postoperative Hip

Total Hip Aspiration for possible infection

Ultrasound-guided aspiration to rule out infection is easily performed and is especially useful in urgent/emergent clinical situations that preclude MSK- or interventional radiology availability. A primary example is the patient in the ICU who cannot be moved to the radiology suite. A resident on-call can perform this procedure very rapidly to obtain an adequate synovial fluid sample for cultures and gram stain. The technique involves standard sterile prepping and draping of the affected hip, along with placing the probe in a sterile sleeve.

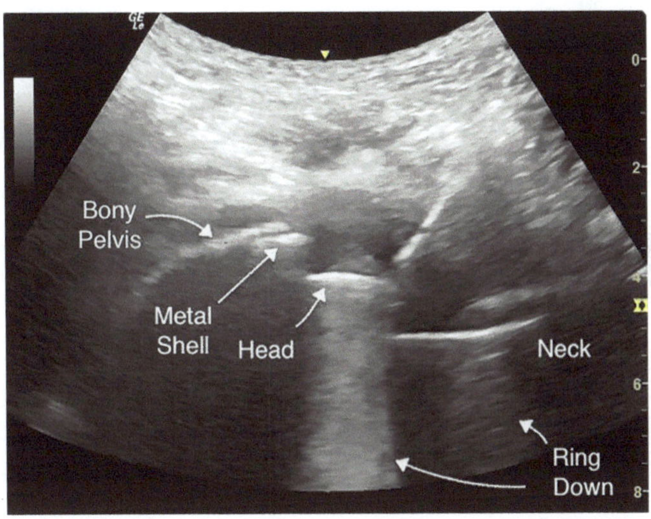

(THA r/o infection)

Figure 5-43: A long-axis view of the femoral neck where the tip of a nerve block needle (Metal Shell) is seen entering the hypoechoic fluid near the head-neck junction. The indentations on the needle allow the examiner to approach obliquely at a steep angle and still maintain visibility. This aspiration was performed in the office and results of the aspirate were found to be aseptic. The ring-down effect deep to metal of the head and neck should also be noted, particularly deep to the head.

Iliopsoas on acetabular shell

Following a total hip arthroplasty, the patient experienced anterior hip pain and weakness in hip flexion. Injection of the iliopsoas bursa transiently, but completely ameliorated the pain for approximately two months. The patient was referred back to his surgeon for re-evaluation and possible revision surgery.

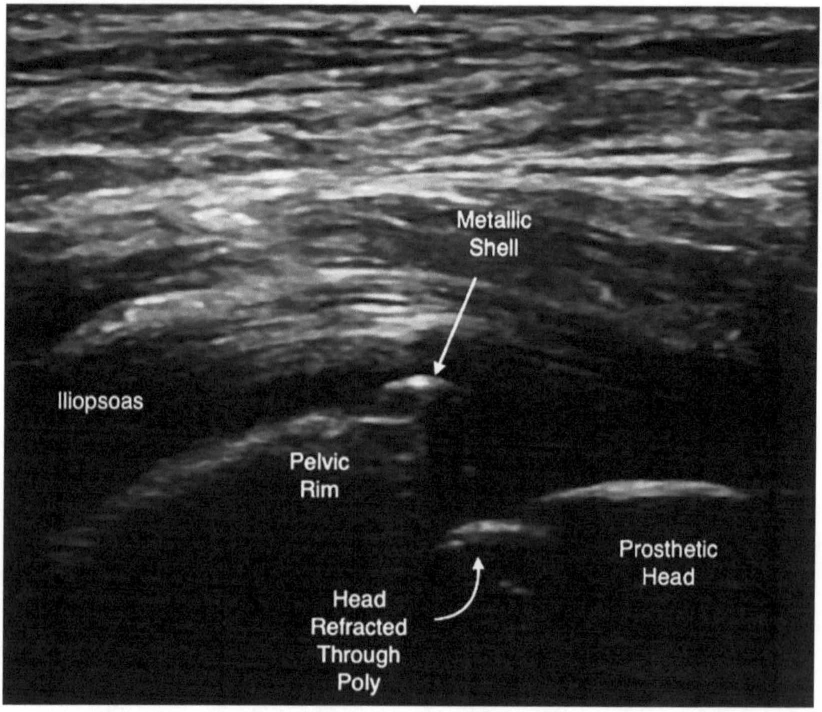

Figure 5-44a

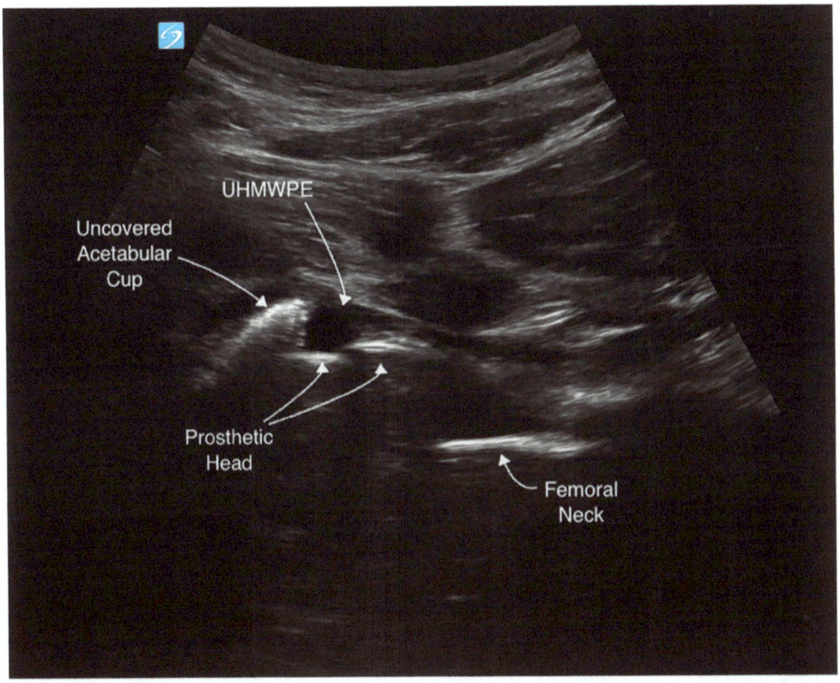

Figure 5-44b

Fig. 5-44a: Long-axis view of psoas tendon impinging on the edge of the metallic acetabular shell. Give the patient's small stature, the metal acetabular shell is susceptible to becoming prominent above the bony rim, which creates friction along the psoas tendon. As seen above, the iliopsoas the tendon is hypoechoic, even when the probe is placed perpendicular to the long axis of its fibers. b: A second patient viewed in the long axis of the femoral neck. He had unrelenting hip pain and weakness in hip flexion since the surgery. The psoas tendon could not be visualized. This orientation gives the best view of the exposed ingrowth metal of the acetabular cup. In addition, it also shows how the refraction by the acetabular poly flattens the image of the head that is deep to the poly.

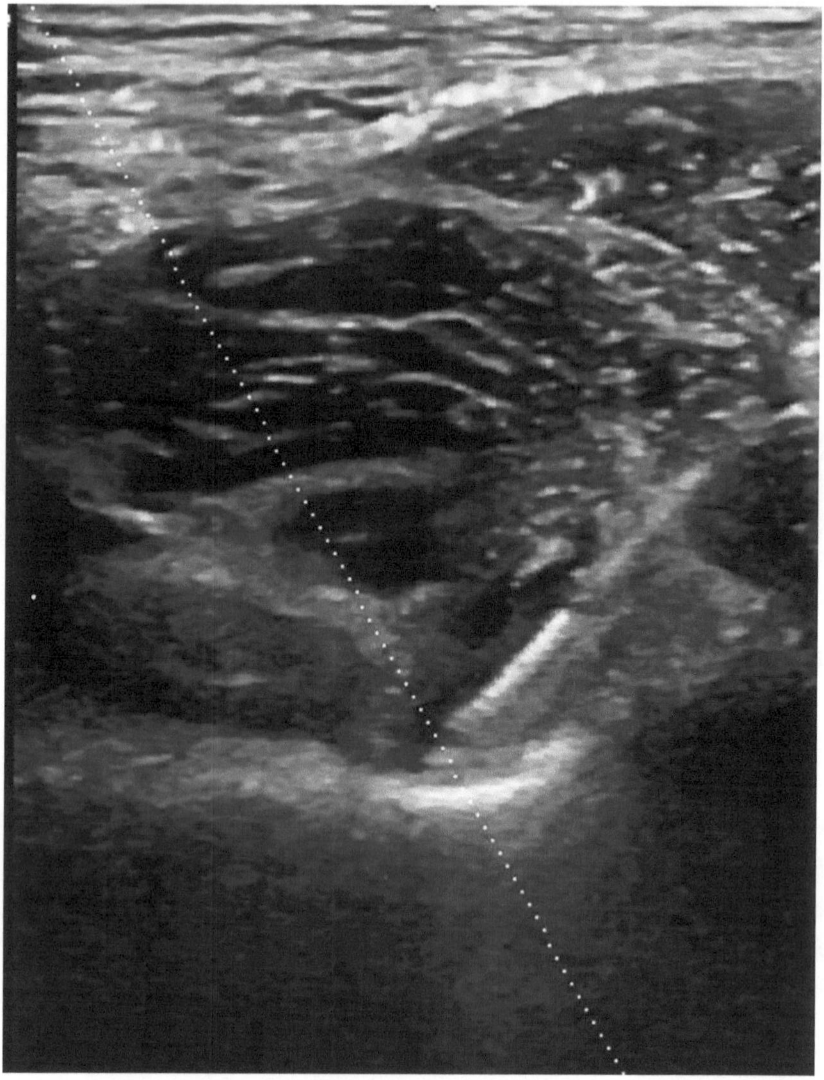

Figure 5-45: The same patient previously shown in Figure5-44a, now in the transverse, or short-axis, view. Here, the bursa on the bony brim of the pelvis is injected in this view with a nerve block needle directed transversely across the body in a lateral to medial direction. Pain relief was instantaneous and complete. This level was chosen because the cortex is easier to visualize than the metal rim. As mentioned previously, be sure to look for the shadow of the needle and anisotropy, as can be seen obscuring the anterior inferior iliac spine in the lower right corner of the above image.

Postoperative view after Hamstring Repair

This repair of the semimembranosus was done about seven months after the original injury. At approximately two weeks after the surgery, a palpable fullness developed within the posterior thigh. Ultrasound was performed to characterize the etiology of the lesion and evaluate post-operative anatomical aberrations, including re-rupture of the repair. The palpable mass was demonstrated to be a hematoma, and the blood served as a nice contrast medium for the sciatic nerve.

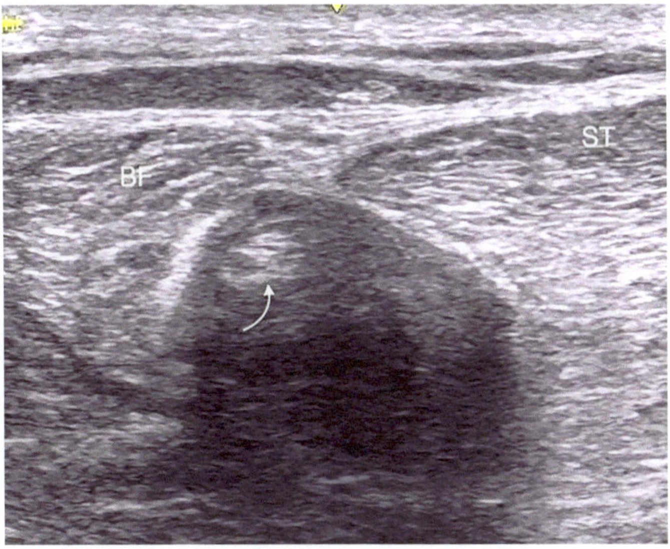

Figure 5-46: The intact semitendinosus (ST) and biceps femoris (BF) and their conjoint tendon arch over the relatively hypoechoic hematoma. The sciatic nerve (curved arrow) is outlined by the fluid.

Interventional Hip Ultrasound

Biplanar localization in ultrasound

Biplanar localization is a fundamental element in placement of needles and other instruments. Ultrasound offers an advantage over other methods in that the instrument of visualization (the probe) does not need to be adjusted and reoriented like a fluoroscope. Hip procedures provide a vivid illustration of this concept.

In selecting the orientation of the probe along the long axis of the femoral neck, we select the orientation of the needle in the frontal plane. Simultaneously, we selected a modified transverse plane that is perpendicular to the frontal plane, just as a true transverse plane would be. A needle observed in this fashion exemplifies biplanar localization.

Hip aspiration and injection.

The femoro-acetabular joint injection is probably the most frequently performed intervention at the hip, and further hip interventions may be regarded simply as variations from this index procedure.

To perform the injection, the patient is first positioned supine. As some patients are uncomfortable in full extension. One or more pillows can be placed behind the knee for comfort without impairing hip visualization. The area is first evaluated with the curvilinear probe (unless the patient is very thin) in the long axis of the femoral neck and head. Figure 5-47 and 5-48

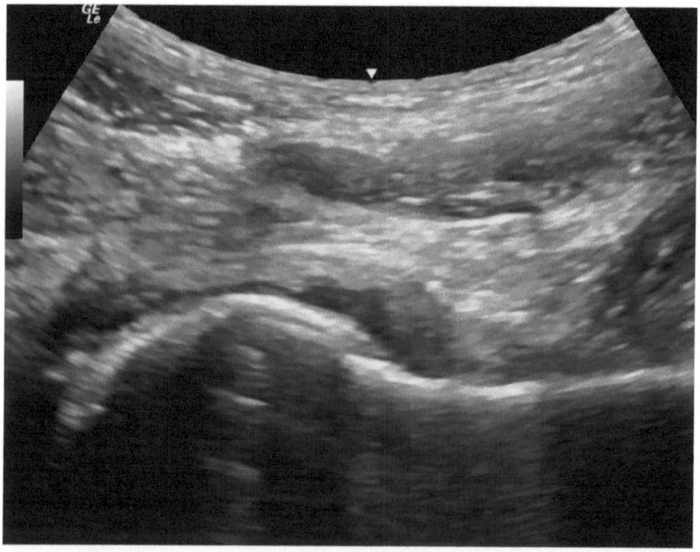

Figure 5-47: This illustration was chosen because the hypoechoic joint fluid nicely outlines the head and neck and depicts the accumulation at our intended target (the head-neck junction). The capsule is also nicely visualized. In most instances, there will not be visible fluid nor such a round head.

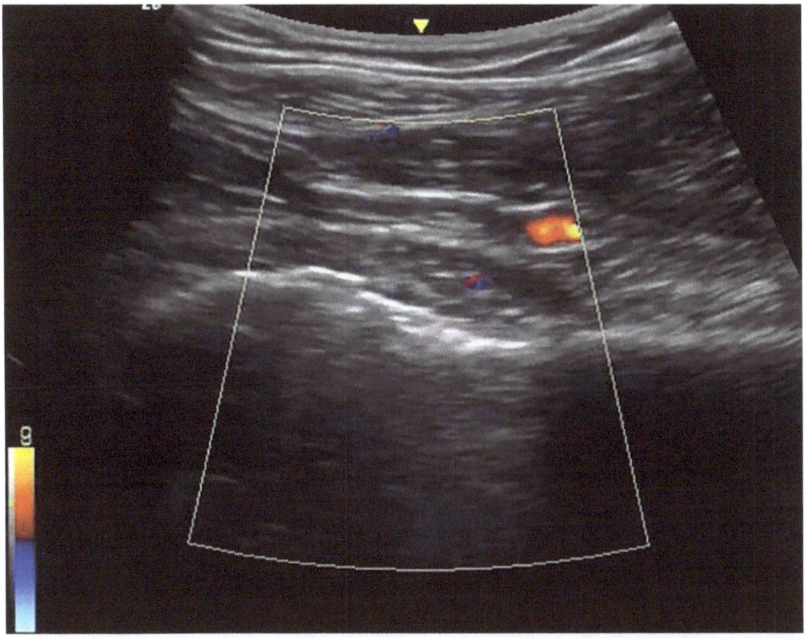

Figure 5-48: In addition to the bony outline, a Doppler exam is performed to look for branches of the lateral femoral circumflex artery. The artery is to be avoided not only for protection of the artery, but also because nerves and vessels travel together. In turn, protecting the artery simultaneously ensures minimization of pain and damage to nervous structures. This view shows an artery that is much larger and closer to the anterior capsule than those usually observed. The referring surgeon should be advised that he or she may encounter it during an arthroplasty procedure.

A needle is selected, medication prepared, and a mixture of corticosteroid and local anesthetic is aspirated into a syringe. A steep, oblique approach from lateral to medial is performed as previously described with the ultrasound nerve block needle. To reiterate, these needles have small indentations on the shaft that ensure visible, even at such an obtuse angle (Figure 5-49). Despite the contours on the needle, needle enhancement software may also be used if available to facilitate the intervention. A 22 G needle is sufficient, however, ultimately, needle length is based on patient physiognomy.

Masks and sterile gloves are worn, the area is prepared with chlorhexidine, the probes held in a sterile cover.

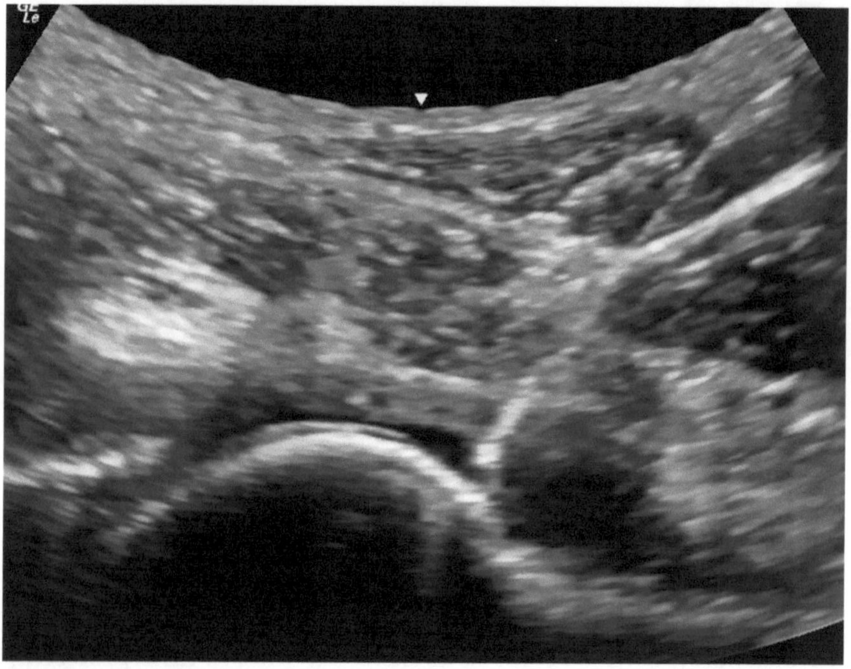

Figure 5-49: This still image shows the steep approach with the needle just prior to injection.

Adjusting to avoid structures.

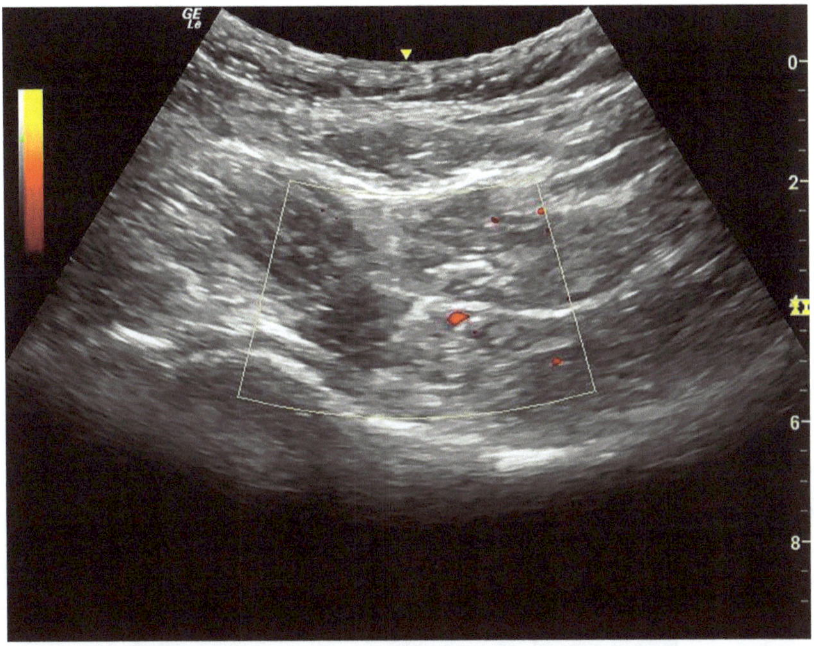

Figure 5-50: To avoid the neurovascular structures, the ultrasonographer can approach at an even steeper angle, or move the lateral end of the probe proximal even as far as a straight transverse approach. As the entry point is moved more cephalad, the neurovascular structures course more laterally, and may vanish from view altogether.

Injection for MRI arthrogram

US is not usually used to inject for MRI arthrogram, but this unusual case allows us to visualize the distribution of fluid. This patient is a very athletic woman demonstrated to suffer from femoro-acetabular impingement. Figure 5-51 and 5-52

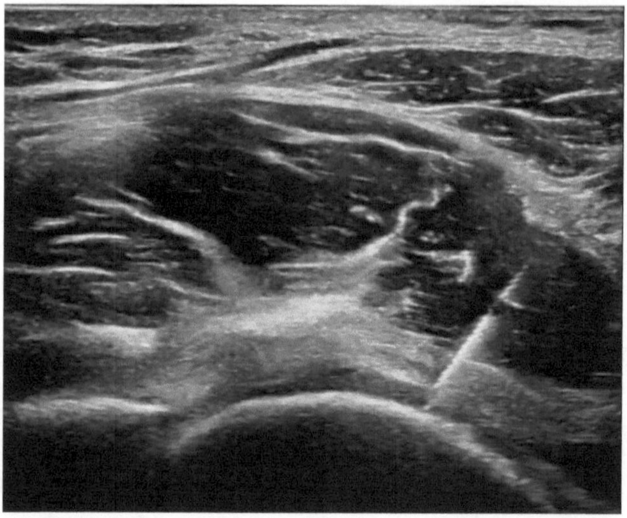

Figure 5-51: This still image depicts the maximum injection volume with the hip joint capsule, which is only slightly elevated from the femoral head.

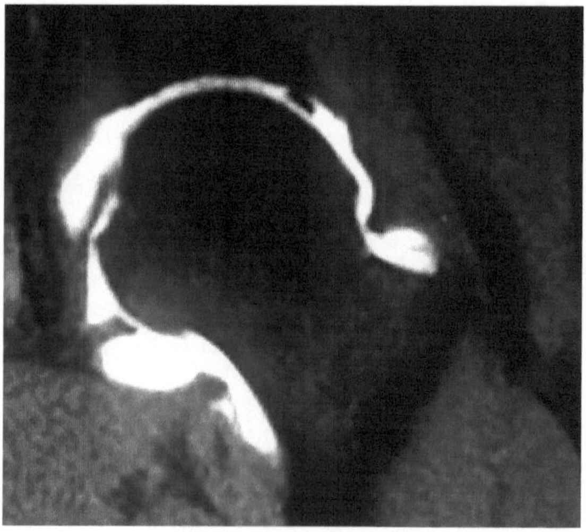

FAI distribution

Figure 5-52: This coronal MRI view of the same patient demonstrates the specific intra-articular locations of fluid accumulation within the femoroacetabular joint capsule. This image illustrates the concept that little fluid accumulates superiorly or anteriorly, as these regions are compressed under the iliofemoral ligament.

Meralgia paresthetica

The lateral femoral cutaneous nerve is superficial enough that it can easily be treated by hydro-dissection or injection. The nerve is located by first identifying the inguinal ligament in the ligament's long axis, and looking just medial to its attachment on the ASIS for the nerve in the short axis.

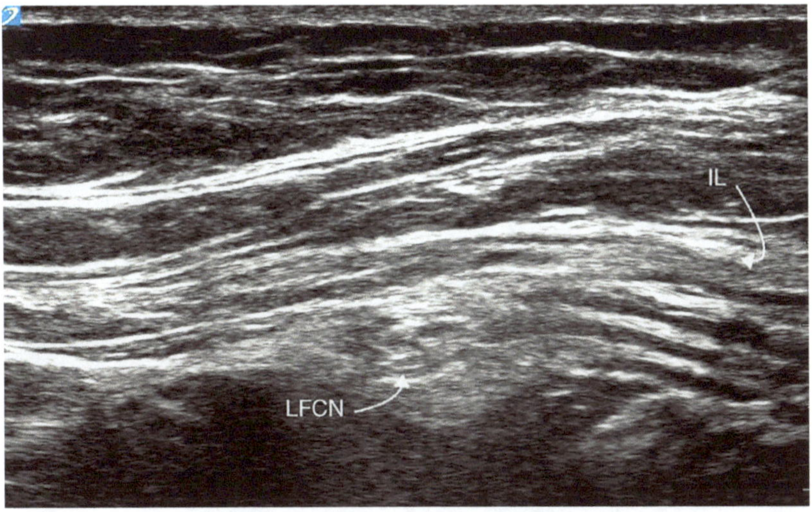

Figure 5-53: The lateral femoral cutaneous nerve (LFCN) is visualized just deep to the inguinal ligament (IL). In this view the lateral side is to the right, longitudinally just distal to the ASIS.

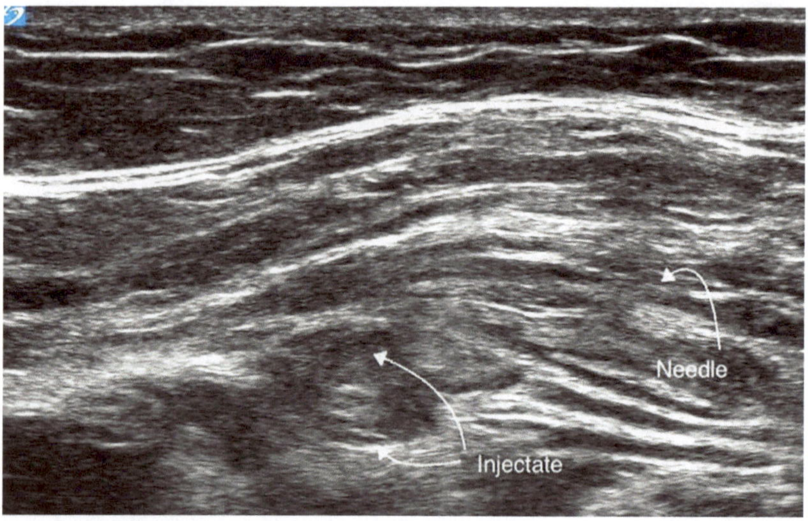

Figure 5-54: The needle approach from the lateral side. The nerve is seen surrounded by lidocaine and steroid.

Ultrasound assistance in arthroscopy

Hip joint.

IT band

Intraoperative ultrasound has developed utility in the placement of arthroscopic portals including: Central femoral acetabular portals, peripheral hip portals, and selecting portals for iliotibial band release and resection.

Intra-articular arthroscopy (Modified Weinrauch Technique)

This set up for hip arthroscopy for both central and peripheral portals diseases is the same as that which the hip arthroscopist would normally use. If the surgeon prefers the lateral position, ultrasound can also be used for portal placement. In hip arthroscopy, ultrasound is essentially only replacing the functionality of the C-arm. Weinrauch recommends the posterior superior portal as the initial portal.

The ultrasound demonstrates to the surgeon the posterior superior femoral head and neck, greater trochanter, capsule, joint, and the ilium. The first portal is usually posterior superior at the level of the top of the trochanter,, and the entry point is marked in standard fashion. A curvilinear probe is used for 2 reasons: first is to obtain deeper visualization for the approach especially in heavier patients; and the second is that a more panoramic view facilitates portal placement.

The exam begins with the posterior trochanteric portal in the following fashion. Once the patient has been placed on the traction table with the involved hip in slight internal rotation and mild flexion. A central post is place in the usual proximal position against the upper inner thigh. This allows a combination of traction and hip adduction to put distraction force on the hip joint. A scout ultrasound view is obtained without and then with traction in the long axis of the lower limb along the line of approach that one will use for the portal. Traction is applied to the lower limb either by a traction device or by using the patient's body as a counterweight in a mild Trendelenburg position. Traction produces distraction of the joint and makes the capsule more visible between the femoral head and labrum. The surgeon can then use this view to observe needle insertion, which is long enough to reach the hip and has a lumen with a large enough caliber to accept a Nitinol wire. A 20-cc syringe of saline is attached to the back of the needle, so the femoral head can still be visualized when fluid enters the joint. The surgical procedure proceeds in the normal fashion after the portals are established. An alternative approach to subluxing the hip is to use a needle through a peripheral portal, see below, on the anterior neck and fill the joint with saline. This allows easier distraction while allowing the head to be visualized.

The development of a peripheral portal is also done with a curvilinear probe. In this case, the anterior femoral head and neck serve as the landmark. This approach is similar to the one described in the section on hip injections. The probe is aligned with the long axis of the neck, and then slid cephalad and caudad to ensure the surgeon is directly over the central, ultrasonically = brightest portion. The needle, which is the same as the one used for the central portals, is about 17G and 3 inches and advanced under ultrasound guidance through the capsule into the joint. For this part of the surgery, traction is not needed or, in fact, desirable.

The ultrasound set up is similar to the standard set up except no C-arm is needed, leaving the surgeon more physical space and subsequent flexibility in creating non-standard planes for observation.

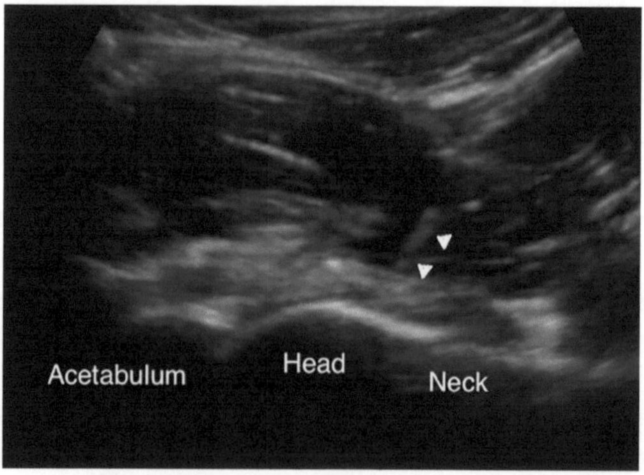

5-55 A

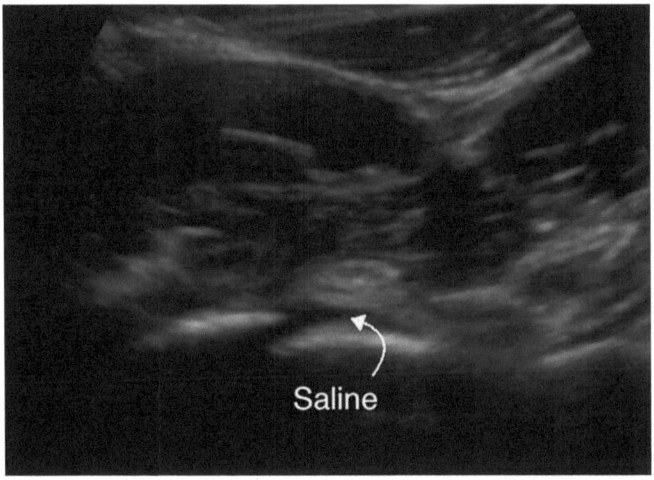

5-55 B

5-55 A and B: A shows the needle (arrowheads) in position to inject. A 20 ml syringe is attached to the needle and the needle is also full of saline. This is to prevent air from entering and blocking the ultrasound waves from striking the head. B. the head has moved distal and lateral so that we just get just a little of the head off center. One might expect more fluid, but it doesn't accumulate very much in this anterior superior area as is shown in figure 5-52

Portal placement for ITB release

Iliotibial band

The scope portal for the iliotibial band resection is created under ultrasound guidance while the more proximal, or instrument portal, is developed under arthroscopic visualization. The curvilinear probe is again place to outline the anatomy around the greater trochanter in short and long axis. This allows placement of the portal at the mid-portion of the iliotibial band in terms of anterior posterior positioning, and somewhat distal to the most prominent portion of the greater trochanter in the longitudinal position. The proximal or instrument portal is then developed under arthroscopic visualization, and a layer of fat is resected off the lateral border of the iliotibial band. Longitudinal release of the iliotibial band is performed with special care not to damage muscles, including the vastus lateralis distally and gluteal tendons proximally. Additional iliotibial band resection and release can be carried out anteriorly and posteriorly, and any inflamed bursa can be resected. At the end of the procedure, a catheter for the continuous release of local anesthetic can be placed under arthroscopic visualization.

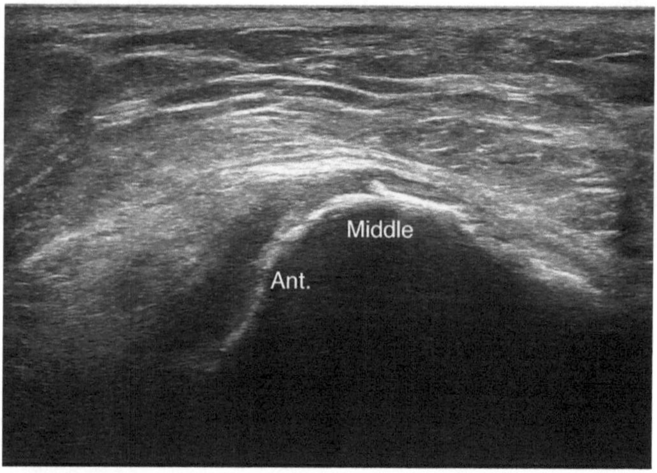

Figure 5-56: A short-axis scout view of the greater trochanter (GT) allows localization of the 'ski chalet' (the angle between the anterior and middle facets), but more importantly, the overlying ITB. This establishes the anterior-posterior location of the entry point.`

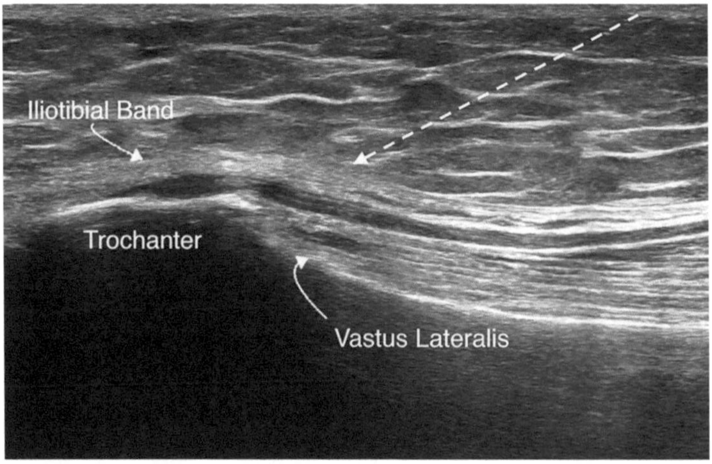

Figure 5-57: A long-axis view showing the bone and the ITB . The desired approach is from distal, so that the ITB can be viewed over the entire area of planned resection. . We want to start our visualization at the lower border of the trochanter. In the heavier patients one starts more distal. Instruments enter through a more superior portal, which is developed with the needle viewed through the arthroscope.

Using adjacent vessels to localize nerves for surgical planning.

The posterior femoral cutaneous nerve (PFCN) is a small nerve in a large region of the body and entrapment is rare. Fortunately, it travels with the inferior gluteal artery, which can serve as a landmark to help locate it. In cases of PFCN entrapment, the surgeon can use color Doppler of the adjacent artery y to localize the nerve and initiate surgical planning. First, the lower edge of the gluteus maximum is found in in the long axis and its lower edge used as a landmark for the incision site. Then, in the short-axis view, Doppler can be used to help locate the artery.

Identifying the nerve by finding the descending gluteal artery can be repeated intraoperatively as well.

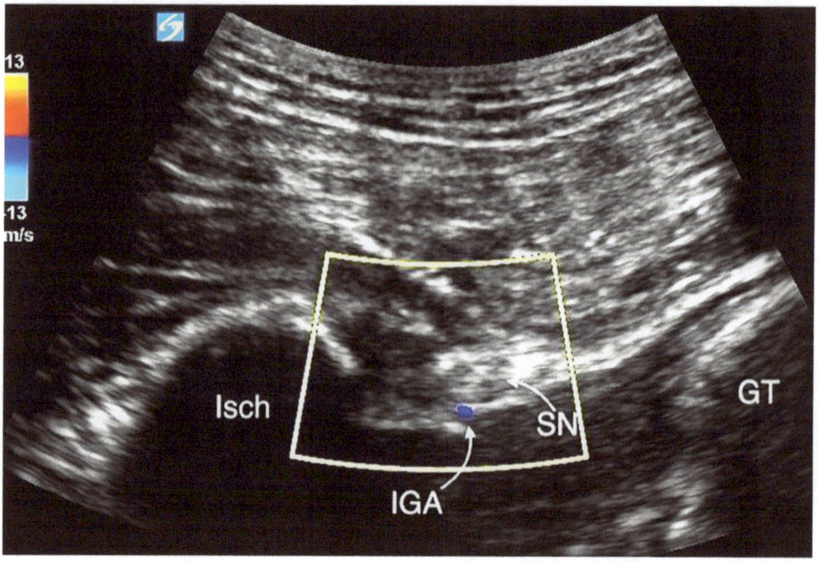

Figure 5-58: Using the inferior gluteal artery (IGA) to find the posterior femoral cutaneous nerve (PFCN), we ultrasonically pick up the artery next to the visible sciatic nerve (SN). Although the PFCN is not itself visible, the IGA travels with it, and can be traced down into the posterior thigh. This allows surgical planning with Doppler in cases of PFCN entrapment, which occurs at the inferior border of the gluteus maximus where the nerve and artery penetrate the fascia. This figure demonstrates finding the artery deep to the gluteus maximus.

Summary

Although the depth of the structures at the hip precludes the use of higher frequency probes, the large size of most of the structures facilitates visualization. Ultrasound turns out to be very useful for the hip surgeon. It should also be noted much of its utility involves some type of intervention. As the technology evolves, we foresee even more practical uses for ultrasound.

References

1. Jacobson, Jon A. Fundamentals of Musculoskeletal Ultrasound Third edition, Elsevier, Philadelphia, 2017

2. Van Holsbeeck, Marnix T and Introcaso, Joseph H, Musculoskeletal Ultrasound third edition. MedEd3D 2015

3. Weinrauch, Patrick . Kermeci, Sharon , Ultrasound-Assisted Hip Arthroscopy, Arthroscopy Techniques April 2014 pp. e255-e259

4. Weinrauch, Patrick . Kermeci, Sharon, Ultrasonography-Assisted Arthroscopic Proximal Iliotibial Band Release and Trochanteric Bursectomy, Arthroscopy Techniques April 2013 pp. e433-e435

Subject Index

Volume 1

Chapter 1. Introduction 1 – 43
- a. History of Ultrasound 3 - 5
- b. Basic Physics of Ultrasound 5 – 7
- c. Echogenicity 7 – 8
- d. Anisotropy 9 – 11
- e. Obtaining the best image 12 – 27
- f. Indications 27
- g. Standard exam 28 – 30
- h. Locating pathology 30 – 37
- i. Interventional Ultrasound 37 – 40
- j. Conclusion 40

Chapter 2 Shoulder
- a. Diagnostic examination 46 – 59
- b. Massive rotator cuff tear 59 – 64
- c. Post-Operative Shoulder 64 – 68
  - a. Cuff repair
  - b. Arthroplasty
- d. Calcific Tendinitis 68 - 72
- e. Pectoralis Major tear 72 – 75
- f. Snapping Scapular bursitis 75
- g. Post-op rotator cuff 76 – 79
- h. Glenohumeral Roughness 79 – 83
- i. Interventional US 84 – 93
  Subacromial; intraarticular; subacromial; biceps and scapulothoracic

Chapter 3 Elbow and Forearm
- a. Introduction 99 – 100
- b. Diagnostic exam
  - a. Anterior elbow 100 – 113
    - i. Distal biceps 107 - 112
      4 approaches
  - b. lateral elbow 114 – 120

c. Medial elbow 120 – 129
d. posterior elbow 129 – 133
e. anterior forearm 133 – 136
f. posterior forearm 137 – 139
c. Pathology
a. distal biceps 140 – 142
b. distal triceps 143 – 145
c. common tendon origins 145 – 147
d. medial ulnar collateral lig. 148 – 149
e. Radial collateral complex 149 – 150
f. Ulnar nerve 150 - 153
g. Median nerve 153 – 154
h. Radial nerve 154 – 156
i. elbow joint space 156 – 157
j. Olecranon bursa 157 – 158
d. Interventions
a. Joint injection 159 – 161
b. Lateral epicondylitis 161 – 163
c. Medial epicondylitis 164
d. Ulnar nerve sheath injection 164 – 166
e. Ulnar collateral ligament 166 – 187
f. radial tunnel injection 167 – 168
g. distal biceps tendon 168 – 169
h. Olecranon bursa aspiration 170
i. biopsy of mass 170 – 171
j. foreign body removal 171
k. nerve blocks 172
e. post op evaluation
a. UCL and Ulnar nerve 172
Chapter 4 Hand and wrist
a. Introduction 185
b. Diagnostic evaluation 186 – 197
a. Wrist volar 186 – 189
b. Wrist dorsal 190 – 192
c. Fingers volar/ dorsal 193
d. Review of volar anatomy 194 – 197

c. Wrist Pathology 198 - 252
a. Carpal tunnel 202 - 234
i. Diagnosis and evaluation 202 - 209
ii. Hydro-dissection 210 – 214
iii. Procedure 215 – 219
iv. Aftercare 219 -221
v. Cases: Fracture; synovitis; reverse palmaris; median artery; artery on the ligament. 222- 234
b. De Quervain Tenosynovitis 235 – 238
c. Wrist masses 239 – 244
d. Extensor carpi ulnaris subluxation 245 – 249
e. Thumb CMC arthritis 249 – 250
d. Radiocarpal injections 251 – 252
e. Finger pathology 253–
a. Foreign bodies 253 – 254
b. Tendon lacerations 255 – 257, 277 - 278
c. Trigger finger 258 – 260
d. Extensor tendon mechanism 261
e. Dupuytren's contracture 261 – 264
f. Finger masses 264 – 270
g. Nailbed tumor 271 – 272
f. Small joint injection 273 - 274
g. Flexor tenosynovitis 274 – 276
h. Trauma 279 – 284
a. Screwdriver to palm 279
b. Assist in fracture 280 – 282
i. Hardware protrusion 280
ii. Post op complications 281 – 282
i. In-Office nerve block 283 – 284
Chapter 5 Hip and thigh 291 – 359
a. Introduction 291 – 292
b. Diagnostic exam 292 – 340
a. Positioning, draping etc 292 - 298
b. Anterior hip 298 – 314
c. Iliopsoas and neuro-vasc. Bundle 304 – 310
d. Anterior Inferior iliac spine 310 – 313

e. Anterior superior iliac spine 313 - 314
f. Lateral hip 314 – 322
g. Posterior hip 323 - 326
h. Posterior hip muscles 327 - 336
c. In-office dynamic exams 336 – 340
a. Snapping psoas 336 – 338
b. Snapping iliotibial band 338 - 340
d. Postoperative Hip 341 – 345
a. Aspiration for infection 341
b. Iliopsoas on acetabular shell 342 - 344
c. S/P hamstring repair 345
e. Intervention 345 – 352
a. Hip 345 – 350
b. Meralgia paresthetica 351 – 352
f. Assist in arthroscopy 352 – 357
g. Using Doppler assist in OR 357 – 358

Volume 2

Chapter 6 Knee and Calf 360 - 463
a. Introduction 360
b. Anatomy and positioning 361 - 396
a. Distal thigh and quadriceps 361- 367
b. Anterior knee 368 - 373
c. Medial knee 373 - 378
d. Lateral knee 378 - 387
e. Posterior knee 388 - 395
f. Leg compartments 396
c. Office diagnostic work 397 - 421
a. MCL injury 397 - 398
b. Meniscus 399 - 400
c. Snapping lateral plica 401
d. Effusions 402 - 404
e. Crystalline arthropathy 405
f. Cysts and cyst-like masses 406 - 409
g. Cyst-like tumor 410 - 411

h. Fungus 412 - 413
i. Quadriceps rupture 414
j. Tendinosis 415 - 417
k. Post TKA tendon pain 418
l. Osgood-Schlatter vs. enthesophyte 419
m. Medial Gastrocnemius Tear 420 - 421
d. Post-operative exam 421 - 429
a. Knee pain after IM nail 422 - 423
b. Meniscus repair pain 424
c. Fabella subluxation 425 - 427
d. Loose PMMA in TKA 428 - 429
e. Intervention – office 430 - 439
a. Injection and aspiration 430 - 433
b. In morbid obesity 434
c. Tendinosis 435
d. Bursae 436 - 438
e. Cellulitis 439
f. US in OR 439 - 457
a. Portal placement in obesity 440 - 441
b. Portal placement in posterior knee 442 - 449
i. PVNS or stiff knee 442 - 446
ii. Loose body 447 - 449
c. Nerve block at the knee 450 - 451
d. Abscess drainage 452 - 455
e. Multiple wounds (dog bite) 456 - 457
g. Preoperative planning 457 - 462
Chapter 7 Foot and ankle 464 - 516
a. Introduction 464 - 465
b. Diagnostic exam 465 - 495
a. Anterior ankle 465 - 467
b. Medial ankle 467 - 476
c. Lateral ankle 476 - 484
d. Posterior ankle heel and calf 485 - 492
e. Forefoot 493 - 495
c. Pathology and treatment 495 - 526

a. Arthritis 495 - 499
i. Tibiotalar joint 495 - 496
ii. Subtalar joint 496 - 497
iii. Midfoot injection 498 - 499
b. Ankle impingement 499
c. Flexor Hallucis longus injection 499 - 500
d. Sinus tarsi syndrome 500 - 501
e. Achilles tendon 502 - 503
i. Hydro-dissection 502 - 503
f. Posterior tibial tendon 504 - 505
g. Peroneal tendons 505 - 507
h. Knot of henry 508 - 507
i. Plantar fascia 507 – 509
j. Interdigital neuromas 510 - 511
k. Foreign bodies 511
l. Tarsal tunnel 511 - 513
m. Superficial peroneal and sural nerves 513 – 515
Chapter 8 Pediatrics and Spine 528 - 613
a. Brief history of US in Pediatric Orthopaedics 529 - 530
b. Hip Dysplasia 532 - 536
c. Other Hip pathology 537 - 537
d. Musculoskeletal infections 537 - 548
a. Septic arthritis 537 - 540
b. Osteomyelitis 541 - 545
c. Pyomyositis 545 - 546
d. Cellulitis and abscesses 546 - 548
e. Infective tenosynovitis 548
e. Fractures and dislocations 548 - 563
a. Distal forearm 549 - 550
b. Screening elbow injuries 550 - 551
c. Proximal humerus fractures 551
d. Clavicle fractures 551
e. Other long bones 551 - 560
f. Other joint dislocations 561 - 563
f. Muscle agenesis 564 - 568

	g. Slipped epiphysis	569
	h. Evaluate fracture healing	570 - 571
	i. Spine diagnoses	570 - 580
	j. Intraoperative spine US	580 - 595
	k. Epidural placement in newborn	595
	l. Analysis of flap vascular anatomy	596 - 600
	m. Conclusion	601
Chapter 9	Integrating ultrasound into your practice	615 - 637
	a. Getting started	616 - 620
	b. Obtaining an ultrasound machine	620 - 631
	c. Financing	632
	d. Coding and reimbursement	632 - 635
	e. Practice integration	635 - 636

www.ingramcontent.com/pod-product-compliance
Lightning Source LLC
LaVergne TN
LVHW062352150926
848178LV00013B/159

* 9 7 8 1 9 6 0 9 9 5 9 5 7 *